Phonological Encoding and Monitoring in Normal and Pathological Speech

This book reports recent research on mechanisms of normal formulation and control in speaking and in language disorders such as stuttering, aphasia and verbal dyspraxia. The theoretical claim is that such disorders result from both deficits in a component of the language production system and interactions between this component and the system that "monitors" for errors and undertakes a corrective behaviour. In particular, the book focuses on phonological encoding in speech (the construction of a phonetic plan for utterances), on verbal self-monitoring (checking for correctness and initiating corrective action if necessary), and on interactions between these processes.

Bringing together sixteen original chapters by leading international researchers, this volume represents a coherent statement of current thinking in this exciting field. The aim is to show how psycholinguistic models of normal speech processing can be applied to the study of impaired speech production. This book will prove invaluable to any researcher, student or speech therapist looking to bridge the gap between the latest advances in theory and the implications of these advances for language and speech pathology.

Robert J. Hartsuiker is Senior Lecturer in the Department of Experimental Psychology, Ghent University (Belgium).

Roelien Bastiaanse is Professor in Neurolinguistics in the Graduate School for Behavioural and Cognitive Neuroscience (BCN), University of Groningen (NE).

Albert Postma is Associate Professor in the Psychological Laboratory, Utrecht University (NE).

Frank Wijnen is Senior Lecturer in the Department of Linguistics, Utrecht Institute of Linguistics, Utrecht University (NE).

Phonological Encoding and Monitoring in Normal and Pathological Speech

Edited by
**Robert J. Hartsuiker, Roelien Bastiaanse,
Albert Postma and Frank Wijnen**

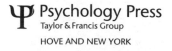 Psychology Press
Taylor & Francis Group
HOVE AND NEW YORK

KH

First published 2005
by Psychology Press
27 Church Road, Hove, East Sussex BN3 2FA

Simultaneously published in the USA and Canada
by Psychology Press
270 Madison Avenue, New York NY 10016

Psychology Press is part of the Taylor & Francis Group

Copyright © 2005 Psychology Press

Typeset in Times by RefineCatch Limited, Bungay, Suffolk
Printed and bound in Great Britain by TJ International Ltd,
Padstow, Cornwall
Cover design by Anú Design

British Library Cataloguing in Publication Data
A catalogue record for this book is available from the British Library

Library of Congress Cataloging-in-Publication Data
Hartsuiker, Robert J., 1968–
   Phonological encoding and monitoring in normal and
pathological speech / Robert J. Hartsuiker . . . [et al.].
      p.   cm.
   Includes bibliographical references and index.
   ISBN 1-84169-262-X
   1. Speech disorders.   2. Linguistics.   I. Title.

RC423.H345   2005
616.85 ′5–dc22   2004012990

ISBN 1-84169-262-X

7/15/15

Contents

PART V
Conclusions and prospects

16 **Phonological encoding, monitoring, and language pathology:
Conclusions and prospects**
FRANK WIJNEN AND HERMAN H. J. KOLK

List of Contributors

Roelien Bastiaanse, Graduate School of Behavioral and Cognitive Neurosciences (BCN), University of Groningen, The Netherlands.

Chris Code, School of Psychology, University of Exeter, UK; School of Communication Sciences and Disorders, University of Sydney, Australia.

Edward G. Conture, CCC-SLP, Department of Hearing and Speech Sciences, Vanderbilt University, Nashville, Tennessee, USA.

Martin Corley, School of Philosophy, Psychology and Language Sciences, University of Edinburgh, UK.

Gary S. Dell, Beckman Institute, University of Illinois at Urbana-Champaign, USA.

Robert J. Hartsuiker, Department of Experimental Psychology, Ghent University, Belgium.

Albert E. Kim, Department of Psychology, University of Washington, Seattle, Washington, USA.

Herman H. J. Kolk, Nijmegen Institute for Cognition and Information, University of Nijmegen, The Netherlands.

Robin J. Lickley, Speech and Language Sciences, Queen Margaret University College, UK.

Ben Maassen, Department of Medical Psychology, Paediatric Neurology, University Medical Center, Nijmegen, The Netherlands.

Heike Martensen, Centre for Psycholinguistics, University of Antwerp, Belgium.

Nadine Martin, Temple University, Philadelphia, Pennsylvania, USA.

Kenneth S. Melnick, CCC-SLP, Communication Sciences & Disorders Department, Worcester State College, Worcester, Massachusetts, USA.

Lian Nijland, Department of Medical Psychology, Paediatric Neurology, University Medical Center, Nijmegen, The Netherlands.

Sieb G. Nooteboom, Utrecht Institute of Linguistics OTS, Utrecht University, The Netherlands.

Ralph N. Ohde, CCC-SLP, Department of Hearing and Speech Sciences, Vanderbilt University, Nashville, Tennessee, USA.

Claudy C. E. Oomen, Psychological Laboratory, Helmholtz Institute, Utrecht University, The Netherlands.

Dirk-Bart den Ouden, Graduate School of Behavioural and Cognitive Neurosciences (BCN), University of Groningen, The Netherlands.

Albert Postma, Psychological Laboratory, Helmholtz Institute, Utrecht University, The Netherlands.

Ardi Roelofs, Max Planck Institute for Psycholinguistics and F.C. Donders Centre for Cognitive Neuroimaging, Nijmegen, The Netherlands.

Melanie Russell, Speech and Language Sciences, Queen Margaret University College, UK.

Nada Vasiç, Utrecht Institute of Linguistics OTS, Utrecht University, The Netherlands.

Frank Wijnen, Utrecht Institute of Linguistics OTS, Utrecht University, The Netherlands.

Preface

Sometimes we speak fluently, without any speech errors, pauses, repetitions, and so on. But on other occasions we are disfluent. This is especially so for speakers with certain speech or language pathologies such as stuttering, apraxia of speech, and aphasia. This book brings together research from various disciplines including speech-language pathology, linguistics, experimental psychology, and cognitive modeling. The aim is to better understand *why* speech is so often disfluent and whether there is *continuum* between "normal speech" and "pathological speech". To do this, we test current proposals about the way speakers plan speech (phonological encoding) and about the way they inspect that speech is still going according to plan (self-monitoring). Our underlying assumption is that studying speech and language pathologies can inform us about normal speech planning, but that theories about normal planning can also inform us about the reasons for pathologies.

This book emanates from a research programme that started in 1996 under the direction of Frank Wijnen, Albert Postma, Roelien Bastiaanse, and Herman Kolk and a subsequent grant awarded to Ben Maassen. Both grants were awarded by NWO, the Netherlands' Organization for Scientific Research. The grant enabled Remca Burger, Nada Vasic, Dirk-Bart den Ouden, Claudy Oomen, Lian Nijland, and Rob Hartsuiker to conduct their research projects, which stood on the basis for several chapters in this volume. We are indebted to NWO for making this possible.

In addition to many fruitful meetings within this Groningen–Nijmegen–Utrecht consortium, we also organised an international workshop at the Max Planck Institute for Psycholinguistics in Nijmegen, 1999. Many of the authors were present at this workshop and presented papers that have led to chapters in the present book. We are very grateful to Pim Levelt for hosting that workshop and to all presenters, discussants, and participants who contributed to it.

Ghent, February 2004

1 Phonological encoding and monitoring in normal and pathological speech

Robert J. Hartsuiker, Roelien Bastiaanse, Albert Postma, and Frank Wijnen

Introduction

Imagine two speakers playing a dialogue game. Both speakers have a map of a fictional terrain full of pine trees, streams, goldmines, huts in which outlaws hide, waterfalls, and even crashed spacecrafts. On one of these maps a route is drawn and the first speaker, the instruction giver, is describing this route to his interlocutor, the instruction follower. The instruction follower attempts to draw the route on his own map (unaware that there are subtle differences between the two maps!). In this game, one can expect utterances such as (1) and (2):[1]

(1) Right. Follow the stream [pause]. Follow the path of the stream right down
(2) Okay, well go between the gold line gold mine and the outlaws' hideout

In (1) the speaker apparently deemed the description "stream" not specific enough. Speech is stopped, there is retracing to "follow", and the more specific description "path of the stream" is produced. In (2), the speaker committed a phonological error. He said "line" instead of "mine". Here, speech is retraced to the first constituent of the compound "goldmine", and the error is repaired. In this case, the repair followed the error without a pause (as opposed to (1) in which there was a perceptible pause).

These examples show that speakers *monitor* themselves when producing spontaneous speech. They detect that sometimes the realised utterance does not confirm to their standards: That is, the utterance, although linguistically well formed, does not contain sufficient information to achieve communicative success as in (1), or the utterance deviates from linguistic standards, as in (2). In both incidents, the detection of such a discrepancy between ideal speech and actual speech has repercussions: The speaker decides to interrupt, and then takes corrective action: The formulation of a self-correction, or a "repair".

One aim of this book is to report recent research on the mechanisms of self-monitoring: How does the self-monitoring system work? What kinds of channels does this system use to detect that is something wrong? How does self-monitoring affect the quality of the actual speech output? What is the role of self-monitoring in various speech pathologies? These, and other relevant questions, were first addressed in the 1980s in publications by Nooteboom (1980) and Levelt (1983). But recently there has been a "new wave" of interest in these issues (e.g. Hartsuiker & Kolk, 1989, 2001; Postma, 2000). The present book is a direct consequence of this renewed attention for monitoring.

Now consider another example, which is taken from a recent article by Clark and Fox Tree (2002). A British academic called Reynard answers (3) to the question: "And he's going to the top, is he?"

(3) Well, Mallet said he felt it would be a good thing if Oscar went.

But this answer is fictitious. It is what a journalist, interviewing Reynard, might have reported in her article. But what Reynard actually said was (4):

(4) well,. I mean this . uh Mallet said Mallet was uh said something about uh you know he felt it would be a good thing if u:h. if Oscar went,

This example shows many interesting phenomena at once. Reynard pauses between words, he produces *fillers*, such as *uh*, *you know*, and *I mean*, he revises phrases (Mallet said Mallet was) and he repeats words (*if if*). In other words, real speech is full of disfluencies (in Clark & Fox Tree's terminology, *performance additions*).

How should we view such incidents? As Clark and Fox Tree point out, in Chomsky's view (1965) these are misapplications of our knowledge of the language. What linguistic theory (and perhaps its sub-discipline psycho-linguistics) should be concerned with is the ideal delivery (3), not an utterance like (4) which is distorted by constraints on performance (random errors, lack of attention). Indeed, in most psycholinguistic studies on sentence com-prehension, the participants will listen to perfectly grammatical sentences such as (3), perhaps containing a syntactic ambiguity, but not to spontaneous utterances such as (4).

The basic tenet of this book is completely different. Indeed, we do consider speech errors and some disfluencies as deviations from a plan. But rather than labelling these incidents as uninteresting, irrelevant for language processing (or even pathological) we study such incidents to gain an understanding of the architecture and mechanisms of normal formulation and control in speaking. Assuming that Reynard wanted to express the message so perfectly conveyed by sentence (3), what mechanisms in his speech production system are responsible for his utterance to come out as (4)? A theoretical claim that is pervasive in this book is that such deviations from ideal are the result of two factors: First, there are occasional derailments in components of the language production system, leading to errors in pre-articulatory speech. Second, there are interactions between the planning process and the self-monitoring system. As a result of these interactions, the speaker engages in corrective behaviour, which directly affects the quality of the utterance (for example, monitoring can shape the pattern of speech errors one observes) or, indirectly introduces phenomena such as self-repairs.

Why do we need two factors in order to explain deviations from plan? It is obvious, both from considering normal spontaneous speech and pathological speech, that speech errors occur. But few theorists have taken into account the fact that errors have an aftermath: The verbal monitoring system continuously inspects self-produced speech and adjusts or corrects if necessary. Many of these monitoring processes occur before speech is articulated. That implies that the end product, overt speech, is a function of both phonological encoding processes and of monitoring. Any valid theory of "normal" speech errors or speech pathologies needs to take monitoring into account.

Another tenet of this book is the continuity thesis. Consider pathologies of language production such as stuttering, aphasia, and apraxia of speech. Each of these pathologies is characterised by (pathologically) many deviations from plan. People who stutter show excessive numbers of disfluencies (part-word repetitions, *b.b.brand*, prolongations, *sssssship*, and so on). People with aphasia are often very disfluent, produce many speech errors, and often leave them uncorrected. The speech of children with developmental apraxia of speech is characterised by many phonological speech errors and with problems in articulation. According to the continuity thesis, these pathological deviations can be explained in a similar way as "normal" deviations. That is, they are the result of deficits to specific components of the language formulation mechanism and of interactions between these components and a mechanism that safeguards the quality of speech: The self-monitoring system.

In this book, we aim at showing how psycholinguistic models of normal processing can be fruitfully applied to speech dysfunction (on the continuity thesis). Furthermore, the detailed analyses of language pathology that will be reported help constrain existing models of normal behaviour. In Chapter 16 (Wijnen & Kolk), the continuity thesis is explicitly evaluated in the light of the contributions to this volume.

Interplay of phonological encoding and self-monitoring

What are these components of language formulation that sometimes go awry? This book will specifically focus on *phonological encoding* in speech (the construction of a phonetic plan for the utterance), on *verbal self-monitoring* (checking for correctness and initiating corrective action if necessary), and on *interactions* between these processes. Let us see how these processes fit in a framework of language production. This is a framework sketched by Levelt (1989) and which is influenced by earlier work by Bock (1982), Fromkin (1971), Garrett (1975), Kempen and Huijbers (1983) and others. This framework is depicted in Figure 1.1.

Levelt (following, for example, Garrett, 1975) divided language production into three major components. First, the conceptualiser provides an interface between thought and language. It has access to the speaker's intentions, knowledge of the world, the current (physical and social) context, and a "model" of the current state of the discourse (who said what earlier in the conversation, what is the main topic, what subtopic is currently in focus, and so on). If the speaker, given this current context, decides to engage in a speech act, he or she will formulate a pre-verbal message. This can be thought of as a

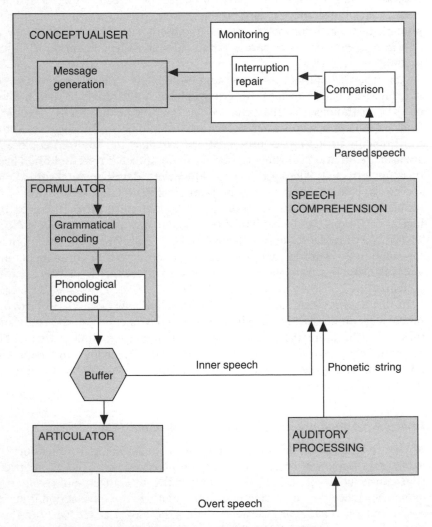

Figure 1.1 Blueprint of the speaker. (Adapted from Levelt, 1989.)

semantic structure, not itself yet language, but containing information that *can* be conveyed by a speech act.

The formulator uses this message to construct a sentence representation. It is subdivided into two components. The first component, grammatical encoding will, select from the mental lexicon words that match the specifications in the message. Based on message properties, this component will also assign grammatical functions to these words and build a phrasal representation, specifying the hierarchical relation between syntactic constituents and their linear order. The second component is phonological encoding. This component uses the sentence-level representation, including the words which have been assigned positions in that representation, and determines (a) the prosody of the sentence, and (b) the phonological form of the words. The latter process includes "spelling out" the phonological segments in the words, determining the metrical structure of these words (e.g. how many syllables? which syllable is stressed?), and assigning the segments to structural positions in these words.

The resulting representation is phonological in nature. But in order for the utterance to be articulated, this representation needs to be translated into the language of motor control. According to some proposals, this latter process yields "articulatory gestures", which specify in an abstract (context-independent) way what patterns of articulatory movements are required. The actual control of motor programming and motor execution is the task of the third component, the articulator.

The right-hand side of the graph sketchily shows speech comprehension, which is subdivided into auditory processing of overt speech (which renders a phonetic string), and speech comprehension proper, which is responsible for word recognition, syntactic analysis, and mapping the syntactic representation onto meaning. The resulting representation, which Levelt (1989) called "parsed speech", feeds into the conceptualiser.

As Figure 1.1 shows, this framework of language processing localises the monitor in the conceptualiser. Our speech reaches the conceptualiser through the speech comprehension system, and there are two channels feeding into this system. We can listen to our own overt speech (using auditory analysis) just as we can listen to anyone else's speech. But we can also "listen" to a representation of speech before it is articulated: Inner speech. This second channel is depicted in the figure as a connection between the articulatory buffer, which temporarily stores the speech plan while it waits for articulation, and the language comprehension system. Both of these feedback loops will reach the conceptualiser, and that system, finally, compares whether our own "parsed speech" matches our intended speech. This view on monitoring is not uncontroversial (see Postma, 2000, for review), and indeed a number of the chapters reported here will report tests of its tenability. Let us zoom in on the phonological encoding and the monitoring components in turn.

Phonological encoding

Figure 1.2 depicts a proposal for phonological encoding, based on Levelt, Roelofs, and Meyer (1999).

The process is illustrated with the encoding of the Dutch word *tijger* (tiger). In this graph, memory representations are depicted with circles, and the flow of processing is depicted with arrows. The first two memory representations, lexical concepts (TIGER(X)) and lemmas (tijger), are not part of phonological encoding proper, but they form the input to the process. Producing a word begins with the appropriate concept for that word (a semantic representation which can be expressed with, specifically, that word), which in turn activates a lexical representation. There is debate on how many levels of lexical representation there are: Levelt et al. (1999) assume there are two levels, lemmas and word forms, but this has been questioned by other authors (Caramazza, 1997; Starreveld & La Heij, 1995), who argue that only one level suffices. For present purposes, we remain agnostic, and depict both, but with lemmas between brackets.

Phonological encoding proper begins with the word form. Most theories of

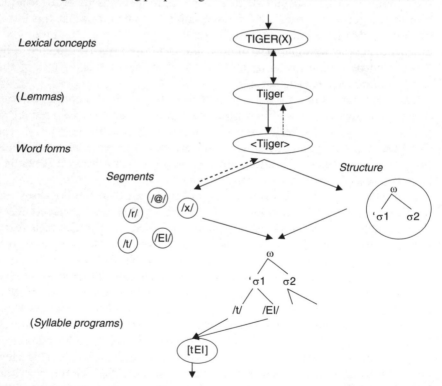

Figure 1.2 Illustration of the process of phonological encoding. (Based on Levelt et al., 1999.)

phonological encoding assume that encoding the word form is divided into two separate processes: One process which retrieves the phonological content of the word (the phonological segments) and one process which retrieves the structure of the word (e.g. the number of syllables, which syllable bears stress). The chapters by Martin (4) and Den Ouden and Bastiaanse (5) focus on the spelling of phonological content in the context of language pathology.

The notion of separately spelling out content and structure is relatively undisputed in the literature. But there is debate about the nature of the structural representation. Does it for example contain a word's CV structure? (see, for example, Hartsuiker, 2002 for review). There is also considerable debate about the nature of activation flow. According to Levelt et al. (1999) the information flows only top down. Other authors argue that there is direct feedback, both from segments to word forms, and from word forms to lemmas (e.g. Damian & Martin, 1999; Dell, 1986; see Vigliocco & Hartsuiker, 2002 for review). This book contributes further to this debate. See, in particular, the chapters by Dell and Kim (2), Nooteboom (10), and Roelofs (3).

What happens after structure and content are separately spelled out? They are put back together again! As Levelt et al. (1999) point out this is paradoxical: What is the point of decomposing a word form in its components and then recomposing it again to a whole? The answer lies in the fact that speakers produce connected speech, not just a string of citation forms. Connected speech has important repercussions for syllabification. If I am saying "give it!" the syllable boundaries do not coincide with the word boundaries (gi – vit). The process of segment-to-frame association therefore works with a number of language-specific syllabification rules, such as the rule for Dutch that as many segments as possible are placed in the onset of a syllable, unless that would make the previous syllable illegal (Booij, 1995). Because the resulting representation is no longer a word (in the sense of a stored representation in the mental lexicon), it is now called a *phonological* word, consisting of a single content word, followed and or preceded by a number of function words.

Based on the phonological word, the programs guiding articulation are determined. Levelt et al. (1999) and Levelt and Wheeldon (1994) made a very specific proposal for how this is done, based on work by Crompton (1982). This proposal assumes a repository of syllable programs, a so-called mental syllabary which would store the most frequent syllables in the language. Thus, articulatory scores for syllables are usually not computed on the fly, but retrieved from a store. Once more we should note that this part of the theory is disputed (see the chapters by Code (7) and by Nijland & Maassen (8) for discussion of this issue).

Self-monitoring

Figure 1.3 depicts a proposal of self-monitoring, based on Levelt's (1983; 1989) perceptual loop theory and an amendment proposed by Hartsuiker and Kolk (2001).

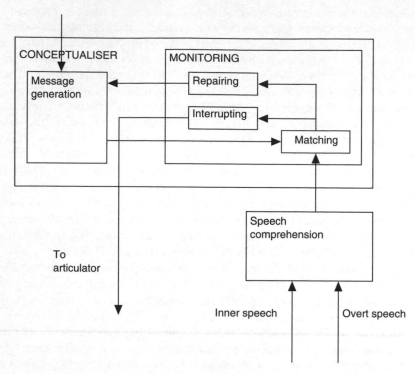

Figure 1.3 Components and information channels involved in self-monitoring.
(Adapted from Hartsuiker and Kolk, 2001.)

There is little doubt that speakers can listen to themselves speak out loud, and scrutinise what they hear. But a central claim of the theory is that there is also an additional channel, which monitors speech before articulation: An internal channel. This claim is supported by a rich set of data (reviewed in Hartsuiker & Kolk, 2001). However, it is less clear *what* the nature of this internal code is. For example, Levelt (1989) assumed it was a phonetic code. In subsequent work (Wheeldon & Levelt, 1995), the claim rather became that it is a phonological code as it unfolds over time: Particularly the product of segment-to-frame attachment, as illustrated in Figure 1.2. However, this amendment means that the monitor has direct access to representations being constructed in production, rather than to an end product of production (Hartsuiker & Kolk, 2001). This conflicts with another assumption of Levelt (1989), that formulation is an automatic process and only end products can reach awareness (Vigliocco & Hartsuiker, 2002).

Second, the perceptual loop theory claims that the internal channel is monitored through the language comprehension system. This is an elegant hypothesis, because it does not postulate any additional machinery: The monitor uses an existing mechanism, which is already there for other purposes. However, this claim is controversial. There are various competing theories, which localise the monitor in the language production system, in a modality-neutral network of linguistic representations, or which even claim there are two internal channels, one perception based and one production based. Unfortunately, none of these proposals is as of yet worked out in great detail (perhaps with the exception of Eikmeyer, Schade, Kupietz, & Laubenstein, 1999). This issue is discussed in the chapters by Oomen, Postma, and Kolk (12), and by Postma and Oomen (9).

An implication of postulating two channels is that there must be a division of labour between them: Some of the errors will be detected by one channel, others by the other. Presently, theories of monitoring leave unspecified what this division is. How many errors are detected by each channel? Which ones? Can the speaker strategically shift between the two channels? This aspect of monitoring is discussed in the chapters by Hartsuiker, Kolk, and Martensen (11) and by Oomen et al (12).

Another claim is that monitoring proper takes place at the level of the conceptualiser. In order to detect that something is wrong with the stream of "parsed speech" that reaches this component, a comparison needs to be made between actual and intended speech. Relatively little is known about the way this process of comparison works (but see Nooteboom, this volume (Chapter 10), for discussion and a specific proposal).

Finally, error detection has an aftermath. The speaker will interrupt herself and attempt to correct the error. In Levelt's (1989) proposal, the coordination between these two processes is governed by the "main interruption rule". That is, the speaker interrupts immediately on error detection and halts all components of language production. Since it takes time to stop action, there will be a short interval during which speech goes on. This interval ends when overt speech is interrupted. That moment marks the beginning of the "editing phase", during which the repair is planned. However, this main interruption rule turns out to be false. Blackmer and Mitton (1991) and Oomen and Postma (2001) showed that repairs often begin immediately on the moment of interruption. This implies that the repair is already planned during the interruption interval. Hartsuiker and Kolk (2001) therefore proposed a modified interruption rule, which conceives of interruption and repair as two parallel processes that *both* start immediately after error detection. They tested this new rule in their computational model of self-monitoring, and showed that they could account for Oomen and Postma's data on the time course of self-interruption and self-repair (however, see Postma & Oomen, this volume (Chapter 9), for a criticism of this proposal).

Interactions between speech production and self-monitoring

The basic claim of this book is that deviations from a "normal" speech plan, both in normal speech and in pathological speech, are a function of both disfunction of the mechanisms that plan speech (in particular of components of the phonological encoder) and of interactions between encoding and the self-monitoring system. We can illustrate this claim with an analogy from astronomy. Suppose you are an astronomer, studying a constellation of stars with your telescope. The image you will register will be a function of the "real" constellation that is out there, but also of properties of the earth's atmosphere that will break the light and distort the true pattern. What you see is *not* what is out there, even if you put your telescope on a high mountain in the Andes so as to minimise atmospheric distortion. You now have two options: Either you mount your telescope on a satellite which you then launch into space (so you bypass the atmosphere), or you build up a theory about the filtering effects of the atmosphere and then, based on that theory, design at telescope that reconstructs the "true" image. Astronomers have taken both options.[2]

If there is an internal self-monitoring system, and all the evidence suggests there is, then we have an analogous problem. What someone says is not what that person planned in the first instance: The true speech plan is filtered first. Since we cannot look at this internal speech plan directly, our job is to go for the second option: To construct a theory about the filtering effects of the monitor and how it interacts with speech planning to yield the speech we actually hear.

An example of such a possible interaction is the lexical bias effect (Baars, Motley, & MacKay, 1975). If speakers produce phonological speech errors (*good gear* instead of *good beer*), these errors tend to be real words (like *gear*) instead of nonwords (like *keer*). This can be explained as follows. As the "wrong" phoneme (/g/ or /m/) occurs in the context, it happens to be highly active when the phonemes for the target word "beer" are spelled out (see Figure 1.2). As a result, the speaker will sometimes choose the wrong phoneme, leading to the incorrect phonological code (*keer* or *gear*). All other things being equal, this means the nonlexical error is as likely as the lexical error. However, the phonological code is inspected by the monitoring system. If we assume that this system uses lexicality (is this a real word?) as a criterion, then it is more likely to detect that *keer* is wrong than that *gear* is wrong. Consequently, it will edit out more nonword errors than lexical errors, so that more lexical error become overt. Hence, we observe a lexical bias effect. Indeed, the monitoring explanation is supported by other experiments reported by Baars and colleagues. (See also Roelofs, this volume (Chapter 3), for similar explanations for other speech error patterns. See Dell & Kim (Chapter 2) and Nooteboom (Chapter 10), this volume, for a critique.)

Another example of interactions between speech planning and self-monitoring, is Kolk's (1995) approach to agrammatism, and Postma and Kolk's (1993) approach to stuttering. Speech in Broca's aphasia is slow, effortful, and characterised by severe limitations in morphosyntaxis (e.g. omission of closed-class material, reduced variety of syntactic structure). Under certain experimental conditions, however, these patients can shift their pattern somewhat, yielding speech that is more fluent, but characterised by more morphosyntactic errors (e.g. substitutions of closed-class elements).

We can explain this by assuming a deficit in grammatical encoding (see Figure 1.1), which leads to severe problems in building up a sentence representation. Because the self-monitoring system is still largely intact (these patients have relatively minor comprehension problems), many of these problems are detected and are repaired internally. But because this leads to so many revisions, resulting speech is slow, effortful, and contains many disfluencies. Furthermore, if the focus of the monitor is shifted away from morphosyntactic problems due to task demands, the pattern changes: In that case, disfluency is traded in for more overt errors. (The issue of self-monitoring in aphasia is given attention in the chapters by Oomen et al. (12) and by Hartsuiker et al. (11).)

According to Postma and Kolk (1993) and Kolk and Postma (1997), a similar interaction underlies stuttering. These authors propose that people who stutter have a deficit in constructing the phonological code, in particular in the selection of the correct phoneme. As a result, the internal speech plan of stutterers contains many speech errors. However, these errors are intercepted by the self-monitoring system, and covertly repaired. This removes the error from the speech plan. Unfortunately, error detection also implies interrupting. Depending on the timing of that process, covert repairing will interrupt the ongoing execution of the speech plan, leading to disfluencies. (This covert repair hypothesis is further explored in Hartsuiker, Kolk, and Lickley (Chapter 15), and Melnick, Conture, and Ohde (Chapter 6). See also Vasic and Wijnen (Chapter 13) and Russell, Corley, and Lickley (Chapter 14) for a new variant of that hypothesis.)

Structure of the book

Part I deals with phonological encoding. The chapters by Dell and Kim (2) and Roelofs (3) both focus on patterns of speech errors and how they can be accounted for in existing models of phonological encoding and their interaction with the monitor. A recurring issue (with opposite conclusions) in these two chapters is whether the data force us to postulate feedback between levels of encoding (see Figure 1.2) or not.

Part II reports research on phonological encoding in language pathology. Martin (Chapter 4) reports an overview of studies on phonological errors in patients with aphasia. She accounts for error patterns using a connectionist framework (see Dell & Kim, Chapter 2), and attempts to localise functional loci of impairment within such a framework. Den Ouden and Bastiaanse (Chapter 5) also report a study on phonological errors in conduction aphasia. They find two distinct patterns and propose that patients can be divided into a subgroup with a specific deficit in phonological encoding mechanisms, and another subgroup that suffers from impairments in working memory, disallowing maintenance of the phonological plan. Melnick, Conture, and Ohde report a study on phonological encoding in children who stutter, in Chapter 6. They tentatively conclude that these children exhibit deficits in phonological planning. However, it is likely that these problems are accompanied by other types of planning difficulty (e.g. semantic and syntactic planning). In Chapter 7, Code reports research on the impact of brain damage on the production of syllables, comparing individuals with, for example, Broca's aphasia and apraxia of speech. He discusses the notion of the syllabary (see Figure 1.2) and pinpoints areas of the brain involved in syllable processing. Nijland and Maassen report a study on developmental apraxia of speech (Chapter 8). These children show a complex pattern of distortion in their phonological production. The authors conclude that the impairment is multifactorial and affects both syllable planning (see Figure 1.2) and motor programming.

Part III reports research on self-monitoring. Postma and Oomen discuss a number of critical issues in theories of the monitor (Chapter 9). This includes the issue on production versus perception based monitoring, a review of studies on monitoring in patients (e.g. with aphasia), and they discuss the possibility of shifts in the division of labour between channels. Nooteboom (Chapter 10) tests a prediction from the perceptual loop theory of monitoring. If lexical bias is a result of self-monitoring, then one should observe it not only in speech error patterns, but also in overt self-corrections. This, however, turns out not to be the case and he suggests a number of alternative accounts. Hartsuiker, Kolk, and Martensen present a model in Chapter 11 that estimates the division of labour between monitoring channels. They conclude that the internal channel does most of the work, and they account for shifts in the division of labour in terms of selective attention.

Part IV applies psycholinguistic models of self-monitoring to language pathology. Oomen, Postma, and Kolk report a case study on self-monitoring in Broca's aphasia (Chapter 12). They conclude that the patient relies exclusively on the internal channel. They also observed a dissociation between error types. Whereas the patient produced few semantic errors and repaired these easily, he produced many phonological errors and had troubles repairing them. This can be explained in two ways: Either there is a production monitor (because there is a direct relationship between impairment and monitoring) or the patient focuses on semantic errors more than on phonological errors. Vasic and Wijnen (Chapter 13) introduce the vicious circle hypothesis of stuttering. They explain the disfluencies observed in stuttering as a result of excessive covert repairing, in effect similarly to the covert repair hypothesis but they attribute this to disfunctional monitoring: The monitor would focus too much on the fluent delivery of the speech plan, leading to interruptions and repairs. In Chapter 14, Russell, Corley, and Lickley test a prediction that follows from Vasic and Wijnen's account: In an experiment in which listeners judged fluent and disfluent speech samples for goodness, they observed that people who stutter judged the fluent samples as better, and the disfluent samples as worse than people who do not stutter did. Finally, Hartsuiker, Kolk, and Lickley tested the covert repair hypothesis. (Chapter 15) They used their model of the time course of self-interruption to simulate the pattern of stuttering for different groups (young children and adults), for different types of word (function words and content words) and for different positions within the phonological word. Their simulations supported the covert repair hypothesis.

In Part V, Wijnen and Kolk evaluate the state of the art on phonological encoding and self-monitoring in normal and pathological speech (Chapter 16). Where are we now, and what lacunae in our knowledge of these processes are left unfilled? Most importantly, what future directions should we take in this field?

Notes

1 The HCRC Map Task (Anderson et al., 1991) corpus is based on this dialogue game. The examples are taken from transcripts of two male speakers in that corpus.
2 The first option was taken by the designers of the Hubble telescope. There is also a project on the way which attempts to construct a telescope that filters out atmospheric distortions (*New Scientist*, December 2001).

References

Anderson, A. H., Bader, M., Bard, E. G., Boyle, E., Doherty, G., Garrod, S., Isard, S., Kowtko, J., McAllister, J., Miller, J., Sotillo, C., Thompson, H. S., & Weinert, R. (1991). The HCRC Map Task Corpus. *Language and Speech, 34*, 351–66.

Baars, B. J., Motley, M. T., & MacKay, D. G. (1975). Output editing for lexical status in artificially elicited slips of the tongue. *Journal of Verbal Learning and Verbal Behavior, 14*, 382–91.

Blackmer, E. R., & Mitton, E. R. (1991). Theories of monitoring and the timing of repairs in spontaneous speech. *Cognition, 39*, 173–94.

Bock, J. K. (1982). Toward a cognitive psychology of syntax: Information processing contributions to sentence formulation. *Psychological Review, 89*, 1–47.

Booij, G. (1995). *The phonology of Dutch.* Oxford: Clarendon Press.

Caramazza, A. (1997). How many levels of processing are there in lexical access? *Cognitive Neuropsychology, 14*, 177–208.

Chomsky, N. (1965). *Aspects of the theory of syntax.* Cambridge, MA: MIT Press.

Clark, H. H., & Fox Tree, J. (2002). Using *uh* and *um* in spontaneous speaking. *Cognition, 84*, 73–111.

Crompton, A. (1982). Syllables and segments in speech production. In A. Cutler (Ed.), *Slips of the tongue and language production* (pp. 109–62). Berlin: Mouton.

Damian, M. F., & Martin, R. C. (1999). Semantic and phonological codes interact in single word production. *Journal of Experimental Psychology: Learning, Memory, and Cognition, 25*, 345–61.

Dell, G. S. (1986). A spreading activation theory of retrieval in sentence production. *Psychological Review, 93*, 283–321.

Eikmeyer, H.-J., Schade, U., Kupietz, M., & Laubenstein, U. (1999). A connectionist view of language production. In R. Klabunde & C. von Stutterheim, (Eds.), *Representations and processes in language production* (pp. 205–36). Wiesbaden: Deutscher Universitäts-Verlag.

Fromkin, V. A. (1971). The non-anomalous nature of anomalous utterances. *Language, 47*, 27–52.

Garrett, M. F. (1975). The analysis of sentence production. In G. H. Bower (Ed.), *The psychology of learning and motivation* (pp. 133–77). New York: Academic Press.

Hartsuiker, R. J. (2002). The addition bias in Dutch and Spanish phonological speech errors: The role of structural context. *Language and Cognitive Processes, 17*, 61–96.

Hartsuiker, R. J., & Kolk, H. H. J. (2001). Error monitoring in speech production: A computational test of the perceptual loop theory. *Cognitive Psychology, 42*, 113–57.

Kempen, G., & Huijbers, P. (1983). The lexicalization process in sentence production and naming: Indirect election of words. *Cognition, 14*, 185–209.

Kolk, H. H. J. (1995). A time-based approach to agrammatic production. *Brain and Language, 50*, 282–303.

Kolk, H. H. J., & Postma, A. (1997). Stuttering as a covert-repair phenomenon. In R. Corlee & G. Siegel (Eds.), *Nature and treatment of stuttering: New directions* (pp. 182–203). Boston: Allyn & Bacon.

Levelt, W. J. M. (1983). Monitoring and self-repair in speech. *Cognition, 14*, 41–104.

Levelt, W. J. M. (1989). *Speaking: From intention to articulation*. Cambridge, MA: MIT Press.

Levelt, W. J. M., Roelofs, A., Meyer, A. S. (1999). A theory of lexical access in speech production. *Behavioral and Brain Sciences, 22*, 1–38.

Levelt, W. J. M., & Wheeldon, L. (1994). Do speakers have access to a mental syllabary? *Cognition, 50*, 239–69.

Nooteboom, S. G. (1980). Speaking and unspeaking: Detection and correction of phonological and lexical errors in spontaneous speech. In V. A. Fromkin (Ed.), *Errors in linguistic performance: Slips of the tongue, ear, pen, and hand* (pp. 87–95). New York: Academic Press.

Oomen, C. C. E., & Postma, A. (2001). Effects of time pressure on mechanisms of speech production and self-monitoring. *Journal of Psycholinguistic Research, 30*, 163–84.

Postma, A. (2000). Detection of errors during speech production: A review of speech monitoring models. *Cognition, 77*, 97–131.

Postma, A., & Kolk, H. H. J. (1993). The covert repair hypothesis: Prearticulatory repair processes in normal and stuttered disfluencies. *Journal of Speech and Hearing Research, 36*, 472–87.

Starreveld, P. A., & La Heij, W. (1995). Semantic interference, orthographic facilitation, and their interaction in naming tasks. *Journal of Experimental Psychology: Learning, Memory, and Cognition, 21*, 686–98.

Vigliocco, G., & Hartsuiker, R. J. (2002). The interplay of meaning, sound, and syntax in sentence production. *Psychological Bulletin, 128*, 442–72.

Wheeldon, L. R., & Levelt, W. J. M. (1995). Monitoring the time course of phonological encoding. *Journal of Memory and Language, 34*, 311–34.

Part I
Theories and models of phonological encoding

2   Speech errors and word form encoding

Gary S. Dell and Albert E. Kim

Abstract

The properties of everyday slips of the tongue provide useful constraints on theories of language production. This chapter focuses on phonological errors, slips that occur during word-form encoding, and argues that these errors are strongly sensitive to familiarity. Unfamiliar word forms are vulnerable to slipping, and the resulting errors are themselves driven toward familiar pronunciations. The influence of familiarity on errors is explained through the learning and processing mechanisms of connectionist models. Specifically, the chapter discusses the effect of target-word frequency on word-form encoding, the role of linguistic structure in shaping what is pronounced, and the hypothesis that phonological errors reflect feedback between planned speech sounds and the mental lexicon.

Introduction

Speech errors, often called "slips of the tongue", come in many shapes and sizes. Sometimes, a speaker incorrectly replaces one word with another. For example, former US president Gerald Ford once saluted the president of Egypt by mislabeling his nation as "Israel". Here the conceptual similarity between *Israel* and *Egypt* derailed Mr Ford. More recently, US president George W. Bush said: "A tax cut is one of the anecdotes to coming out of an economic illness". He meant to say "antidotes". In this case, the similarity in pronunciation between *anecdote* and *antidote* is a factor in the error. Not all errors involve the speaker saying the wrong word. Sometimes, the slip is just a mispronunciation, such as when President Bush said, "prescription drugs will be an ingritable part of the program". "Integral" was likely the intended word.

Speaking is clearly a complex task, both for presidents and ordinary people. Before we can actually articulate sounds, we must plan our utterance. We must retrieve words from lexical memory, organize them into a grammatically correct sequence, and identify the pronunciation of the words in the sequence. In this chapter, we focus on the last part of this process, planning the pronunciations of words, or *word-form encoding*. The kinds of error that occur during word-form encoding are *phonological errors*. Bush's saying "ingritable" for *integral* would be a phonological error. Our central theme is that such errors are governed by familiarity. Unfamiliar word forms are vulnerable to slipping, and the resulting errors themselves are driven toward familiar pronunciations.

There are many kinds of phonological errors. Some, the contextual or movement errors, involve the ordering of the components of words. Most often, the wrongly ordered components correspond to single phonemes as in "lork yibrary" for *York library*. It is not uncommon, however, for groups of phonemes such as consonant clusters to slip ("flow snurries" for *snow flurries*). Moreover, the features of phonemes themselves can slip as well, as in "glear plue" for *clear blue*, in which the unvoiced feature of the /k/ in *clear* switched places with the voiced feature of the /b/ in *blue*, turning the /k/ into a /g/ and the /b/ into a /p/. Not only do movement errors vary with respect to the size of the slipping components, they also vary in the nature of the movement. The examples just given are all *exchanges* of particular units (see Nooteboom, this volume, Chapter 10). The other common movement errors are *anticipations* ("cuff of coffee" for *cup of coffee*) and *perseverations* ("beef needle" for *beef noodle*), in which either an upcoming or previous speech component is spoken at the wrong time.

Errors in which there is no clear movement also occur. In these *noncontextual errors*, sounds can be erroneously deleted, added, or replaced by other sounds (e.g., *department* spoken as "jepartment"). There are also errors that are hard to categorize because the error is just too complex. Mr. Bush's "ingritable" for *integral* error appears to be, in part, an exchange of /t/ and /gr/. But the error also includes the addition of a syllable, and the main stress was shifted from the first syllable of *integral* to the second syllable of "ingritable."

Phonological errors provide insight into the process of word-form encoding. Consider the "ingritable" example. Why did this happen? We will set aside explanations such as nervousness or lack of sleep. Although such systemic factors undoubtedly affect the chance of error, they are not, by themselves, informative about language production. Instead, we will focus on characteristics of the error, itself, specifically, the low frequency of the target word *integral*, the fact that the error string "ingritable" is structurally well formed, and the possibility that "ingritable" reflects contamination from familiar words such as *incredible*. More generally, this chapter will discuss the effects of target word frequency on word-form encoding, the role of linguistic structure in shaping what is pronounced, and finally, the hypothesis that phonological errors reflect feedback between planned speech sounds and the mental lexicon. What these three issues have in common is that they point to the role of familiarity on errors, both the familiarity of the target word and the influence of familiar phonological forms on the error string.

We will seek explanations for these error phenomena by appealing to mechanisms found in *connectionist models* of lexical retrieval (e.g., Dell, 1986; Plaut, McClelland, Seidenberg, & Patterson, 1996; Seidenberg &

McClelland, 1989). Connectionist models, sometimes called neural-network or parallel-distributed-processing models, compute by using a network of simple processing units that send numeric, as opposed to symbolic, signals to one another, much as neurons do. Because of this, connectionist models are often said to be "neurally inspired". However, this characterization should not be overstated. The models largely aim to account for behavioral data rather than facts about brain anatomy and physiology, and this is most certainly true for connectionist models of language (Christiansen & Chater, 1999).

For our purposes, the most important property of these models is that they are naturally sensitive to experience. Hence, they may be able to give a good account of familiarity effects on phonological errors.

There are four crucial aspects of connectionist models: Their architecture, their initial representations, their processing assumptions, and their learning assumptions. The architecture concerns the form of the network. For example, in Seidenberg and McClelland's (1989) model of reading printed words aloud, the architecture contained three layers of units: Input, hidden, and output. The input layer coded the orthography of the words to be pronounced. The input had connections to the hidden layer, and the hidden layer connected to the output, which represented the pronunciations of the words. The initial representations are the assumptions about how the input and output are coded. For example, Seidenberg and McClelland's output units corresponded to sequences of three phonological features.

The processing assumptions of a connectionist model characterize how activation spreads through the network. Spreading activation is how the model computes its output from its input. More formally, each unit possesses an activation level, a number representing the extent to which that unit participates in the processing. Changes in activation are determined by the *activation rule*, a rule that updates each unit's activation level. This level is a function of the net input, the summed activation delivered to the unit from units that are connected to it. A connectionist model's learning assumptions govern how the strengths, or weights, of the connections among the units change as a function of the model's experience. Learning usually involves training, the presentation of input/output pairs that represent the task at hand. For Seidenberg and McClelland's (1989) reading aloud model, the network would be presented with the input orthographic activation pattern for a word and that word's desired phonological output. This would occur several times for each word with the more common words receiving the most training. The learning algorithm for this model was *backpropagation*. For each experience with a word, activation spreads from the input to the hidden layer and ultimately to the output layer. The activation levels of the output units are then compared to the desired output pattern. To the extent that there is a discrepancy, the connection weights are changed to reduce that discrepancy. More generally, connectionist learning algorithms gradually modify the weights in the network so that the network accomplishes its task as well as it can for the input/output pairs that it is trained on.

Many connectionist models of language can be divided into two families, with different approaches to learning and representation. In "localist" networks, each unit codes a whole concept, such as the meaning of a word. Localist networks also tend not to have learning components; the weights on connections between units are stipulated. These models accomplish most of their explanatory work through their choices of architecture and processing assumptions. We refer to models of this sort in the section entitled "framed-based models" and in the final section "speech errors and phonological-lexical feedback". In the rest of the chapter, we refer mainly to "distributed" networks, where each concept is represented as a pattern of activation distributed across many units. These models tend to focus on learning algorithms and how such networks acquire complex aspects of speech production behavior from exposure to statistical regularities in linguistic experience.

For word-form encoding in production, the task is to create the pronunciation of words. So, in connectionist terms, the output would be a representation of pronunciation across a set of units in a network. For some models, this representation is articulatory (Plaut & Kello, 1999). Most models, however, view the output of word-form encoding as more abstract, such as an ordered set of phonemes (Dell, Schwartz, Martin, Saffran, & Gagnon, 1997; Shattuck-Hufnagel, 1979), phonetic syllables (Roelofs, 1997), or phonological features (e.g., Anderson, Milostan & Cottrell, 1998; Dell, Juliano, & Govindjee, 1993). The input to word-form encoding is somewhat more difficult to characterize. Theories of language production distinguish word-form encoding from grammatical encoding (Levelt, Roelofs, & Meyer, 1999). The former is concerned with the pronunciation of words, and the latter with selecting these words in accordance with the message to be conveyed and the grammar of the language. Given this distinction, the input to word-form encoding would be the output of grammatical encoding, which is assumed to be a set of words, ordered and arranged into phrases, with the words represented in terms of their grammatical rather than phonological properties. The lexical representations associated with grammatical encoding are often called *lemmas* (Kempen & Huijbers, 1983; Levelt et al., 1999). In short, word-form encoding starts with lemmas, symbols that identify words and indicate their grammatical properties, and ends up with a representation of the words' sound forms.

In the remaining three sections of this chapter, we discuss word-form encoding from a connectionist perspective. Our goal is to explain the three previously mentioned speech error phenomena: The vulnerability of low frequency words to error, the structural well-formedness of the errors, and error effects that suggest feedback from the phonological to the lexical levels.

Word frequency

Everyone's intuition is that common words are easy to say and rare words are difficult. This intuition is correct. Stemberger (1983) examined a large collection of phonological slips and found that less familiar words such as *integral* were particularly subject to error. In an analysis of naturally occurring word blends such as "herrible" for *horrible/terrible*, Laubstein (1999) reported that the words involved tended to be uncommon and, moreover, for blends involving phonologically similar targets (like "herrible"), the more frequent of the blending words contributed more to the output. Dell (1990) used an experimental procedure and found that initial consonant exchanges were three times more likely in low-frequency word pairs (*vogue pang* spoken as "pogue vang") than in high-frequency pairs (*vote pass* spoken as "pote vass"). Frequency effects are apparent in the phonological errors of aphasic speakers (e.g., Martin, Saffran, & Dell, 1996), in incidences of tip-of-tongue (TOT) states (Harley & Bown, 1998), and in a variety of production tasks in which the dependent variable is speed rather than errors (e.g., Griffin & Bock, 1998; Jescheniak & Levelt, 1994).

So, we know that word frequency matters. By itself, this fact does not provide much information about word production. Any reasonable theory would accord with the claim that common words are more accurately spoken. A more compelling issue is that of where frequency effects are located in the system. Recall that production theory distinguishes between the lexical representations in grammatical encoding (lemmas), and those involved in word-form encoding. More specifically, we can distinguish between lemma access and word-form access. Is the advantage of high-frequency words associated with lemma access, word-form access, or both? The evidence that we have reviewed is more consistent with word-form access. The speech-error evidence concerns phonological errors, slips in which the word's form is disrupted. These can be unambiguously assigned to word-form encoding and, hence, the presence of frequency effects on these errors associates frequency with word-form representations. Similarly, the finding that TOT states occur primarily with uncommon words also implicates word form as the locus of frequency effects. TOTs are often associated with successful access of a word's grammatical properties (Caramazza & Miozzo, 1997, Vigliocco, Vinson, Martin, & Garrett, 1999), but not the word's phonological properties. Consequently, some TOT blockage occurs in accessing word forms, again associating frequency effects with forms.

Other evidence for the claim that word frequency effects are felt during the access of word forms rather than lemmas comes from studies of homophones. Homophone pairs (e.g., *we* and *wee*) share their forms, but not their lemmas. Thus, by studying the production of homophones, researchers can disentangle the influence of the frequency of the lexical item from its form. Dell (1990) found that low-frequency homophones (e.g., *wee*) had the same phonological error rate as their high-frequency mates (e.g., *we*) and suggested that the low-frequency word inherits the invulnerability to error of its mate. Similarly, Jescheniak and Levelt (1994) found that response latencies for producing the low-frequency member of a homophone pair were similar to those for high-frequency words matched to the frequency of the high-frequency member of the pair, and faster than those for words matched to the low-frequency member. From these results, it can be concluded that the frequency of the word form, more so than the lemma, matters in production.

Why is word frequency felt primarily during the access of a word's form? Specifically, why not during lemma access? Connectionist models may have an answer to this question. Consider the representations that are involved in lexical access. The input can be thought of as a set of activated semantic feature units. Words with similar meanings such as CAT and LION would share units. The output representation would code for word form in some manner. Words that are similar in their phonological form (CAT and SAT) would share units.

We must also hypothesize the existence of an intermediate representation between word meaning and word form. This representation is required for two reasons. First, it is needed for computational reasons. The relation between word meaning and word form is largely arbitrary. CAT and LION share semantic, but not formal properties. CAT and SAT share form, but not semantics. Because there is little correlation between meaning and form, the mapping from semantic features to word form is not *systematic*. A consequence of this lack of systematicity is that one cannot go *directly* from the semantic units of a word to the correct phonological units. More precisely, there exist no semantic-to-form weights that enable the mapping to be achieved for all words. There must be at least one intermediate hidden layer. Hidden units compute nonlinear combinations of semantic units to create representations that are more systematically related to phonology.

The other motivation for a representation that mediates between word meaning and form is the need to represent the grammatical properties of words, such as whether a word is a noun or a verb (syntactic class), or more specific properties, such as whether a verb takes a direct object. These properties are essential for determining how words are placed in sentences. The lemma representations that we referred to earlier contain this kind of information. Several production theorists have specifically proposed that lemmas are intermediate between lexical-semantic and lexical-form representations (e.g., Dell et al., 1997; Levelt et al., 1999; see, however, Caramazza, 1997). Evidence for this proposal comes from studies showing that a word's grammatical properties are activated after its semantic properties, but before its phonological properties (e.g., Schmitt, Schiltz, Zaake, Kutas, & Münte, 2001; Van Turennout, Hagoort, & Brown, 1997; 1998).

Thus we see that a representation that is sensitive to the grammatical properties of lexical items must mediate between semantics and word form. What would such a representation be like? In modern production theories, lemma-level representations consist of a unit that uniquely identifies the lexical item and links to other units that represent grammatical properties of item (e.g., Dell et al., 1997; Levelt et al., 1999). If such representations were to be acquired by connectionist learning algorithms, they would contain similar information, but the representations would be distributed, that is, each lemma would be a pattern of activation across a great many units. Moreover, these "distributed lemmas" would reflect semantic as well as the grammatical properties of the lexical item. For example, the representation of BOY would be sensitive to the fact that it functions as a noun (e.g., can come after THE) and that it is singular (cannot come after THESE). However, it would also be sensitive to semantic properties that are predictive of other words in the utterance (e.g., it can serve as the subject of verbs of cognition). This is because the distributional properties of lexical items, which are the basis for grammatical categories, are correlated with their semantic properties. Connectionist learning algorithms naturally pick up on whatever correlations are present in the linguistic input.

Thus far, we have hypothesized that lexical access involves a chain from semantics to (distributed) lemma and from lemma to phonological form. Now we are ready to locate word frequency in this chain. In general, connectionist models are naturally sensitive to frequency through their learning assumptions. Each time a model produces a word, it increases the strength of the connections between activated units at the semantic level and the proper units at the lemma level. The same process occurs between the lemma units and the phonological units. The result is that the words that are often produced are produced more accurately and fluently.

This process would seem to locate frequency effects during both the semantics-to-lemma and the lemma-to-form mappings. It turns out, however, that much of the frequency effect will inhabit the lemma-to-form mapping. This is because the semantics-to-lemma relationship is more systematic than the lemma-to-form one. Consider the semantically related words, CAT and LION. Their distributed lemmas are also similar to one another. Both are singular count nouns. More generally, both would have similar distributional properties. The same point can be made for verbs. The more similar in meaning any two verbs are, the more similar are their distributional constraints such as their subcategorization frames (Fisher, Gleitman, & Gleitman, 1991). Although semantically similar words are not required to have similar distributional constraints, on average they do, and that is what makes the semantics-to-lemma mapping a fairly systematic one. The lemma-to-form mapping is, in contrast, largely unsystematic. Words with similar forms (e.g., CAT and SAT) are unlikely to have similar syntactic functions. Although there are cases of systematic lemma-form mappings due to derivational morphology (e.g., words ending in *-ment* will often be nouns), it is fair to say that, at least in languages such as English, this factor is a minor one limited largely to the ends of word forms.

The systematicity of the mapping is important because the frequency with which a particular item is trained matters more when the mapping is unsystematic than when it is systematic. This is the "frequency by regularity interaction" emphasized in discussions of connectionist models of reading (Plaut et al., 1996; Seidenberg & McClelland, 1989). Networks (and people) show a strong word-frequency effect when reading words that are not regularly spelled, but little or no effect when the words are regular. So, a less common but regularly spelled word such as MODE can be read aloud as quickly as a common one such as NINE. When words are not regularly spelled, however, frequency makes a big difference. The common word LOSE is easy, but the uncommon one DEAF is difficult. In reading models, regular words represent systematic mappings. -ODE is always pronounced as *owed*. Consequently, even though the model receives little training on the uncommon word MODE, the fact that MODE is regular means that the components of its mapping (-ODE = *owed*) receive training from other words such as CODE or RODE. Thus, an uncommon item that belongs to a systematically related set of items does not suffer from its low-frequency status. The other items make up for it. In this manner, connectionist models explain the frequency by regularity interaction.

From this analysis, we can see why word frequency will matter less in accessing a lemma than it will in accessing a word's phonological form. The systematicity of the semantics-to-lemma mapping implies that the frequency with which a particular word is experienced is unimportant. But because the word's form cannot be predicted from the characteristics of its lemma, success in accessing form is much more dependent on how often that particular mapping has been experienced.

In this way, connectionist assumptions can explain the data suggesting that frequency effects in production are associated primarily with the access of phonological form. More generally, connectionist learning and representational assumptions allow us to understand why experience is such a powerful factor in word form encoding. If the word *integral* is not very familiar, we should expect to have trouble retrieving its form even if we have a clear sense of what it means.

In the following section, we move from the target words involved in phonological errors (e.g., *integral*) to the characteristics of the error strings themselves. Even though the error strings are often nonwords (e.g., "ingritable"), they are familiar in the sense that they follow the phonological constraints of the language being spoken. To explain the effect of these constraints, we will have to discuss specific mechanisms in models of word-form encoding.

Speech errors and phonological structure

Speech errors tend to be phonologically well formed. That is to say, erroneous speech almost never contains phonological sequences that do not normally occur in the language. For example, in English, no word begins with [dl]; that is, [dl] is *phonotactically illegal* in onset position. Consequently it would be highly unusual for a speech error to create such a sequence. Violations do occur – Stemberger (1983) noted the occurrence of "dlorm" for *dorm* – but they are rare. Stemberger found that over 99 per cent of his phonological errors were well formed.

Structural regularities appear to shape errors in at least two ways. First, movement errors tend to involve interference between structurally identical pieces of phonological material – syllable onsets replace other onsets, and codas replace codas. For instance, in the error *a reading list* spoken as "a leading list" (Fromkin, 1971), the onset /l/ occurs in the wrong word but not in the wrong syllable position. Second, syllable structure appears to influence the "detachability" of phonological material. Syllable onsets are more likely than codas to participate in errors (Vousden, Brown, & Harley, 2000). And when an adjacent vowel and consonant are both replaced, the sequence is more likely to be VC than CV (Nooteboom, 1973; Shattuck-Hufnagel, 1983). The latter pattern appears to involve the widely hypothesized sub-syllabic division between onset and rhyme; VC sequences often constitute a rhyme, while CV sequences never form such a unit. In this section, we will discuss three different approaches to accommodating such evidence of linguistic knowledge in language production.

Frame-based models

Frame-based models separate language production into components of content and structure (Dell, 1986; 1988; Hartsuiker, 2002; Shattuck-Hufnagel, 1979; Stemberger, 1990). Units of phonological content (phonemes) and structural frames are retrieved independently during production, and the content units are inserted into slots within the frames. The frames enforce the phonological rules of the language.

One example of this approach is the spreading activation model of Dell (1988, Figure 2.1), which adopts structural assumptions from Stemberger (1983; 1990).

The model is composed of two networks of units, a lexical network, which contains word and phoneme units, and a structural network, which contains wordshape units (e.g., CVC) and phoneme category units (e.g., Ci, V, Cf). (See Hartsuiker, 2002, for an implemented variant of this model using syllable structures instead of wordshapes.) At the start of word-form access, the selected word unit sends activation to its constituent phoneme units. This causes the word's phonemes to become more active than other phonemes in the lexicon. The selected word unit also activates a wordshape unit. The wordshape unit activates a sequence of phoneme category units, and each phoneme category unit sends activation to a class of phoneme units in the lexical network. Thus, phonemes are connected to both lexical and structural sources of activation. A phoneme is selected for output when it receives sufficient activation from both the current word unit and the current phoneme category unit. This process is subject to structural constraints, which are built into the model's architecture. First, the phoneme category units are activated in rule-based sequences (e.g., CVC, but not CCCC). Second, phoneme units are segregated into categories, each of which receives activation from only one phoneme category unit (e.g., onset-/k/ is different from coda-/k/). The process is illustrated by the production of the first sound in

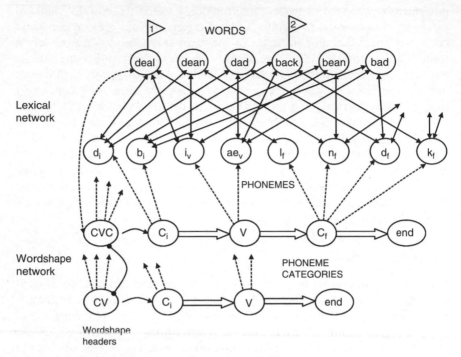

Figure 2.1 Frame-based model of word-form encoding. (From Dell, 1988.)

"cat". The word unit CAT excites three phonemes: onset-/k/, vowel-/ae/, and coda-/t/. CAT also activates the CVC wordshape, which triggers the sequence Ci, V, Cf. At the first step in this sequence, CAT and Ci are both activated. In general, onset-/k/ will be activated more highly than any other phoneme in the language, because it is the only phoneme to receive activation from both CAT and Ci.

The structural aspects of the model lead directly to syllable position effects in speech errors. One way for phonological errors to occur is through antici-patory activation of upcoming words. During the production of "cat food", for instance, the word unit FOOD receives anticipatory priming while the model is producing CAT. This activity spreads to phonemes connected to FOOD (onset-/f/, vowel-/u/, coda-/d/), creating the potential for errors. How-ever, these phonemes will never receive activation sufficient for selection without structural support. When the Ci unit is activated, onset-/f/ may be a candidate for selection, but coda-/d/ will not. Thus, movement errors preserve syllable position.

A major strength of the frame-based approach is a connection to well-developed formal theories of phonology. The phoneme categories and the restrictions on their ordering directly embody phonological rules, such as *syllable → onset nucleus coda.* Such rules are motivated by a wide range of phonological phenomena in a variety of languages, including many of the most robustly reported patterns of speech error. Other rules, such as restrictions on consonant cluster formation (/st/ but not /ts/ pre-vocalically), can be incorporated into frame-based models by elaborating the wordshape network. The straightforwardness of this incorporation of linguistic structure makes the models explicit and comprehensible.

At the same time, the explicit stipulation of rules sidesteps important issues. The imposition of categories on phonemes, causes a loss of generality: The onset /p/ and coda /p/ are treated with independent, slot-specific representations, even though they belong to the same phoneme by most accounts. More generally, explicit linguistic rules may be theoretically unwieldy in that they introduce domain-specific mechanisms rather than explaining language production in terms of general principles of learning and cognition.

Connectionist accounts

The deepest weakness of the frame-based approach may be a general inappropriateness of formal rule-based approaches. Frame-based accounts have difficulty explaining exceptions to the rules that sometimes occur. Beyond isolated exceptions are many indications that phonotactic constraints are graded, or probabilistic. Studies of experimentally induced speech errors have shown that the ability of a phoneme to intrude on another is affected by phoneme frequency and transitional frequencies (Levitt & Healy, 1985). Dell, Reed, Adams, and Meyer (2000) found that phonotactic constraints on speech errors span a continuum of strength, ranging from language-wide "rules" to weaker tendencies, which were acquired during participation in an experimental task. Probabilistic phonotactic constraints are also seen in language comprehension by both adults and infants (Jusczyk, Luce, & Charles-Luce, 1994) and in distributional analyses of language (Kessler & Treiman, 1997). The graded nature of phonotactic constraints seems to extend even into the domain of clear violations. Native speakers of English will find /pnik/ feels easier to produce than /ngih/, even though both sequences are "illegal".

Connectionist learning systems provide a natural account for such "quasi-regular" patterns. Structural effects emerge within the system from experience with many similar patterns. Both rule-like patterns and idiosyncratic "exceptions" are accommodated within a single system of statistical knowledge (cf. Seidenberg & McClelland, 1989). The most radical form of this approach views all structure as emergent, avoiding any explicit separation of linguistic structure from content. The model of Dell et al. (1993) explores this perspective. The model is a simple recurrent network (SRN) (Elman, 1990; Jordan, 1986), which learns to map a static lexical representation to a temporal sequence of feature-based phoneme descriptions, using backpropagation learning. Activation feeds forward from input to output via a hidden layer, and the hidden layer receives a copy of its previous activation state as feedback (see Figure 2.2).

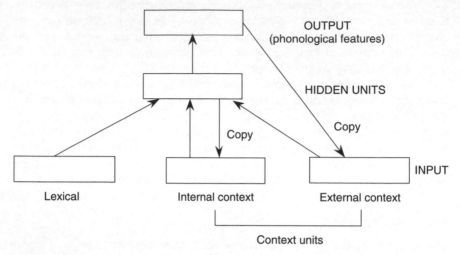

Figure 2.2 A simple-recurrent-network model of word-form encoding. (Dell et al., 1993.)

The recurrent feedback causes the production of each phoneme to be influenced by prior context. The model learns to produce vocabularies of 50–400 words (although only the 50-word vocabularies are learned perfectly). If noise is used to create errors, the errors exhibit some structural effects. Structural effects emerge as a result of the model's sensitivity to frequency and similarity in combination with the structure of the training vocabulary. For instance, the model produces VC errors over twice as often as CV errors, mirroring the syllable constituent effects just described. This arises because VC sequences are more redundant in the training vocabulary; individual VC sequences occur more frequently in the vocabulary than CV sequences (e.g., *run, gun, son*). Each training exposure to a sequence causes adjustments to the model's connections weights, and the model acquires a bias to produce VC sequences as units. For similar reasons, the model's errors tend to be phonologically well formed. For example, the model would be less likely to produce *nun* as the illegal "ngun" than the legal "nung". The model's operation can be understood as following familiar well-worn trajectories in the space defined by the output units. Training sends the model along some trajectories and groups of similar trajectories more often than others, and the model's output tends to stay close to well-worn paths.

While the SRN exhibits structural regularities without resort to explicit rules, this approach is incomplete in several ways. First, the model's vocabulary is a small corpus of short words. There is some possibility that a larger vocabulary would be either harder to learn accurately or that subtler structural regularities may exist, which exceed the SRN's learning capacities. Even with a simple vocabulary, the regularities that the model showed were less strong than those of normal speakers. Another flaw is the lack of any movement errors in the model's output. The majority of speech errors do involve movement. The model explains asymmetries in the degree to which various pieces of phonological material may be vulnerable to error, but provides no account of why a phoneme might move to a different syllable or word in the utterance, either in anticipation, perseveration, or exchange.

A hybrid model

A remaining challenge for connectionist accounts of language production is to understand how connectionist mechanisms can produce structural phenomena without simply imposing linguistic structure by stipulation. It is important here to understand the role of similarity in the emergence of structural regularities in connectionist models. In the Dell et al. (1993) model, consonants and vowels have very dissimilar output representations, and this plays a critical role in the model's ability to learn structural regularities involving those two categories. By contrast, the syllable-structural categories of onset and coda do not correspond to obvious phonological feature-based groupings of phonemes (both categories can be filled by consonants of almost any sort, with the exception of phonemes like /ng/ and /h/). If the model is to acquire knowledge of such abstract regularities as *syllable → onset nucleus coda*, it must induce something resembling the categories onset and coda. The difficulty of doing this is suggested by the fact that the model's errors were slightly less regular than human errors. One way to extend the SRN approach is to elaborate the model's descriptions of phonological events in a way that adds structurally relevant dimensions of similarity.

Kim (2001) implements an SRN with several differences from the Dell et al. (1993) architecture. The most important difference is that the output representation of each segment includes both phonological and structural features. The structural features encode information about the location of the current segment within a larger syllabic context. For instance, the structural features for /s/ in *mask* would indicate that the current segment is in coda position, with one consonant to its right, inside a CVCC syllable. The structural features represent each segment along dimensions that are relevant to abstract structural regularities.

The model's task is complex in two ways. First, the addition of structural features adds complexity to the model's output layer, compared to phonological features only. Second, the vocabulary acquired by the model is substantially more complex than that of most other models of phonological encoding: 1200 words, ranging in length from one to three syllables. The complexity of the task provides a strong test of the learning capacities of simple recurrent networks.

In addition to adding new complexities to the model's task, however, the new components have far-reaching effects on how the model learns to perform its main task of producing phonological features. We compared the model to one with the same architecture, but for which the task of outputting structural features was removed. Comparing *only* phonological feature output, the structural features model learned faster and more accurately than the no-structural features model. This occurred even though the structural features model performs a mapping of greater complexity with the same amount of processing resources (hidden units).

The model learns to create states with structural properties, which provide a system of landmarks within each word, aiding in the production of phonological features. Structural feature sequences are highly regular, and the model therefore learns to produce structural features with greater ease and accuracy than phonological features. Early in training, the model begins producing structurally related activation patterns in the hidden layer. These patterns are incorporated into the model's recurrency-based contextual representation, where they provide highly reliable information about where the model is in the production of a word. This information is used by the model to guide the production of both structural and phonological features. It is so useful that the model can produce both structural and phonological features more quickly and accurately than it can produce phonological features alone.

The model embodies a lexicalist perspective toward the relationship between linguistic structure and content: structural information is stored and retrieved alongside phonological features in the lexicon rather than being imposed by extra-lexical rules. This lexicalist perspective helps explain a number of phenomena in which structural regularities are shaped by the idiosyncratic properties of individual items of lexical content. For instance, the model learns that /ng/ occurs only as a syllable coda, while /h/ occurs only as an onset. It also learns weaker patterns, such as a tendency for /b/ to occur in onset positions and for /n/ to occur as a coda. These are all structural constraints that are shaped by the behavior of individual phonemes in the model's vocabulary.

In a typical run with 300 hidden units, the model produces errors once in a thousand phonemes, a level of accuracy that is within the range of normal human performance. As with the Dell et al. (1993) model, larger quantities of speech errors can be induced by adding noise to the model's operation, and these show a strong tendency to obey the phonotactic constraints of English. In addition to knowledge of phonotactics, however, the model also appears to be influenced by abstract structural knowledge. For instance, the model occasionally makes errors that alter the shape of the word by adding or deleting phonological material:

> *frustrations* → f r ax s t r ey eh sh ih n z "frustrayetions"
> *percentage* → p er z eh n ih jh "perzenage"

In *frustrations*, a syllable is added, while in *percentage*, a consonant cluster is simplified. The vast majority of such wordshape errors are syllabically well-formed utterances (e.g., errors like *percentage* → p er s eh n t jh are very rare). Within-word phoneme exchanges also occur. Although not common, existing

specimens appear to involve knowledge of syllable position (e.g., *trumpet* →
p r eh m t ih t).

The model, like that of Dell et al. (1993), describes the production of a
single word and thus cannot explain structural effects in between-word
movement errors. We are currently exploring ways of extending the model to
account for movement errors. Critically, the inclusion of structurally relevant
dimensions of similarity in the output representations, along with phenomena we have already observed, suggest that the model may provide new
insights into the nature of structural effects in speech errors.

Thus, we see that there are a variety of approaches to explaining structural
effects in phonological speech errors. Frame-based approaches have been
around the longest and have much support. However, they stipulate, rather
than explain, the effects of linguistic structure on errors, and they do not have
motivated accounts of the probabilistic nature of structural influences on
errors or the role of learning in word-form encoding. In this respect at least,
hybrid connectionist models have promise.

Speech errors and phonological-lexical feedback

As we have seen, models of word-form encoding specify how lexical representations send activation to phonological units. The question that we now
consider is whether activation flows in the reverse direction as well, from
word-form units to lexical representations.

Although this kind of feedback has often been considered as an explanation for certain familiarity and similarity effects on errors (e.g., Dell &
Reich, 1981), the existence of such feedback is controversial. Indeed in the
most complete model of lexical access in production (Levelt, Roelofs, &
Meyer, 1999), phonological-lexical feedback is not permitted. After reviewing
the feedback hypothesis, we will consider some of the arguments against it.

To make things specific, we examine phonological-lexical feedback in the
lexical access model described in Dell et al. (1997) (see Figure 2.3).

Its network contains layers of semantic features, words (or lemmas), and
phonemes, and the connections between layers are excitatory and run in
both directions. These bidirectional connections make the model *interactive.*
Activation flows both in top-down (semantics to phonemes) and bottom-
up (phonemes to semantics) directions. Here, we are concerned with the
bottom-up feedback from phonemes to words and how that impacts
processing.

This model makes the usual assumption that lexical access involves both
lemma and word-form access. Lemma access begins with a jolt of activation
to the semantic features of the sought after word. Activation spreads
throughout the network for a fixed period of time according to an activation
rule that includes random noise. Then, the most activated word unit of the
proper syntactic category is selected. So, if the target lemma is to serve as the
head of a noun phrase, only nouns can be selected. As a result of the noisy

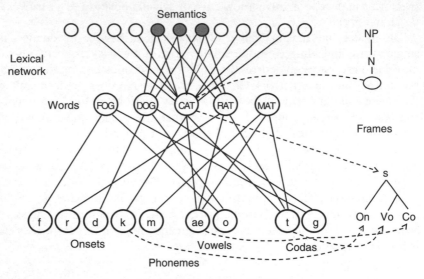

Figure 2.3 Lexical access model. (From Dell et al., 1997.)

spreading activation process, words other than the target have some chance of being selected. For example, if CAT is the target, semantic neighbors of CAT such as DOG gain some activation from semantic units shared with CAT. This explains semantic substitution errors such as when President Ford said "Israel" instead of "Egypt". More importantly, however, the model allows for phonological neighbors such as MAT to become activated during lemma access. This happens because of phoneme-to-word feedback. The target CAT sends activation to its phoneme units, /k/, /ae/, and /t/, and these in turn feed back to words possessing these phonemes. In this way, a word such as MAT can become activated and, if sufficiently so, can be selected creating a formally-related word substitution. We will use the term *malapropism* for these kinds of errors (Fay & Cutler, 1977). President Bush's "anecdote" for "antidote" error is a real-life example. As we will see, some empirical tests of phoneme-to-word feedback make use of the properties of malapropisms.

Word-form access follows lemma access in the model and begins with a jolt of activation to the selected word unit. The timing of this jolt is controlled by syntactic processes. Then, activation spreads throughout the network in the same way as during lemma access, with activation flowing in both top-down and bottom-up directions. Word-form access is concluded by the selection of the most activated phonemes. These are then linked to the slots in a phonological frame. The errors that occur during word-form access are phonological errors. They occur when the wrong phonemes are more active than the correct ones. The erroneously activated phonemes could be active because they belong to a previous word, or a future word, leading to perseverations or anticipations, respectively. Phonological errors could make nonwords such as "lat" or "cag" for CAT, or they might create words, such as "mat" or "sat". Notice that phonological errors that create words are, on the surface, similar to malapropisms; a word is replaced by a formally similar word. However, malapropisms are hypothesized to occur during lemma access and are supposed to belong to the same syntactic class as the target (e.g., Bush's "anecdote" for "antidote" is the substitution of a noun for a noun). Phonological errors that happen to create words during word-form access are, according to the model, not required to match the target word's class.

There are three error phenomena that have been attributed to phoneme-word feedback. These are the *mixed-error effect, the syntactic class effect in malapropisms*, and the *lexical bias effect* in phonological errors. The mixed-error effect concerns semantic substitution errors, which happen during lemma access. In the model, such errors are more likely when the erroneous word also shares phonemes with the target. These mixed errors exhibit semantic and formal relations simultaneously. For example, everything else being equal, RAT would be a more likely error than MOUSE for the target CAT. Mixed errors such as RAT for CAT are especially promoted because the word unit for RAT gains activation from the bottom-up spread of activation from phonemes shared with the target. A purely semantic neighbor such as MOUSE does not have this source of activation.

It is clear that models with phoneme-word feedback predict that mixed errors should be especially likely. But is this true of real speakers? It seems to be. The mixed error effect has been demonstrated in natural errors (Dell & Reich, 1981; Harley, 1984) and in experimental settings in which speakers name pictures (Ferreira & Griffin, 2003; Martin, Gagnon, Schwartz, Dell, & Saffran, 1996; Martin, Weisberg, & Saffran, 1989). These demonstrations have specifically shown that the influence of word form on semantic errors is greater than what would be expected by chance. Moreover, the effect is present in some aphasic patients' lexical errors, specifically in those whose semantic errors reflect damage to lemma access, but who have relatively intact access to word form (Foygel & Dell, 2000; Rapp & Goldrick, 2000). So, the studies with patients allow us to associate the mixed error effect with a derailment of a lemma access process that is influenced by phonological information. In other words, the data support the hypothesis that, during lemma access, phonological forms are activated and feed back to the lemma-level decisions.

The syntactic category effect on malapropisms concerns nonsemantic word substitutions that share form with the target, for example MAT or SAT for the target CAT. As we explained earlier, in the model, these errors happen during lemma access as a result of phoneme-word feedback (true malapropisms) and during word-form access. If there is a genuine tendency for malapropisms during lemma access, they should be syntactically constrained. For example, if the target is a noun, the error should be as well. Thus, the model predicts that a collection of nonsemantic form-related substitutions should match their targets' syntactic class in excess of chance (e.g., errors like the noun MAT for noun CAT should be common). Such a result would implicate phoneme-word feedback by showing that the level at which syntactic information is important, the lemma level, is also influenced by word form.

The evidence for the syntactic category effect on malapropisms is reasonably clear. For the errors of normal speakers, form-related word substitutions are highly constrained to belong to the category of the target (Fay & Cutler, 1977). For errors of aphasic speakers, the situation is similar to that for mixed errors. Some patients show the effect and others do not, and the patients that do, have impaired lemma access along with relatively good access to word form (Dell et al., 1997; Gagnon, Schwartz, Martin, Dell, & Saffran, 1997). These results support the claim that phoneme-word feedback is operating.

The final source of evidence for phoneme-word feedback is the lexical bias effect. Unlike the mixed-error or malapropism effect, lexical bias concerns phonological errors. The claim is that phoneme-word feedback makes phonological errors create words. For example, consider the anticipation error "flow flurries" for *snow flurries*. Although the error is clearly the movement of the /fl/ cluster from *flurries* to *snow*, the fact that *flow* is a lexical item is hypothesized to increase the chance of the error. This is because the activation of *flow*'s phonemes is enhanced by feedback. Bottom-up feedback converges on the word unit for *flow*, activating it, which in turn reinforces the activation of its phonemes. If the potential error did not correspond to a word, this extra boost of activation would not occur.

The evidence for lexical bias comes from natural errors (Dell & Reich, 1981; Nooteboom, this volume, Chapter 10) and from experimental studies (Baars, Motley, & MacKay, 1975; Barch, 1993; Dell, 1986; 1990; Frisch & Wright, 2002). For example, Baars et al. compared the rate of initial consonant exchanges that created words such as *dumb seal* spoken as "some deal" to that of exchanges that created nonwords such as *dump seat* spoken as "sump deat". The slips with word outcomes were more than twice as likely as those with nonword outcomes. Dell (1986; 1990) replicated this effect, but found that it did not occur when speech was exceedingly fast, and suggested that a fast speech rate was too fast for feedback to have an effect. It is important to note that, in all of these studies, the lexical bias effect is only a statistical bias. Nonword outcomes are quite common in phonological speech errors. Clearly, President Bush's "ingritable" for *integral* error was not a word outcome. Nonetheless, even nonword outcomes may reflect phoneme-word feedback. Schwartz, Wilshire, Gagnon, and Polansky (2004) suggested that the nonword errors of aphasic patients exhibit contamination from the target's formal neighbors. In fact, Bush's error could be an example from a normal speaker. Perhaps the encoding of the phonemes of *integral* led, via feedback, to the activation of *incredible*, resulting in a blend of the two. In the absence of a systematic study of these errors, however, this interpretation is speculative.

Thus, we have seen that some speech-error phenomena support the claim of interactive feedback between phonemes and words. However, as we mentioned before, this proposal is a controversial one. We will now list some arguments against the feedback hypothesis (see Levelt et al., 1991; Levelt et al., 1999; Roelofs, this volume, Chapter 3) and respond to them.

It is unclear whether phoneme-word feedback benefits production. An original motivation for feedback during production was that such connections are needed for word recognition. However, the claim that the connections used in recognition and production are the same has been challenged by neuropsychological data suggesting that these abilities can be dissociated (e.g., Nickels & Howard, 1995). Hence, there seems to be no remaining purpose for the feedback connections. The response to this argument has been to note that feedback does serve an important function (Dell et al., 1997). It is to the speaker's advantage to choose a lemma whose form will be subsequently easy to retrieve. Word-phoneme feedback biases lemma access so that lemmas with retrievable forms are selected. Feedback thus prevents the speaker from being lost in TOT blockages. For example, if the phonological form of *liar* is more accessible than that of *prevaricator*, feedback will favor the selection of *liar*. Without feedback, the inaccessibility of the form of *prevaricator* would be unable to guide the production system to the word that is easier to say.

The evidence for feedback just comes from properties of speech errors. The point is that the processes involved in incorrect utterances may differ from those in correct ones. For example, perhaps normally phoneme-word feedback does not occur. When the production process is derailed, such feedback may occur. Thus one would only see evidence for feedback from errors. Our response is twofold. First, the situation described is implausible, particularly if the mechanism for feedback transmission is connections among representational units. Why and how does the system keep these connections inoperative until an impending error? Second, there is evidence for feedback that does not come from the properties of errors. Word-form encoding is more accurate for words in dense formal neighborhoods (Gordon, 2000; Harley & Bown, 1998; Vitevitch, 2002). For example, Harley and Bown found that words with more neighbors were less vulnerable to TOTs. One interpretation of these results is that target phonemes of words with many neighbors gain activation because the feedback process allows activation to reverberate between the lexical units of the neighbors and the target phonemes. Although this interpretation is not compelled by the results, it is consistent with them.

The lexical bias effect can be explained by self-monitoring instead of feedback. The process whereby speakers detect and correct their errors also occurs prior to the articulation of a potential error. This *prearticulatory editing* is more likely to detect and eliminate errors that create nonwords and hence the emitted errors are more likely to be words than nonwords (Baars et al., 1975). We agree that there is overwhelming evidence for both prearticulatory and overt detection and correction of speech errors. This volume reviews that evidence. But there is little evidence that the lexical bias effect is caused by such a process. The one source of evidence that is cited is the demonstration by Baars et al. (1975) that lexical bias was reduced when all the targets in the experimental list were nonwords. This finding is somewhat more consistent with a strategic editing explanation for the effect than one based on automatic spreading activation. However, the report of the experiment actually provided no statistical evidence that the lexical bias effect was significantly smaller with the nonword lists. Numerically, there was a lexical bias with both word and nonword lists. (It was only significant for the word list.) In fact, there is specific evidence that lexical bias is *not* caused by editing. Barch (1993) used the experimental method of Baars et al. and demonstrated that normal controls and schizophrenic patients have equivalent lexical bias, with word error outcomes outnumbering nonword outcomes by about three to one. However, the patients had demonstrable deficits in monitoring and correcting overt errors compared to the controls. Nooteboom (this volume, Chapter 10) showed that the lexical bias present in a natural error collection was not a function of output editing because overt self-corrections showed no lexical bias. In general, the lexical bias effect can be dissociated from the editing processes that occur with overt speech errors. This dissociation renders the explanation that lexical bias results from an internal form of this kind of editing less likely.

The mixed-error and malapropism effects can also be explained by self-monitoring instead of feedback. The idea is that mixed errors and form-related errors that occur at lemma access can be explained by postulating that the process of monitoring for and correcting errors is more likely to filter out errors that are not formally related to their targets than errors that are. So, if the target is CAT, the potential errors RAT or MAT are less likely to be caught than DOG or RUG. As a result, errors of lemma access that share form with the target are over-represented in error corpora. This is indeed a possible explanation. However, we note that the monitoring explanation is post hoc and underspecified in contrast to the feedback account. Moreover, the feedback explanation uniquely predicts which aphasic patients would exhibit the mixed-error and malapropism effects (Dell et al., 1997). Potentially, the monitoring explanation could be developed to predict these or related data (see particularly Roelofs, this volume, Chapter 3). At least one precise account of monitoring exists (Hartsuiker & Kolk, 2001), but it has not been developed in this direction.

The mixed-error effect can be explained by cascading instead of feedback. This proposal (Levelt et al., 1999) is that on occasion, the target and one or more intruder words undergo word-form encoding (cascading). The intruder words will be semantically related to the target, such as DOG or RAT for CAT. The mixed-error effect emerges because intruders that share sounds with the target will be more likely to be encoded. The target sounds reinforce the mixed intruder, while a purely semantic intruder gets no such benefit. This is an interesting explanation. But it remains to be seen whether it can account for the data. Rapp and Goldrick (2000) compared feedback accounts of the mixed-error effect with cascaded accounts in computational models of aphasic performance. Only the feedback accounts were able to reproduce the data patterns. Because the cascaded models locate the mixed-error effect at word-form access instead of lemma access, the models cannot account for the joint patterns of mixed errors and other phonological errors such as nonwords. However, Rapp, and Goldrick made specific assumptions about the models and so it remains possible that other kinds of cascaded models could do the job.

Word recognition does not involve word-phoneme feedback; why should word production? This observation reflects the MERGE model of word recognition (Norris, McQueen, & Cutler, 2000), which seeks to explain lexical effects in speech perception without feedback from lexical units to phonemes or other sublexical units. In response, we note, first, that the feedback issue is as controversial in recognition as it is in production. There are, to us, noteworthy demonstrations of lexical-sublexical feedback in speech perception (e.g., Samuel, 1997). Second, MERGE actually does allow a flow of activation from word to phoneme units in order to account for interactive effects. It just does not hypothesize that these phoneme units are identical to those that provide the direct evidence for lexical items. Assuming that MERGE is correct, its implications for feedback in word production are simply unclear.

In summary, we see that the arguments against phoneme-word feedback in word-form encoding vary in their merit. Some of the alternative explanations for the feedback error effects have potential, but that potential is only beginning to be realized by the development of precise explanations. To us, phoneme-word feedback remains the most promising explanation because it is simple, it explains a variety of effects, and there is no clear contrary evidence that we are aware of.

Conclusions

Speech errors are a rich source of data. As Fromkin (1973) puts it, they provide a "window into linguistic processes" (p. 43). Here, we claim that this window is particularly revealing of the processes involved in word-form encoding. What they reveal is an encoding mechanism that is highly sensitive to experience and to structure. And their study paves the way for the development of explicit models.

Acknowledgements

This research was supported by NSF SBR 98–73450 and NIH DC-00191. We thank Rob Hartsuiker, Frank Wijnen, Zenzi Griffin, and Ulrich Schade for helpful comments and Judy Allen for work on the manuscript.

References

Anderson, K., Milostan, J., & Cottrell, G. W. (1998). Assessing the contribution of representation to results. In *Proceedings of the Twentieth Annual Meeting of* the Cognitive Science Society (pp. 48–53). Mahwah, NJ: Lawrence Erlbaum Associates, Inc.

Baars, B. J., Motley, M. T., & MacKay, D. G. (1975). Output editing for lexical status in artificially elicited slips of the tongue. *Journal of Verbal Learning and Verbal Behavior, 14,* 382–91.

Barch, D. M., (1993). *Communication disorder and language production.* University of Illinois PhD dissertation.

Caramazza, A. (1997). How many levels of processing are there in lexical access? *Cognitive Neuropsychology, 14,* 177–208.

Caramazza, A., & Miozzo, M. (1997). The relation between syntactic and phonological knowledge in lexical access: Evidence from the 'tip-of-the-tongue' phenomenon. *Cognition, 64,* 309–43.

Christiansen, M. H., & Chater, N. (1999). Connectionist natural language processing: The state of the art. *Cognitive Science, 23,* 417–37.

Dell, G. S. (1986). A spreading activation theory of retrieval in language production. *Psychological Review, 93,* 283–321.

Dell, G. S. (1988). The retrieval of phonological forms in production: Tests of predictions from a connectionist model. *Journal of Memory and Language, 27,* 124–42.

Dell, G. S. (1990). Effects of frequency and vocabulary type on phonological speech errors. *Language and Cognitive Processes, 5,* 313–49.

Dell, G. S., Juliano, C., & Govindjee, A. (1993). Structure and content in language production: A theory of frame constraints in phonological speech errors. *Cognitive Science, 17,* 149–95.

Dell, G. S., Reed, K. D., Adams, D. R., & Meyer, A. S. (2000). Speech errors, phonotactic constraints, and implicit learning: A study of the role of experience in language production. *Journal of Experimental Psychology: Learning, Memory, and Cognition, 26,* 1355–67.

Dell, G. S., & Reich, P. A. (1981). Stages in sentence production: An analysis of speech error data. *Journal of Verbal Learning and Verbal Behavior, 20,* 611–29.

Dell, G. S., Schwartz, M. F., Martin, N., Saffran, E. M., & Gagnon, D. A. (1997). Lexical access in aphasic and nonaphasic speakers. *Psychological Review, 104,* 801–38.

Elman, J. L. (1990). Finding structure in time. *Cognitive Science, 14,* 179–211.

Fay, D., & Cutler, A. (1977). Malapropisms and the structure of the mental lexicon. *Linguistic Inquiry, 8,* 505–20.

Ferreira, V. S., & Griffin, Z. M. (2003). Phonological influences on lexical (mis)selection. *Psychological Science, 14,* 86–90.

Fisher, C., Gleitman, H., & Gleitman, L. R. (1991). On the semantic content of subcategorization frames. *Cognitive Psychology, 23,* 331–92.

Foygel, D., & Dell, G. S., (2002). Models of impaired lexical access in speech production. *Journal of Memory and Language, 43,* 182–216.

Frisch, S. A., & Wright, R. (2002). The phonetics of phonological speech errors: An acoustic analysis of slips of the tongue. *Journal of Phonetics, 30,* 139–62.

Fromkin, V. A. (1971). The non-anomalous nature of anomalous utterances. *Language, 47,* 27–52.

Fromkin, V. A. (1973). *Speech errors as linguistic evidence.* The Hague: Mouton.

Gagnon, D. A., Schwartz, M. F., Martin, N., Dell, G. S., & Saffran, E. M. (1997). The origins of formal paraphasias in aphasics' picture naming. *Brain and Language, 59,* 450–72.

Gordon, J. K. (2000). *Aphasic speech errors.* McGill University PhD dissertation.

Griffin, Z. M., & Bock, J. K. (1998). Constraint, word frequency, and the relationship between lexical processing levels in spoken word production. *Journal of Memory and Language, 38,* 313–38.

Harley, T. A. (1984). A critique of top-down independent levels models of speech production: Evidence from non-plan-internal speech errors. *Cognitive Science, 8,* 191–219.

Harley, T. A., & Bown, H. E. (1998). What causes a tip-of-the-tongue state? Evidence for lexical neighbourhood effects in speech production. *British Journal of Psychology, 89,* 151–74.

Hartsuiker, R. J. (2002). The addition bias in Dutch and Spanish phonological speech errors: The role of structural context. *Language and Cognitive Processes, 17,* 61–96.

Hartsuiker, R. J., & Kolk, H. H. J. (2001). Error monitoring in speech production: A computational test of the perceptual loop theory. *Cognitive Psychology, 42,* 113–57.

Jescheniak, J. D., & Levelt, W. J. M. (1994). Word frequency effects in speech production: Retrieval of syntactic information and phonological form. *Journal of Experimental Psychology: Learning, Memory, and Cognition, 20,* 824–43.

Jordan, M. I. (1986). Attractor dynamics and parallelism in a connectionist sequential machine. In *Proceedings of the Eighth Annual Conference of the Cognitive Science Society* (pp. 531–46). Hillsdale, NJ: Lawrence Erlbaum Associates, Inc.

Jusczyk, P. W., Luce, P. A., & Charles-Luce, J. (1994). Infants' sensitivity to phonotactic patterns in the native language. *Journal of Memory and Language, 33,* 630–45.

Kempen, G., & Huijbers, P. (1983). The lexicalization process in sentence production and naming: Indirect election of words. *Cognition, 14,* 185–209.

Kessler, B., & Treiman, R. (1997). Syllable structure and the distribution of phonemes in English syllables. *Journal of Memory and Language, 37,* 295–311.

Kim, A. E. (2001). *A connectionist, lexicalist model of phonological encoding.* Presented at 14th annual CUNY Conference on Human Sentence Processing. Philadelphia, PA.

Laubstein, A. S. (1999). Word blends as sublexical substitutions. *Canadian Journal of Linguistics, 44,* 127–48.

Levitt, A. G., & Healy, A. F. (1985). The roles of phoneme frequency, similarity, and availability in the experimental elicitation of speech errors. *Journal of Memory and Language, 24,* 717–33.

Levelt, W. J. M., Roelofs, A., & Meyer, A. S. (1999). A theory of lexical access in speech production. *Behavioral and Brain Science, 21,* 1–38.

Levelt, W. J. M., Schriefers, H., Vorberg, D., Meyer, A. S., Pechmann, T., & Havinga, J. (1991). The time course of lexical access in speech production: A study of picture naming. *Psychological Review, 98,* 122–42.

Martin, N., Gagnon, D. A., Schwartz, M. F., Dell, G. S., & Saffran, E. M. (1996). Phonological facilitation of semantic errors in normal aphasic speakers. *Language and Cognitive Processes, 11,* 257–82.

Martin, N., Saffran, E. M., & Dell, G. S. (1996). Recovery in deep dysphasia: Evidence for a relation between auditory-verbal STM capacity and lexical errors in repetition. *Brain and Language, 52,* 83–113.

Martin, N., Weisberg, R. W., & Saffran, E. M. (1989). Variables influencing the occurrence of naming errors: Implications for models of lexical retrieval. *Journal of Memory and Language, 28,* 462–85.

Nickels, L., & Howard, D. (1995). Aphasic naming: What matters? *Neuropsychologia*, *33*, 1281–303.

Nooteboom, S. G. (1973). The tongue slips into patterns. In V. Fromkin (Ed.), *Speech errors as linguistic evidence* (pp. 87–95). The Hague: Mouton.

Norris, D., McQueen, J. M., & Cutler, A. (2000). Merging information in speech recognition: Feedback is never necessary. *Behavioral and Brain Sciences*, *23*, 299–370.

Plaut, D. C., & Kello, C. T. (1999). The emergence of phonology from the interplay of speech comprehension and production: A distributed connectionist approach. In B. MacWhinney (Ed.), *The emergence of language*. Mahwah, NJ: Lawrence Erlbaum Associates, Inc.

Plaut, D. C., McClelland, J. L., Seidenberg, M. S., & Patterson, K. (1996). Understanding normal and impaired word reading: Computational principles in quasi-regular domains. *Psychological Review*, *103*, 56–115.

Rapp, B., & Goldrick, M. (2000). Discreteness and interactivity in spoken word production. *Psychological Review*, *107*, 460–99.

Roelofs, A. (1997). The WEAVER model of word-form encoding in speech production. *Cognition*, *64*, 249–84.

Samuel, A. G. (1997). Lexical activation produces potent phonemic percepts. *Cognitive Psychology*, *32*, 97–127.

Schmitt, B. M., Schiltz, K., Zaake, W., Kutas, M., & Münte, T. F. (2001). An electrophysiological analysis of the time course of conceptual and syntactic encoding during tacit picture naming, *Journal of Cognitive Neuroscience*, *15*, 510–22.

Schwartz, M. F., Wilshire, C. E., Gagnon, D. A., & Polansky, M. (2004). The origins of nonword phonological errors in aphasics'picture naming. *Cognitive Neuropsychology*, *21*, 159–86.

Seidenberg, M. S., & McClelland, J. L. (1989). A distributed developmental model of visual word recognition and naming. *Psychological Review*, *96*, 523 68.

Shattuck-Hufnagel, S. (1979). Speech errors as evidence for a serial-order mechanism in sentence production. In W. E. Cooper & E. C. T. Walker (Eds.), *Sentence processing: Psycholinguistic studies presented to Merrill Garrett* (pp. 295–342). Hillsdale, NJ: Lawrence Erlbaum Associates, Inc.

Shattuck-Hufnagel, S. (1983). Sublexical units and suprasegmental structure in speech production planning. In P. F. MacNeilage (Ed.), *The Production of Speech* (pp. 109–136). New York: Springer Verlag.

Stemberger, J. P. (1983). *Speech errors and theoretical phonology: A review*. Indiana University Linguistics Club.

Stemberger J. P. (1990). Wordshape errors in language production. *Cognition*, *35*, 123–57.

Van Turennout, M., Hagoort, P., & Brown, C.M. (1997). Electrophysiological evidence on the time course of semantic and phonological processes in speech production. *Journal of Experimental Psychology: Learning, Memory, and Cognition*, *23*, 787–806.

Van Turennout, M., Hagoort, P., & Brown, C. M. (1998). Brain activity during speaking: From syntax to phonology in 40 milliseconds. *Science*, *280*, 572–4.

Vigliocco, G., Vinson, D. P., Martin, R. C., & Garrett, M. F. (1999). Is 'count' and 'mass' information available when the noun is not? An investigation of tip of the tongue states and anomia. *Journal of Memory and Language*, *40*, 534–58.

Vitevitch, M. S. (2002). The influence of phonological similarity neighbourhoods on speech production. *Journal of Experimental Psychology: Learning, Memory, and Cognition, 28*, 735–47.

Vousden, J. I., Brown, G. D. A., & Harley, T. A. (2000). Serial control of phonology in speech production: A hierarchical model. *Cognitive Psychology, 41*, 101–75.

3 Spoken word planning, comprehending, and self-monitoring: Evaluation of WEAVER++

Ardi Roelofs

Abstract

During conversation, speakers not only talk but they also monitor their speech for errors and they listen to their interlocutors. Although the interplay among speaking, self-monitoring, and listening stands at the heart of spoken conversation, it has not received much attention in models of language use. This chapter describes chronometric, error, and aphasic evidence on spoken word planning and its relations with self-monitoring and comprehending, and it uses the evidence to evaluate WEAVER++, which is a computational model of spoken word production that makes the relations explicit. The theoretical claims implemented in WEAVER++ are contrasted with other theoretical proposals.

Speaker as listener

Speakers not only talk but they also listen to their interlocutors' speech and they monitor their own speech for errors. This chapter describes empirical evidence on spoken word planning and its relationships with comprehending and self-monitoring. It uses the evidence to evaluate WEAVER++ (Levelt, Roelofs, & Meyer, 1999a; Roelofs, 1992, 1997a, 2003a), which is a computational model of spoken word production that makes the interplay among planning, comprehending, and monitoring explicit. The claims implemented in WEAVER++ are contrasted with other theoretical approaches. It is argued that the interplay among speaking, comprehending, and self-monitoring is not only of interest in its own right, but that it also illuminates classic issues in spoken word production.

This chapter consists of two parts. The first part reviews relevant empirical evidence and it explains what claims about spoken word planning, comprehending, and self-monitoring are implemented in WEAVER++. This model assumes that word planning is a staged process that traverses from conceptual preparation via lemma retrieval to word-form encoding. Comprehending spoken words traverses from forms to lemmas and meanings. Concepts and lemmas are shared between production and comprehension, whereas there are separate input and output representations of word forms. After lemma retrieval, word planning is a strictly feedforward process. Following Levelt (1989; see also Hartsuiker, Kolk, & Lickley, this volume; Chapter 14), WEAVER++ assumes two self-monitoring routes, an internal and an external one, both operating via the speech comprehension system. Brain imaging studies also suggest that self-monitoring and speech comprehension are served by the same neural structures (e.g., McGuire, Silbersweig, & Frith, 1996; Paus, Perry, Zatorre, Worsley, & Evans, 1996). The external route involves listening to self-produced speech, whereas the internal route involves evaluating the speech plan. Self-monitoring requires cognitive operations in addition to speech comprehension. For example, lexical selection errors may be detected by verifying whether the lemma recognized in inner speech corresponds to the lexical concept prepared for production, which is an operation specific to self-monitoring. The self-monitoring through speech comprehension assumed by WEAVER++ is shown to be supported by a new analysis performed on the self-corrections and false starts in picture naming by 15 aphasic speakers reported by Nickels and Howard (1995).

The second part of the chapter applies WEAVER++ to findings that were seen as problematic for feedforward models (e.g., Damian & Martin, 1999; Rapp & Goldrick, 2000): The statistical overrepresentation of mixed semantic-phonological speech errors and the reduced latency effect of mixed distractors in picture naming. The mixed error bias is the finding that mixed semantic-phonological errors (e.g., the erroneous selection of *calf* for *cat*, which share the onset segment and, in American English, the vowel) are statistically overrepresented, both in natural speech-error corpora and in picture naming experiments with aphasic as well as nonaphasic speakers (Dell & Reich, 1981; Martin, Gagnon, Schwartz, Dell, & Saffran, 1996). The bias is also called the "phonological facilitation of semantic substitutions." Rapp and Goldrick (2000) observed that the presence of a mixed error bias depends on the impairment locus in aphasia. The bias occurs with a post-conceptual deficit (as observed with patients P.W. and R.G.B., who make semantic errors in word production only) but not with a conceptual deficit (as observed with patient K.E., who makes semantic errors in both word production and comprehension). The mixed-distractor latency effect is the finding that mixed semantic-phonological distractor words in picture naming (e.g., the spoken word CALF presented as a distractor in naming a pictured cat; hereafter, perceived words are referred to in uppercase) yield less interference than distractors that are semantically related only (distractor DOG), taking the facilitation from phonological relatedness per se (distractor CAP) into account (Damian & Martin, 1999; Starreveld & La Heij, 1996).

Elsewhere, it has been discussed how WEAVER++ deals with other speech error tendencies such as the bias towards word rather than non-word error outcomes (Roelofs, 2004a, 2004b), and with aphasic phenomena such as modality-specific grammatical class deficits and the finding that semantic errors may occur in speaking but not in writing, or vice versa (Roelofs, Meyer,

& Levelt, 1998). Nickels and Howard (2000) provide a general evaluation of the model in the light of a wide range of findings on aphasia. Here, I focus on the mixed-error bias, its dependence on the locus of damage in aphasia, and the mixed-distractor latency effect. I argue that these findings are not problematic for WEAVER++ but, on the contrary, support the claims about the relations among speaking, comprehending, and monitoring in the model. According to WEAVER++, mixed items (e.g., *calf* in naming a cat) are weaker lexical competitors than items that are semantically related only (e.g., *dog*), because they co-activate the target (*cat*) as a member of their speech comprehension cohort. Therefore, compared with items that are semantically related only, mixed items are more likely to remain unnoticed in error monitoring (yielding more mixed-speech errors) and, as distractors, they have a smaller effect on latencies (yielding less semantic interference). The simulations reported by Roelofs (2004a, 2004b) and reviewed here showed that WEAVER++ not only accounts for the mixed-distractor latency effect, but also for the mixed-error bias and the influence of the impairment locus in aphasia. The assignment of the mixed-distractor latency effect to properties of the speech comprehension system by the model is shown to be supported by recent chronometric studies, which revealed that there are semantic effects of word-initial cohort distractors in picture naming (Roelofs, submitted-a) and that there is no reduced latency effect for mixed rhyme distractors (Roelofs, submitted-b).

An outline of the WEAVER++ model

WEAVER++ distinguishes between conceptual preparation, lemma retrieval, and word-form encoding, with the encoding of forms further divided into morphological, phonological, and phonetic encoding (Roelofs, 1992, 1997a). During conceptual preparation, a lexical concept is selected and flagged as goal concept (e.g., the concept of a cat in naming a pictured cat). In lemma retrieval, a selected concept is used to activate and select a lemma from memory, which is a representation of the syntactic properties of a word, crucial for its use in sentences. For example, the lemma of the word *cat* says that it is a noun. Lemma retrieval makes these properties available for syntactic encoding. In word-form encoding, the selected lemma is used to activate and select form properties from memory. For example, for *cat*, the morpheme <cat> and the segments /k/, /æ/ and /t/ are activated and selected. Next, the segments are rightward incrementally syllabified, which yields a phonological word representation. Finally, a motor program for [kæt] is recovered. Articulation processes execute the motor program, which yields overt speech. Figure 3.1 illustrates the stages. Lemma retrieval and word-form encoding are discrete processes in that only the word form of a selected lemma becomes activated.

After lemma retrieval, word planning happens in a strictly feedforward fashion, with feedback only occurring via comprehension (Roelofs, 2004b).

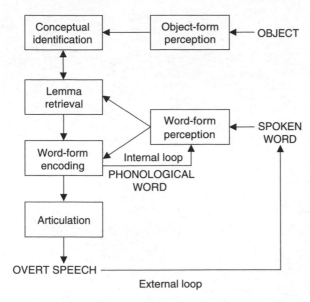

Figure 3.1 Flow of information in the WEAVER++ model during the planning, comprehending, and self-monitoring of spoken words.

Comprehending spoken words proceeds from word-form perception to lemma retrieval and conceptual identification. A perceived word activates not only its lemma, but also in parallel, its output form. Self-monitoring is achieved through the speech comprehension system. There exist internal and external self-monitoring routes, as illustrated in Figure 3.1. The external route involves listening to self-produced overt speech, whereas the internal route includes monitoring the speech plan by feeding a planned phonological word representation, specifying the syllables and stress pattern, back into the speech comprehension system.

Word planning involves retrieval of information from a lexical network. There are three network strata, shown in Figure 3.2. A conceptual stratum represents the concepts of words as nodes and links in a semantic network. A syntactic stratum contains lemma nodes for words, such as *cat*, which are connected to nodes for their syntactic class (e.g., *cat* is a noun, N). A word-form stratum represents the morphemes, segments, and syllable programs of words. The form of monosyllables such as *cat* presents the simplest case with one morpheme <cat>, segments such as /k/, /æ/, and /t/, and one syllable program [kæt]. Polysyllables such as *feline* have their segments connected to more than one syllable program; for *feline*, these program nodes are [fi:] and [laIn]. Polymorphemic words such as *catwalk* have one lemma connected to more than one morpheme; for *catwalk* these morphemes are <cat> and <walk>. For a motivation of these assumptions, I refer to Levelt (1989), Levelt et al. (1999a, 1999b), Roelofs (1992, 1993, 1996, 1997a, 1997b, 1997c,

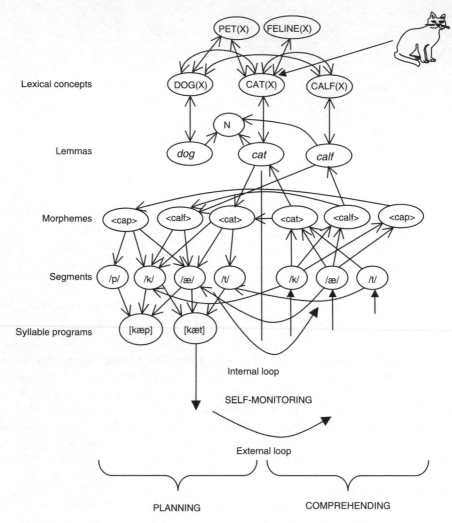

Figure 3.2 Fragment of the production and comprehension networks of the WEAVER++ model.

1998, 1999, 2003a), Roelofs and Meyer (1998), and Roelofs, Meyer, and Levelt (1996, 1998).

Information needed for word production is retrieved from the network by spreading activation. For example, a perceived object (e.g., a cat) activates the corresponding concept node (i.e., CAT(X); hereafter, propositional functions denote lexical concept nodes). Activation then spreads through the network following a linear activation rule with a decay factor. Each node sends a proportion of its activation to the nodes it is connected to. For example, CAT(X) sends activation to other concepts such as DOG(X) and to its lemma node *cat*. Selection of nodes is accomplished by production rules. A production rule specifies a condition to be satisfied and an action to be taken when the condition is met. A lemma retrieval production rule selects a lemma after it has been verified that the connected concept is flagged as goal concept. For example, *cat* is selected for CAT(X) if it is the goal concept and *cat* has reached a critical difference in activation compared to other lemmas. The actual moment of firing of the production rule is determined by the ratio of activation of the lemma node and the sum of the activations of all the other lemma nodes. Thus, how fast a lemma node is selected depends on how active the other lemma nodes are.

A selected lemma is flagged as goal lemma. A morphological production rule selects the morpheme nodes that are connected to the selected lemma (<cat> is selected for *cat*). Phonological production rules select the segments that are connected to the selected morphemes (/k/, /æ/, and /t/ for <cat>) and incrementally syllabify the segments (e.g., /k/ is made syllable onset: onset(/k/)) to create a phonological word representation. Phonological words specify the syllable structure and, for polysyllabic words, the stress pattern across syllables. Finally, phonetic production rules select syllable-based motor programs that are appropriately connected to the syllabified segments (i.e., [kæt] is selected for onset(/k/), nucleus(/æ/) and coda(/t/)). The moment of selection of a program node is given by the ratio of activation of the target syllable-program node and the sum of the activations of all the other syllable-program nodes (thus, the selection ratio applies to lemmas and syllable programs).

To account for interference and facilitation effects from auditorily presented distractor words on picture naming latencies, Roelofs (1992, 1997a) assumed that information activated in a speech comprehension network activates compatible segment, morpheme, and lemma representations in the production network (see Figure 3.2). Covert self-monitoring includes feeding the incrementally constructed phonological word representation from the production into the comprehension system. An externally or internally perceived word activates a cohort of word candidates, including their forms, lemmas, and meanings.

Evidence for comprehension cohorts

The assumption implemented in WEAVER++ that a cohort of word candidates is activated during spoken word recognition is widely accepted in the comprehension literature. Cohort models of spoken word recognition such as the seminal model of Marslen-Wilson and Welsh (1978) claim that, on the basis of the first 150 milliseconds or so of the speech stream, all words that are compatible with this spoken fragment are activated in parallel in the mental lexicon. The activation concerns not only the forms but also the syntactic properties and concepts of the words. For example, when an American English listener hears the spoken word fragment CA, a cohort of words including *cat, calf, captain* and *captive* becomes activated. Other models of spoken word recognition such as TRACE (McClelland & Elman, 1986) and Shortlist (Norris, 1994) make similar claims.

Evidence for the multiple activation of lexico-semantic representations of words during word recognition comes from cross-modal semantic priming experiments. For example, Zwitserlood (1989) asked participants to listen to spoken words (e.g., CAPTAIN) or fragments of these words (e.g., CAPT). The participants had to take lexical decisions to written probes that were presented at the offset of the spoken primes. The spoken fragments facilitated the lexical decision to target words that were semantically related to the complete word as well as to cohort competitors. For example, CAPT facilitated the response to SHIP (semantically related to *captain*) and also to GUARD (semantically related to *captive*).

Multiple activation appears to involve mainly cohort competitors. Several studies (e.g., Connine, Blasko, & Titone, 1993; Marslen-Wilson & Zwitserlood, 1989) have shown that when the first segments of a spoken non-word prime and the source word from which it is derived differ in more than two phonological features (such as place and manner of articulation, e.g., the prime ZANNER derived from MANNER), no priming is observed on the lexical decision to a visually presented probe (e.g., STYLE). Marslen-Wilson, Moss, and Van Halen (1996) observed that a difference of one phonological feature between the first segment of a word prime and its source word leads to no cross-modal semantic priming effect. In an eye-tracking study, Allopenna, Magnuson, and Tanenhaus (1998) observed that, for example, hearing the word COLLAR (a rhyme competitor of *dollar*) had much less effect than hearing DOLPHIN (a cohort competitor of *dollar*) on the probability of fixating a visually presented target dollar (a real object). Thus, the evidence suggests that in spoken word recognition there is activation of cohort competitors, whereas there is much less activation of rhyme competitors, even when they differ in only the initial segment from the actually presented spoken word or non-word.

Evidence for phonological words in inner speech

The assumption implemented in WEAVER++ that phonological words are monitored rather than, for example, articulatory programs (e.g., [kæt]) or strings of segments (e.g., /k/, /æ/, and /t/) was motivated by a study conducted by Wheeldon and Levelt (1995). The participants were native speakers of Dutch who spoke English fluently. They had to monitor for target speech segments in the Dutch translation equivalent of visually presented English words. For example, they had to indicate by means of a button press (yes/no) whether the segment /n/ is part of the Dutch translation equivalent of the English word WAITER. The Dutch word is *kelner*, which has /n/ as the onset of the second syllable, so requiring a positive response. All Dutch target words were disyllabic. The serial position of the critical segments in the Dutch words was manipulated. The segment could be the onset or coda of the first

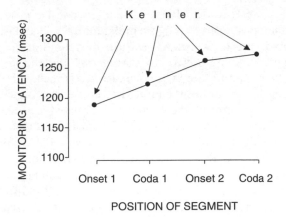

Figure 3.3 Mean monitoring latencies (in msec) as a function of the position of the target segment observed by Wheeldon and Levelt (1995).

syllable, or the onset or coda of the second syllable. If a rightward incrementally generated phonological word representation is consulted in performing self-monitoring, an effect of serial position is to be expected. Such an effect was indeed empirically obtained. Monitoring latencies increased with the serial position of the segments within the word, as illustrated in Figure 3.3.

In order to experimentally verify whether phonological words rather than phonetic motor programs are monitored, participants had to perform the segment-monitoring task while simultaneously counting aloud, which is known to suppress the maintaining of phonetic representations. The monitoring latencies were longer with the counting task, but the seriality effect was replicated. This suggests that monitoring involves a phonological rather than a phonetic representation. Finally, to assess whether monitoring involves a syllabified representation rather than a string of segments, participants had to monitor for target syllables. The target syllable corresponded to the first syllable of the Dutch word or it was larger or smaller. For example, the target syllable was CA or CAP and the first syllable of the Dutch word was CA or CAP. If phonological words are monitored, which are syllabified, then a syllable match effect should be obtained, whereas if a string of segments is monitored, the syllabic status of the segments should not matter. The experiment yielded a clear syllable match effect. Syllable targets were detected much faster when they exactly matched the first syllable of the words than when they were larger or smaller. This suggests that phonological words rather than strings of segments are monitored.

Evidence from self-corrections and false starts

Independent support for the involvement of planned phonological words in self-monitoring comes from a new analysis that I performed on the patient data reported by Nickels and Howard (1995). The data consist of the responses in a picture-naming task from 15 aphasic individuals. Each aphasic speaker named 130 black and white drawings. As measures of self-monitoring, Nickels and Howard counted the attempted self-corrections and the false starts made by the patients in naming the pictures. False starts included all those responses where an initial portion of the target was correctly produced but with production being stopped before the word was completed (e.g., saying 'ka' when the target was *captain*). The presence of false starts was taken to specifically reflect internal feedback and monitoring. Nickels and Howard computed the correlations between the proportion of trials that included phonological errors, self-corrections and false starts, on the one hand, and the performance on three tasks involving speech perception (auditory synonym judgement, auditory lexical decision, and auditory minimal-pair discrimination), on the other hand, and found no significant correlations. They argued that this challenges the idea of self-monitoring through speech comprehension. However, the absence of significant correlations may also mean that the three speech perception tasks are not good indicators of the patients' self-monitoring abilities (see Nickels, 1997, for discussion). Most aphasic individuals performed close to ceiling on the three auditory input tasks. Furthermore, auditory synonym judgement and minimal-pair discrimination ask for input buffering of two perceived words, something that is not crucial for the type of monitoring proposed.

According to the proposed monitoring view, the capacity to feed back and evaluate planned phonological word representations via the comprehension system should be critical to self-monitoring. Interestingly, Nickels and Howard (1995) report the speakers' scores on a task that seems to tap into this capacity, namely homophone judgement from pictures, but they did not include this measure in their analyses. The homophone judgement task involves the selection of two homophone items from a triad of pictures (e.g., hair, hare, and steak). Performing this task minimally involves silently generating the sound form of the name of one of the pictures and then evaluating which of the other two pictures this sound form also correctly names. Thus, this task contains all the processing components that are presumed to be involved in the internal monitoring of a speech plan. To test whether this capacity is indeed involved in the speakers' self-monitoring, I computed the correlations between self-corrections and false starts and the performance on the homophone task.

I first confirmed that the total number of semantic errors made by the aphasic speakers in the picture-naming task was negatively correlated with their ability to perform auditory synonym judgements. On the synonym task, the speakers are presented with pairs of spoken words and they are required to judge whether the words are approximately synonymous. The correlations were indeed highly significant (high imageability words: $r = -.63, p = .01$; low imageability words: $r = -.91, p = .001$). Interestingly, the total number of semantic errors made by each speaker was also negatively correlated with their performance on the homophone task ($r = -.77, p = .001$). The higher the score on this task, the lower the number of semantic errors. This suggests that the ability to evaluate a phonological representation is a precondition for (lexical/semantic) error detection. Moreover, there were positive correlations between performance on the homophone task and the proportion of phonological self-corrections and false starts. The correlation was higher for the false starts ($r = .64, p = .01$) than for the self-corrections ($r = .47, p = .08$), suggesting that the homophone task captures a capacity that is more heavily engaged in internal than in external monitoring. Thus, the capacity to silently generate word forms and to evaluate them with respect to their meaning is positively correlated with the number of false starts and, to a lesser extent, the number of self-corrections of the patients. This supports the idea that self-monitoring of speech may be performed by feeding back phonological word representations to the comprehension system and evaluating the corresponding meaning.

Accounting for mixed-error bias

When *cat* is intended, the substitution of *calf* for *cat* is more likely than the substitution of *dog* for *cat* (Dell & Reich, 1981; Martin et al., 1996), taking error opportunities into account. On the standard feedback account, the mixed-error bias arises because of production-internal feedback from segment nodes to lexical nodes within a lexical network. Semantic substitution errors are taken to be failures in lexical node selection. The word *calf* shares phonological segments with the target *cat*. So, the lexical node of *calf* receives feedback from these shared segments (i.e., /k/ and /æ/), whereas the lexical node of *dog* does not. Consequently, the lexical node of *calf* has a higher level of activation than the lexical node of *dog*, and *calf* is more likely involved in a selection error than *dog*.

The mixed-error bias does not uniquely support production-internal feedback, however (Rapp & Goldrick, 2000; 2004). Rapp and Goldrick (2000) demonstrated by means of computer simulation that the error bias may occur at the segment rather than the lexical level in a feedforward cascading network model. So, production-internal feedback is not critical. Likewise, Levelt et al. (1999a) argued that the mixed-error effect occurs in WEAVER++ when the lemma retrieval stage mistakenly selects two lemmas rather than a single one. In a cascading model, activation automatically spreads from one level to the other, whereas in a discrete multiple-output model the activation is restricted to the selected items. Both views predict a mixed error bias. The bias occurs during word planning in WEAVER++, because the sound form of a target like *cat* speeds up the encoding of the form of an intruder like *calf* but not of an intruder like *dog*. Therefore, the form of *calf* is completed faster than the form of *dog*, and *calf* has a higher probability than *dog* of being produced instead of *cat*. The assumption of multiple output underlying certain speech errors is independently supported by word blends, like a speaker's integration of the near-synonyms *close* and *near* into the error "clear". Dell and Reich (1981) observed the mixed-error bias also for blends.

Levelt et al. (1999a) argued that a mixed-error bias is also inherent to self-monitoring. Monitoring requires attention and it is error prone. It has been estimated that speakers miss about 50 percent of the errors they make (Levelt, 1989). The more the error differs from the target, the better it should be noticeable. In planning to say "cat" and monitoring through comprehension, the lemma of the target *cat* is in the comprehension cohort of an error like *calf* (fed back through comprehension), whereas the lemma of the target *cat* is not in the cohort of the error *dog*. Consequently, if the lemma of *calf* is mistakenly selected for the goal concept CAT(X), there is a higher probability that the error remains undetected during self-monitoring than when the lemma of *dog* is mistakenly selected. Thus, the mixed error bias arises from the design properties of the internal self-monitoring loop.

Rapp and Goldrick (2000) rejected a self-monitoring account of the mixed error bias by arguing that "not only does it require seemingly needless reduplication of information, but because the specific nature of the mechanism has remained unclear, the proposal is overly powerful" (p. 468). However, on the account of self-monitoring through the speech comprehension system, as implemented in WEAVER++, there is no needless reduplication of information. The form representations in word production differ from those in comprehension, but this distinction is not needless because it serves production and comprehension functions. Furthermore, the reduplication is supported by the available latency evidence (see Roelofs, 2003b, for a review). Moreover, the distinction explains dissociations between production and comprehension capabilities in aphasia.

Under the assumption that word production and perception are accomplished via the same form network, one expects a strong correlation between production and comprehension accuracy, as verified through computer simulations by Dell, Schwartz, Martin, Saffran, Gagnon, (1997) and Nickels and Howard (1995). However, such correlations are not observed empirically for form errors (e.g., Dell et al., 1997; Nickels & Howard, 1995). Therefore, Dell et al. (1997) also made the assumption for their own model that form representations are not shared between production and perception, in spite of the presence of backward links in their production network, which might have served speech comprehension. Thus, the assumption implemented in WEAVER++ that form representations are not shared between word production and comprehension is well motivated.

Rapp and Goldrick (2000) argued that the mechanism achieving self-monitoring "has remained unclear" (p. 468). However, because the effect of spoken distractors has been simulated by WEAVER++ (Roelofs, 1997a) and self-monitoring is assumed to be accomplished through the speech comprehension system, the required mechanism is already computationally specified to some extent in the model. Technically speaking, self-monitoring in WEAVER++ is like comprehending a spoken distractor word presented at a large post-exposure stimulus onset asynchrony (SOA), except that the spoken word is self-generated. In addition, self-monitoring via the speech comprehension system requires cognitive operations to detect discrepancies between selections made in production and comprehension. Lexical selection errors may be detected by verifying whether the lemma of the recognized word is linked to the target lexical concept in production. Errors in lexical concept selection may be detected by verifying whether the lexical concept of the recognized word is linked to the conceptual information derived from the to-be-named object. WEAVER++ implements such verification operations by means of condition-action production rules. Errors in planning and self-monitoring occur when production rules mistakenly fire. The probability of firing by mistake is a function of activation differences among nodes (cf. Roelofs, 1992, 1997a, 2003a).

WEAVER++ employs verification both in self-monitoring and in planning the production of spoken words. Verification in planning achieves that lemmas are selected for intended lexical concepts, morphemes for selected lemmas, segments for selected morphemes, and syllable programs for the syllabified segments. However, whereas verification in word planning happens automatically, verification that achieves self-monitoring is attention demanding. It is unlikely that in self-monitoring, the system can attend simultaneously to all aspects of the speech and at the same time equally well to the internal and external speech. Instead, if internal speech is monitored, external speech is monitored less well. This may explain dissociations between error and repair biases (cf. Nooteboom, this volume, Chapter 10). Thus, although verification in word planning may be seen as a kind of automatic monitoring, it should be distinguished from the operations involved in a speaker's self-monitoring through the speech comprehension system, which are attention demanding.

Computer simulations by Roelofs (2004a) demonstrated that self-monitoring in WEAVER++ suffices to explain the mixed error bias and its dependence on the functional locus of damage in aphasia. The simulations showed that when the lemma of *calf* is mistakenly selected and monitored by feeding its sound form into the speech comprehension system (the internal monitoring loop), the activation level of the lemma of *cat* is increased because of the form overlap with *calf*. However, when the sound form of *dog* is fed back, the activation of the lemma of *cat* is not increased. As a result, the difference in activation between the lemmas of *cat* and *calf* is greater than that between the lemmas of *cat* and *dog*. Consequently, a speaker is more likely to believe that the form of the target *cat* has correctly been prepared for production with the error *calf* than with the error *dog*. By contrast, the simulations showed that the activation of CAT(X) is not much affected by whether a form-related or unrelated item is fed back via the speech comprehension system. Thus, the mixed error bias in WEAVER++ arises at the level of lemmas but not at the level of lexical concepts.

Consequently, a wrong selection of a lexical concept node in naming a picture because of a conceptual deficit (as observed with patient K.E.) has an equal probability of being caught when the wrong concept has a form-related (*calf*) or a form-unrelated (*dog*) name. In contrast, a wrong selection of a lemma for a correctly selected lexical concept because of a post-conceptual deficit (as observed with patients P.W. and R.G.B.) has a greater probability of being caught when the wrongly selected word has a form-unrelated (*dog*) than a form-related (*calf*) name. Thus, whether a mixed error bias occurs in WEAVER++ depends on the locus of the lesion: The bias occurs with a post-conceptual deficit but not with a conceptual deficit, in agreement with the observations by Rapp and Goldrick (2000).

Accounting for the mixed-distractor latency effect

In testing for production-internal feedback in spoken word production, Damian and Martin (1999) and Starreveld and La Heij (1996) looked at semantic and form effects of spoken and written distractor words in picture naming. Naming latency was the main dependent variable. They observed that the distractors yielded semantic and form effects on picture-naming latencies, and jointly, the effects interacted. For example, the naming of a picture of a cat was interfered with by the semantically related distractor DOG compared with an unrelated distractor, and the naming was facilitated by the phonologically related distractor CAP relative to an unrelated distractor. The semantic interference effect was smaller when target and distractor were phonologically related (distractor CALF versus distractor CAP) than when they were unrelated in form (distractor DOG versus distractor DOLL). This is the mixed-distractor latency effect. According to Damian and Martin (1999), the semantic relatedness and form relatedness of distractors influence successive word-planning stages, namely lexical selection and sound form retrieval (see also Levelt et al., 1999a). Therefore, according to Damian and Martin, the interaction between semantic relatedness and form relatedness of distractors in picture naming suggests that there exists production-internal feedback from sounds to lexical items. According to Starreveld and La Heij (1996), the interaction suggests that semantic and form relatedness influence the same stage in word production. In their view, lexical selection and sound retrieval are one and the same process.

However, in the light of the mixed error bias, the reduced-latency effect of mixed distractors raises an interesting problem. The latency findings suggest that there is less competition from mixed items than from items that are semantically related only (hence faster latencies), whereas on the standard production-internal feedback account, the speech error data suggest more competition for mixed items (hence the larger number of errors). On the feedback account, the mixed-error bias occurs because production-internal feedback of activation makes the lexical node *calf* a stronger competitor than *dog* in planning to say "cat," which is exactly opposite to what an explanation of the latency effect of mixed distractors would seem to require. The latency data suggest that *calf* is a weaker competitor than *dog* in planning to say "cat." Thus, the challenge for models is to account for both the error and the latency findings.

Starreveld and La Heij (1996) proposed a new word production model without lemmas (cf. Caramazza, 1997) to account for the mixed-distractor latency finding. Their model consists of concept nodes directly connected to unitary phonological word-form nodes. Computer simulations by Starreveld and La Heij showed that their model could account for the mixed-distractor latency effect. Semantic relatedness and form relatedness both affect phonological word-form node selection in the model and therefore the effects interact. However, although the model can capture the latency effect, it fails on the mixed error bias. In planning to say "cat", the phonological word-form nodes of *calf* and *dog* also become active, but *calf* attains the same level of activation as *dog*. This is because there are no segment nodes in the model that are shared between *cat* and *calf*, and their phonological word-form nodes are not connected.

Furthermore, according to the model of Starreveld and La Heij (1996), the reduction of semantic interference and the pure phonological effect necessarily go together. Because semantic relatedness and form relatedness both have their effect through the activation of phonological word-form nodes, a reduction of semantic interference for mixed distractors is only observed in the context of pure form facilitation from phonologically related distractors. Similarly, on the production internal feedback account (Damian & Martin, 1999), semantic and form relatedness interact because activation of production forms spreads back to the level at which semantic effects arise, namely the level of lexical selection. Therefore, a reduction of semantic interference for mixed distractors should only be observed in the context of facilitation from form-related distractors. However, this is not supported empirically. Damian and Martin (1999) presented the spoken distractors at three SOAs. The onset of the spoken distractor was 150 msec before picture onset (SOA = −150 msec), simultaneously with picture onset, or 150 msec after picture onset. They observed semantic interference at the SOAs of −150 and 0 msec, and phonological facilitation at the SOAs of 0 and 150 msec. The mixed distractors yielded no semantic interference at SOA = −150 msec and facilitation at the later SOAs, exactly like the form-related distractors. Thus, the reduction of semantic interference for mixed distractors was already observed at an SOA (i.e., SOA = −150 msec) at which there was no pure phonological facilitation.

Compared to the unrelated distractors, the form effect at SOA = −150 msec was 5 msec, and the effect of form and mixed distractors combined was 2 msec. The point here is not that form related distractors may not yield facilitation at SOA = −150 msec (e.g., Meyer & Schriefers, 1991, and Starreveld, 2000, obtained such an early effect, whereas Damian & Martin, 1999, did not), but that there may be a temporal dissociation between mixed effects and phonological effects. This suggests that the mixed semantic-phonological effect and the pure form effect are located at different word planning levels, namely the lemma and the word-form level, respectively, as argued by Roelofs et al. (1996).

The assignment of the semantic and form effects to different planning levels is independently supported by the finding that cohort and rhyme competitors yield differential effects in spoken word recognition tasks, whereas they yield similar form effects in picture naming (see Roelofs, 2003b, for an extensive discussion). Whereas form-based activation of cohort competitors in spoken word comprehension is observed (e.g., Zwitserlood, 1989), this does not hold for rhyme competitors when the first segment of the rhyme competitor is more than two phonological features different from the target (e.g., Allopenna et al., 1998; Connine et al., 1993; Marslen-Wilson & Zwitserlood, 1989). In contrast, cohort and rhyme distractors yield form effects of similar size in picture naming (Collins & Ellis, 1992; Meyer & Schriefers, 1991; Meyer & Van der Meulen, 2000), even when they are one complete syllable different from the target.

Meyer and Schriefers (1991) observed that when cohort and rhyme distractors are presented over headphones during the planning of monosyllabic picture names (e.g., the spoken distractors CAP or HAT presented during planning to say the target word "cat"), both distractors yield facilitation compared with unrelated distractors. Also, when cohort and rhyme distractors (e.g., METAL or VILLAIN) are auditory presented during the planning of disyllabic picture names (e.g., "melon"), both distractors yield facilitation too. When the difference in time between distractor and target presentation is manipulated, the SOA at which the facilitation is first detected differs between the two types of distractors. In particular, the onset of facilitation is at an earlier SOA for cohort than for rhyme distractors (i.e., respectively, SOA = −150 msec and SOA = 0 msec). At SOAs where both effects are present (i.e., 0 and 150 msec), the magnitude of the facilitation effect from cohort and rhyme distractors was the same in the study of Meyer and Schriefers (1991). Collins and Ellis (1992) and Meyer and Van der Meulen (2000) made similar observations.

To summarize, the evidence suggests that in spoken word recognition there is some but not much lexical activation of rhyme competitors differing in only the initial segment with a critical word. This contrasts with the findings from spoken distractors in picture naming, where cohort and rhyme distractors word yield comparable amounts of facilitation, even when the target and distractor are one syllable different (i.e., the spoken distractor VILLAIN facilitates the production of the target *melon*).

The difference between the findings from cross-modal priming studies in the spoken word recognition literature (Allopenna et al., 1998; Connine et al., 1993; Marslen-Wilson et al., 1996; Marslen-Wilson & Zwitserlood, 1989) and the findings from spoken distractors in picture naming (Collins & Ellis, 1992; Meyer & Schriefers, 1991; Meyer & Van der Meulen, 2000) is explained if one assumes that spoken distractor words do not activate rhyme competitors at the lemma level but speech segments in the word-form production network. Roelofs (1997a) provided such an account, implemented in WEAVER++, and reported computer simulations of the effects. On this account, METAL and VILLAIN activate the segments that are shared with *melon* to the same extent (respectively, the segments of the first and second syllable), which explains the findings on picture naming of Meyer and Schriefers (1991). At the same time, METAL activates the lemma of *melon* whereas VILLAIN does not, which accounts for the findings on spoken word recognition of Connine et al. (1993), Marslen-Wilson and Zwitserlood (1989), and Allopenna et al. (1998). Cohort activation (because of begin relatedness) does not have to result in facilitation of lemma retrieval for production in the WEAVER++ model, unless there is also a semantic relationship involved (reducing the semantic interference from mixed distractors).

I argued that the mixed-error effect can at least partly be attributed to self-monitoring in WEAVER++. If in planning to say "cat", the lemma of *calf* is selected instead of the lemma of *cat* and the form of *calf* is fed back through the speech comprehension system, the lemma of *cat* is in the comprehension cohort of the error *calf*. However, if, in planning to say "cat", the lemma of *dog* is selected instead of the lemma of *cat*, then the lemma of the target *cat* is not in the cohort of the error *dog*. Hence, the lemma of *cat* is more active when activation from the word form of the error *calf* is fed back via the comprehension system than when activation from the form of the error *dog* is fed back, and the error *calf* for *cat* is more likely to remain unnoticed in self-monitoring than the error *dog* for *cat*. On this account, the lemma of *calf* is a weaker competitor than the lemma of *dog* in planning to say "cat". That *calf* is a weaker competitor than *dog* in planning to say "cat" also accounts for the mixed distractor latency effect in WEAVER++ (cf. Roelofs et al., 1996), except that the latency effect results from comprehension of the speech of others (i.e., spoken distractor words) rather than from self-monitoring.

The mixed distractor CALF yields less interference than the distractor DOG, because the lemma of the target *cat* is primed as a spoken cohort member during hearing the distractor CALF but not during hearing DOG. Thus, WEAVER++ explains why there is a reduction of semantic interference and an increased change of misselection for mixed items. In summary, according to WEAVER++, mixed items are weaker competitors rather than stronger competitors because of the activation dynamics. Therefore, selection failures concerning mixed items are more likely to remain unnoticed in error monitoring and mixed items have less effect as spoken distractors on latencies in WEAVER++, in agreement with the speech error data and the production latency findings.

Computer simulations by Roelofs (2004a) demonstrated that WEAVER++ exhibits the latency effect of mixed distractors. Damian and Martin (1999) observed empirically that at SOA = −150 msec, the semantically related distractor DOG yielded interference in planning to say "cat", but the mixed distractor CALF yielded no interference, even though there was no pure form facilitation from CAP at this SOA. This was also the effect that the auditory distractors had on lemma retrieval in WEAVER++ simulations. At SOA = −150 msec in the simulations, the distractor DOG yielded interference in planning to say "cat" but the mixed distractor CALF yielded no interference, even though there was no pure form facilitation from CAP at this SOA. Thus, form relatedness affected lemma retrieval in case of semantic relatedness even when it yielded no pure form facilitation in lemma retrieval (cf. Levelt et al., 1999b). After both lemma retrieval and word-form encoding in the simulations, there were main effects of semantic and phonological relatedness, and jointly the effects interacted, as empirically observed. The results of the simulations were identical with and without comprehension-based feedback. Thus, self-monitoring in WEAVER++ does not affect latency fits of the model.

Cohort effects on mixed errors and production latencies

If the error biases arise during self-monitoring that is accomplished through the speech comprehension system, cohort effects on errors are to be expected. In particular, initial segment overlap between target and intruder should be critical. Dell and Reich (1981) indeed observed that the mixed error effect in their corpus of spontaneous speech errors was strongest for first segment overlap, and much less strong for second, third, or fourth segment overlap. Martin et al. (1996) replicated this seriality finding for picture naming, both with normal and aphasic speakers.

The claim that the mixed-distractor latency effect arises because of comprehension cohorts rather than because of activation feedback within the production system leads to a few new predictions concerning latencies. First, given the finding of Zwitserlood (1989) that word-initial fragments suffice to yield semantic effects in spoken word comprehension, initial fragments of spoken distractor words should yield semantic interference in picture naming, even when a fragment does not uniquely identify a word. In contrast, Damian and Martin (1999) and Starreveld (2000) argued that such effects of fragments cannot occur in a picture-word interference task. According to them, semantic effects of spoken distractors only occur when the spoken-word recognition system has "settled into a state in which only one candidate (corresponding to the distractor) is activated" (Starreveld, 2000, p. 518). Damian and Martin (1999) expressed the same view: "Semantic access in auditory word recognition critically depends on when lexical uniqueness is achieved" (p. 351). If lexical uniqueness is required to obtain a semantic effect, then the interaction between semantic and form effects cannot be a comprehension cohort effect: The cohort account assumes that CA suffices to activate the lemmas of *cat* and *calf*. Second, given that rhyme competitors are not much activated in speech comprehension (Allopenna et al., 1998; Connine et al., 1993), replicating the study of Damian and Martin (1999) with rhyme competitors should yield additive rather than interactive effects of semantic and phonological relatedness.

The predictions about the spoken fragments and the rhyme distractors have been confirmed recently (Roelofs, submitted-a, -b). The upper panel of Figure 3.4. shows the semantic and phonological effects of word-initial fragments. Participants had to name, for example, a pictured tiger while hearing PU (the first syllable of the semantically related word *puma*), TI (phonologically related, the first syllable of the target *tiger*), or an unrelated syllable. The figure shows that fragments such as PU yielded semantic interference and that

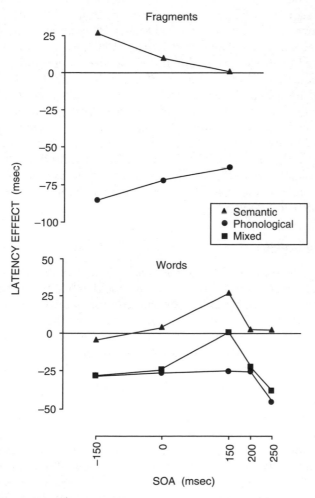

Figure 3.4 Latency effect (in msec) of semantically related, phonologically related, and mixed spoken distractors relative to unrelated distractors in picture naming as a function of SOA (in msec).

fragments such as TI produced phonological facilitation, the first finding supporting the cohort assumption.

The lower panel of Figure 3.4 shows the semantic, phonological, and mixed effects when the form-related and mixed items are rhyme competitors of the target. The mixed distractors were matched for semantic and phonological relatedness to the semantically related and the phonologically related distractors, respectively. Participants had to name, for example, a pictured dolphin while hearing SPARROW (semantically related), MUFFIN (phonologically related), ROBIN (mixed), or an unrelated word. The distractors yielded semantic and form effects, and together, the effects were additive, unlike the interactive effects from cohort distractors observed by Damian and Martin (1999). The semantic and form effects occurred at a positive SOA, presumably because the onset of the critical rhyme fragment determined the SOA in the experiment following Meyer and Schriefers (1991). By contrast, with the fragments and in the study of Damian and Martin (1999), the onset of the distractor determined the SOA. The additivity of the effects poses difficulty to models with production-internal feedback. Production-internal feedback of activation from the mixed rhyme distractor ROBIN should activate the target *dolphin*, just like the cohort distractor CALF activates the target *cat*. Therefore, the reduced latency effect should also be obtained for mixed rhyme distractors, contrary to the empirical findings. Importantly, the fact that the phonologically related rhyme distractor MUFFIN facilitated the production of *dolphin* suggests that the form overlap of rhyme distractors did have an effect, replicating earlier studies (Collins & Ellis, 1992; Meyer & Schriefers, 1991; Meyer & Van der Meulen, 2000).

Summary and conclusions

Aphasic and nonaphasic speakers listen to their own talking and they prevent and correct many of the errors made in the planning and actual production of speech. To account for this type of output control, models need to make assumptions about self-monitoring. I have explained the relations among planning, comprehending, and self-monitoring of spoken words in WEAVER++, a feedforward word-production model that assumes self-monitoring through comprehension-based feedback (Roelofs, 2004a, b). The self-monitoring through comprehension of the model was shown to be supported by a new analysis of the self-corrections and false starts in picture naming by 15 aphasic speakers. Furthermore, the model explained findings that seemingly require production-internal feedback: the mixed-error bias and its dependence on the locus of damage in aphasia, and the reduced latency effect of mixed distractors. Finally, the attribution of the mixed-distractor latency effect to comprehension cohorts by the model was shown to be supported by recent experimental research, which revealed semantic effects of word-initial cohort distractors and the absence of a reduced latency effect for mixed rhyme distractors. To conclude, the interplay among speaking, comprehending, and self-monitoring is not only of interest in its own right, but it also illuminates classic issues in production.

References

Allopenna, P. D., Magnuson, J. S., & Tanenhaus, M. K. (1998). Tracking the time course of spoken word recognition using eye movements: Evidence for continuous mapping models. *Journal of Memory and Language, 38,* 419–39.

Caramazza, A. (1997). How many levels of processing are there in lexical access? *Cognitive Neuropsychology, 14,* 177–208.

Collins, A., & Ellis, A. (1992). Phonological priming of lexical retrieval in speech production. *British Journal of Psychology, 83,* 375–88.

Connine, C. M., Blasko, D. G., & Titone, D. (1993). Do the beginnings of spoken words have a special status in auditory word recognition? *Journal of Memory and Language, 32,* 193–210.

Damian, M. K., & Martin, R. C. (1999). Semantic and phonological codes interact in single word production. *Journal of Experimental Psychology: Learning, Memory, and Cognition, 25,* 345–61.

Dell, G. S., & Reich, P. A. (1981). Stages in sentence production: An analysis of speech error data. *Journal of Verbal Learning and Verbal Behavior, 20,* 611–29.

Dell, G. S., Schwartz, M. F., Martin, N., Saffran, E. M., & Gagnon, D. A. (1997). Lexical access in aphasic and nonaphasic speakers. *Psychological Review, 104,* 801–38.

Levelt, W. J. M. (1989). *Speaking: From intention to articulation.* Cambridge, MA: MIT Press.

Levelt, W. J. M., Roelofs, A., & Meyer, A. S. (1999a). A theory of lexical access in speech production. *Behavioral and Brain Sciences, 22,* 1–38.

Levelt, W. J. M., Roelofs, A., & Meyer, A. S. (1999b). Multiple perspectives on word production. *Behavioral and Brain Sciences, 22,* 61–75.

Marslen-Wilson, W., Moss, H. E., & van Halen, S. (1996). Perceptual distance and competition in lexical access. *Journal of Experimental Psychology: Human Perception and Performance, 22,* 1376–92.

Marslen-Wilson, W. D., & Welsh, A. (1978). Processing interactions and lexical access during word recognition in continuous speech. *Cognitive Psychology, 10,* 29–63.

Marslen-Wilson, W. D., & Zwitserlood, P. (1989). Accessing spoken words: The importance of word onsets. *Journal of Experimental Psychology: Human Perception and Performance, 15,* 576–85.

Martin, N., Gagnon, D. A., Schwartz, M. F., Dell, G. S., & Saffran, E. M. (1996). Phonological facilitation of semantic errors in normal and aphasic speakers. *Language and Cognitive Processes, 11,* 257–82.

McClelland, J. L., & Elman, J. (1986). The TRACE model of speech perception. *Cognitive Psychology, 18,* 1–86.

McGuire, P. K., Silbersweig, D. A., & Frith, C. D. (1996). Functional neuroanatomy of verbal self-monitoring. *Brain, 119,* 907–17.

Meyer, A. S., & Schriefers, H. (1991). Phonological facilitation in picture-word interference experiments: Effects of stimulus onset asynchrony and types of interfering stimuli. *Journal of Experimental Psychology: Learning, Memory, and Cognition, 17,* 1146–60.

Meyer, A. S., & Van der Meulen, F. F. (2000). Phonological priming effects on speech onset latencies and viewing times in object naming. *Psychonomic Bulletin & Review*, 7, 314–19.

Nickels, L. (1997). *Spoken word production and its breakdown in aphasia*. Hove: Psychology Press.

Nickels, L., & Howard, D. (1995). Phonological errors in aphasic naming: Comprehension, monitoring, and lexicality. *Cortex*, *31*, 209–37.

Nickels, L., & Howard, D. (2000). When the words won't come: Relating impairments and models of spoken word production. In L. Wheeldon (Ed.), *Aspects of language production* (pp. 115–42). Hove, UK: Psychology Press.

Norris, D. (1994). Shortlist: A connectionist model of continuous speech recognition. *Cognition*, *52*, 189–234.

Paus, T., Perry, D. W., Zatorre, R. J., Worsley, K. J., & Evans, A. C. (1996). Modulation of cerebral blood flow in the human auditory cortex during speech: Role of motor-to-sensory discharges. *European Journal of Neuroscience*, *8*, 2236–46.

Rapp, B., & Goldrick, M. (2000). Discreteness and interactivity in spoken word production. *Psychological Review*, *107*, 460–99.

Rapp, B., & Goldrick, M. (2004). Feedback by any other name is still interactivity: A reply to Roelofs (2004). *Psychological Review*, *111*, 573–8.

Roelofs, A. (1992). A spreading-activation theory of lemma retrieval in speaking. *Cognition*, *42*, 107–42.

Roelofs, A. (1993). Testing a non-decompositional theory of lemma retrieval in speaking: Retrieval of verbs. *Cognition*, *47*, 59–87.

Roelofs, A. (1996). Serial order in planning the production of successive morphemes of a word. *Journal of Memory and Language*, *35*, 854–76.

Roelofs, A. (1997a). The WEAVER model of word-form encoding in speech production. *Cognition*, *64*, 249–84.

Roelofs, A. (1997b). A case for nondecomposition in conceptually driven word retrieval. *Journal of Psycholinguistic Research*, *26*, 33–67.

Roelofs, A. (1997c). Syllabification in speech production: Evaluation of WEAVER. *Language and Cognitive Processes*, *12*, 657–93.

Roelofs, A. (1998). Rightward incrementality in encoding simple phrasal forms in speech production: Verb-particle combinations. *Journal of Experimental Psychology: Learning, Memory, and Cognition*, *24*, 904–21.

Roelofs, A. (1999). Phonological segments and features as planning units in speech production. *Language and Cognitive Processes*, *14*, 173–200.

Roelofs, A. (2003a). Goal-referenced selection of verbal action: Modeling attentional control in the Stroop task. *Psychological Review*, *110*, 88–125.

Roelofs, A. (2003b). Modeling the relation between the production and recognition of spoken word forms. In A. S. Meyer & N. O. Schiller (Eds.), *Phonetics and phonology in language comprehension and production: Differences and similarities* (pp. 115–158). Berlin: Mouton.

Roelofs, A. (2004a). Error biases in spoken word planning and monitoring by aphasic and nonaphasic speakers: Comment on Rapp and Goldrick (2000). *Psychological Review*, *111*, 561–72.

Roelofs, A. (2004b). Comprehension-based versus production-internal feedback in planning spoken words: A rejoinder to Rapp and Goldrick (2004). *Psychological Review*, *111*, 579–80.

Roelofs, A. (submitted-a). *Word-initial cohort effects of spoken distractors in picture naming.*

Roelofs, A. (submitted-b). *Autonomous stages in planning the production of spoken words: Evidence from semantic and form effects of rhyme distractors in picture naming.*

Roelofs, A., & Meyer, A. S. (1998). Metrical structure in planning the production of spoken words. *Journal of Experimental Psychology: Learning, Memory, and Cognition, 24*, 922–39.

Roelofs, A., Meyer, A. S., & Levelt, W. J. M. (1996). Interaction between semantic and orthographic factors in conceptually driven naming: Comment on Starreveld and La Heij (1995). *Journal of Experimental Psychology: Learning, Memory, and Cognition, 22*, 246–51.

Roelofs, A., Meyer, A. S., & Levelt, W. J. M. (1998). A case for the lemma-lexeme distinction in models of speaking: Comment on Caramazza and Miozzo (1997). *Cognition, 69*, 219–30.

Starreveld, P. A. (2000). On the interpretation of context effects in word production. *Journal of Memory and Language, 42*, 497–525.

Starreveld, P. A., & La Heij, W. (1996). Time-course analysis of semantic and orthographic context effects in picture naming. *Journal of Experimental Psychology: Learning, Memory, and Cognition, 22*, 896–918.

Wheeldon, L. R., & Levelt, W. J. M. (1995). Monitoring the time course of phonological encoding. *Journal of Memory and Language, 34*, 311–34.

Zwitserlood, P. (1989). The locus of the effects of sentential-semantic context in spoken-word processing. *Cognition, 32*, 25–64.

Part II

Pathologies of phonological encoding

4 An interactive activation account of aphasic speech errors: Converging influences of locus, type, and severity of processing impairment

Nadine Martin

Abstract

This chapter reviews recent empirical and computational investigations that provide accounts of aphasic speech errors within an interactive activation model of word processing. Studies addressing two areas of investigation are reviewed: Comparisons of normal and pathological error patterns and changes in error patterns after recovery. These studies are discussed as illustrations of current perspectives on factors that influence the occurrence of speech errors in aphasia including locus of impairment (i.e., what linguistic representations are affected), type of processing impairment (e.g., slowed activation or too rapid decay) and severity of impairment.

The study of word-processing impairments has a long history in cognitive neuropsychology. Various theoretical frameworks have been used to account for mechanisms underlying word retrieval and their breakdown in aphasia. In this chapter, I will review some recent accounts of word processing and its impairment that have been framed within interactive activation (IA) models of word processing.

Aphasia is an acquired language impairment caused by neurological disease (e.g., progressive aphasia) or injury (e.g., cerebral vascular accidents or head injury). It can affect both comprehension and production of speech and language. A common symptom of production impairment is the occurrence of speech errors. Speakers with aphasia often produce the wrong words or sounds of a word or the incorrect sequence of words within a sentence or sounds within a word. Normal speakers also produce speech errors, but far fewer than speakers with aphasia. The study of normal speech errors has contributed much to our understanding of the mechanisms that underlie speech and language production (e.g., Dell, 1986; Fromkin, 1971; Garrett, 1975; Harley, 1984; Stemberger, 1985). In conjunction with other approaches to the study of cognitive processes underlying speech and language (e.g., time course studies, Schriefers, Meyer, & Levelt 1990), speech error analyses have guided the development of cognitive models of language. As these models developed, aphasiologists were quick to use them as frameworks within which to evaluate the breakdown of language in aphasia (Schwartz, 1987). In due course, they also used language data from aphasic subjects to test these models (Howard & Franklin, 1988). It is at this point in the history of cognitive neuropsychology that this chapter begins. The enterprises of applying cognitive models to explain the breakdown of language in aphasia and in turn using those data to test these same models have contributed much to our understanding of the cognitive organization of word processing and language more generally.

Cognitive neuropsychological research in the 1970s and 1980s focused on revealing the structural organization of word processing, leading to the development of structural "box and arrow" models that identify the cognitive representations of language (e.g., phonological, semantic, morphological) and pathways by which linguistic information is processed. In the 1980s, models with "connectionist" architectures were developed, providing another framework within which to investigate aphasic impairment. Connectionist models expanded on structural models' identification of information processing pathways by postulating hypothetical constructs of processing (e.g., spreading activation, inhibition, connection strength). These concepts and models allowed researchers to address questions of *how* linguistic representations are processed, and in this respect, expanded the domain of empirical data that can be used test theories. For example, connectionist architectures have been used to explore the effects of impairment severity on task performance (Schwartz & Brecher, 2000) and to predict changes in error patterns associated with recovery from impairment (Martin, Saffran, & Dell, 1996). Additionally, most connectionist models (and recently some discrete stage models, e.g., Laine, Tikkala, & Juhola, 1998) are computationally instantiated. This tool is especially useful when predicting behavior of dynamic systems. Although the use of computational models in studies of normal and aphasic language processing is in its early stages, the advances made in the last decade with this approach should mark the beginning of a new wave of investigations that focus on dynamic aspects of language processing.

In what follows, I will review some recent studies that address two current issues concerning the organization of word retrieval processes and their breakdown in aphasia: (1) How do aphasic speech errors compare with normal speech errors? and (2) how do patterns of aphasic error change with recovery? For each topic, I will provide an overview of recent empirical and computational studies to illustrate approaches that IA models use to address these issues. These studies also should illustrate some current thinking about factors that influence the occurrence of speech errors in aphasia: locus of linguistic impairment (i.e., whether semantic or phonological representations of words are affected), type of processing impairment (e.g., slowed activation or too rapid decay) and severity of impairment. They should also help the reader to gain some appreciation of the challenges involved in studying the breakdown of word retrieval processes in aphasia and the contribution of IA models to our understanding of cognitive processes underlying word retrieval.

A computational model can be lesioned in ways that mimic cognitive impairments resulting from neurological damage. A theory's validity can be examined by comparing performance of brain damaged subjects on a particular task with that of the computational model that is presumably lesioned in the same way. Although our characterizations of cognitive impairments (site and type of lesion) still require refinement, this method of comparing human and computational model performance shows great promise as a means of developing and testing theories of cognition (see also Dell & Kim, this volume, Chapter 2). To date, the most common language task studied using this empirical-computational approach is word retrieval. This is because computational models and subjects (i.e., human speakers) both produce concrete data on a word retrieval task: A distribution of responses across a number of response categories (correct, semantic errors, phonological errors, etc.). The distributions predicted by the model can be compared to those of the subjects, enabling a clear test of a theory's assumptions.

How do aphasic speech errors compare to normal speech errors?

Aphasic individuals produce a range of error types that in many ways resemble those that are produced by non-aphasic speakers. Clearly, they produce more errors than normal speakers do, but it remains an empirical question whether their error patterns are qualitatively different as well. On the surface, there are both similarities and differences.

Both aphasic and non-aphasic speakers produce word substitutions that are semantically and/or phonologically related or even unrelated to the intended utterance. They also both produce nonword errors that are phonologically related to the target word. It would be quite unusual, however, for a normal speaker to produce a nonword error that is not related phonologically to the target word. And yet, some aphasic speakers produce such errors in great quantity. This observation could be held as evidence that aphasic errors are qualitatively different from normal speech errors. An alternative view is that such errors arise from normal error mechanisms under conditions of severe impairment.

From corpora of speech errors collected by a number of researchers (e.g., Fromkin, 1971; Garrett, 1975; Harley, 1984) we know that the most common type of word retrieval error by normal speakers is the semantic substitution (e.g., tomorrow → yesterday), followed by phonologically related word substitution (horse → house) or phonologically related nonword error (e.g., bell → /brEl/) errors. This distribution reflects the sums of errors collected from many unimpaired speakers. Aphasic speakers are studied individually more often than not, and from this practice, we know that patterns of error distribution in word retrieval tasks vary in this population. While some aphasic speakers produce many semantic errors and few, if any, phonological errors, others produce many phonological errors and fewer semantic errors. And, some fail to give any response at all even though they are familiar with the item to be named. These different error patterns can be grossly linked with frontal versus posterior neurological damage and, in cognitive terms, with damage to semantic, lexical and phonological processing operations.

It is possible that among normal speakers there is individual variation in error patterns that, like the aphasic speakers, deviate from the common distribution of speech errors (semantic > phonologically related word > phonologically related nonword). We do not know this, because we study normal speech errors combined from many different speakers, an approach necessitated by the low rate of speech errors produced by individual normal speakers. This question is relevant, however, to the issue of qualitative comparisons of normal and aphasic language because, as noted above, not all aphasic speakers show the "normal" error pattern. If we amassed speech errors produced by a large population of aphasic speakers, it is conceivable that the sum total of errors would fall into the same distribution of errors collected from normal speakers. Conversely, if we evaluated many individual speakers without aphasia, collecting samples of their errors over many communication instances, we might find variations in individual error patterns. For example, some normal speakers might tend to make phonological errors more than semantic errors and vice versa. The challenge for cognitive theorists is to develop a model of normal word retrieval that can produce these various error patterns when lesioned in ways that presumably mimic the cognitive damage resulting from brain damage. In the next sections, I will review one such model that postulates continuity between the known normal speech error pattern (semantic errors > phonological word errors > phonological nonword errors) and aphasic speech error patterns and attributes deviations of aphasic error patterns from the normal pattern to variations in the severity of impairment to word activation processes.

Using an interactive activation model of normal word processing to investigate aphasic speech

One of the first investigations of aphasic speech errors to use an IA model of normal word processing as its theoretical frame of reference was a study by Schwartz, Saffran, Dell, and Bloch (1994). They compared the rates and distribution of errors produced by a jargon aphasic, FL, with those of normal speakers (from the London-Lund corpus of speech errors, Garnham, Shillcock, Brown, Mill, & Cutler, 1982) and found similar relative proportions of open- and closed-class errors in the two corpora. However, within the class of lexical substitutions, FL was inclined to produce a much higher rate of unrelated word substitutions (e.g., gone → caught). Schwartz et al. (1994) and Bloch (1986) argued that discrete two-stage models of word retrieval (e.g., Garrett, 1982) could not account for certain aspects of FL's pattern of error. In particular, FL produced few formal paraphasias (sound-related word errors, e.g., food→ fuse). In a discrete two-stage model, these occur at the stage when the phonological code of a lemma is retrieved from a word-form inventory. At the same time, FL produced many phonologically related non-word errors (e.g., speak → /spisbid/), which presumably occur post-lexically when the phonological code guides retrieval of the word's phonological representations. Thus, an account of FL's word retrieval impairment within a discrete stage model of word retrieval would have to assume that FL suffered from severe deficits at all stages of word retrieval except for a second pass through the lexicon to retrieve the word form. Viewed within the two-stage model this conclusion seemed somewhat counterintuitive.

Schwartz et al. (1994) used an interactive spreading activation theory of word retrieval (Dell, 1986; Dell & O'Seaghdha, 1992) to account for the error patterns of FL. In its simplest form, this model has three layers of representation, semantic, lexical and phonological. Activation spreads across (but not within) levels of representation, in a series of feedforward and feedback activation cycles (Figure 4.1). The spread of activation is regulated by two parameters, connection strength (the rate of activation spread) and decay rate (the rate of activation decline toward resting level). Noise and the number of time steps to production are additional parameters. This is a competitive activation model with no inhibitory connections during retrieval. Spreading activation primes the intended word and related word representations and at the time of retrieval, the most activated word representation (usually the intended utterance) is retrieved and the activation of this word representation is inhibited.

Schwartz et al. (1994) accounted for FL's error pattern (few phonologically related word errors, many sound errors and a high rate of perseverations) by

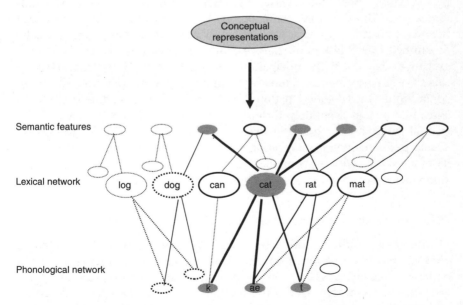

Figure 4.1 An interactive activation model of single word production. (Adapted from Dell and O'Seaghdha, 1992.)

assuming that the connection strength parameters of word retrieval were impaired.[1] In the unimpaired production system, phonologically related word errors occur when spreading activation primes phonological nodes and feeds back to the lexical network to maintain activation of the targeted lexical node ("cat" in Figure 4.1). This feedback also activates phonologically related lexical nodes ("mat" in Figure 4.1). Normally, these competitors would not be retrieved, but if the target node's activation is compromised in some way, their probability of retrieval increases. When connection strength is reduced the spread of feedback activation from phonological to lexical levels would be insufficient to activate phonologically related lexical competitors. Consequently, nonword phonological errors, which occur at the post-lexical phonological encoding stage, would predominate. Perseverations would also increase under conditions of weakened connection strength, because the residual activation of words already retrieved would be better able to compete with weakened activation of the current "target" lexical node, even when connection strength is reduced to all nodes.

Schwartz et al. (1994) also examined rates of anticipations (e.g., "I would cook and food the food") and perseverations (e.g., "from the doctors that I've learned now, they had my doctors open for . . .") in normal speakers and FL. They found that while normal speakers tended to produce more anticipations than perseverations, FL was more inclined toward the opposite pattern. In a companion study, Schwartz et al. (1994) also investigated effects of practice on performance of tongue twisters by normal speaking subjects. They showed that this variable, as predicted by the model, would reduce the rate of perseveration errors that occurred in production of the tongue twister sentences (e.g., Brad's burned bran buns). When normal speakers produced these utterances, the rates of perseverations were initially high but gradually diminished over 8 blocks of trials. A similar pattern was observed with full exchanges, but not with anticipations. Schwartz et al. (1994) characterized this shift in performance as moving from a "bad" error pattern (with weak connections) to a "good" pattern (with sufficient connection strength to spread activation accurately throughout the lexical network). Thus, when normal subjects utter tongue twisters for the first time the conditions are similar to a reduction in connection strength. Practice increases the familiarity of the system with the combinations of sounds and words and presumably strengthens activation connections associated with those combinations.

Other processing impairments in an interactive activation model

Martin, Dell, Saffran, and Schwartz (1994) used Dell's (1986; Dell & O'Seaghdha, 1992) IA model to investigate the naming and repetition error patterns of a patient, NC, who suffered from an acute aphasia secondary to a cerebral aneurysm. His speech production was fluent with semantic errors and phonological word and nonword errors. Auditory comprehension was severely impaired, and reading comprehension was only mildly affected. NC's error pattern had two features of interest: he produced semantic errors in single word repetition (known as "deep dysphasia") and, in speech production, he produced a relatively high rate of formal paraphasias (sound-related whole word substitutions). These error patterns are noteworthy because they deviate from the normal error pattern and have been reported in only a few cases (e.g., Blanken, 1990; Howard & Franklin, 1988).

For the moment, I will focus on the naming error patterns of NC compared to FL. Whereas FL produced few formal paraphasias and many nonword phonological errors in naming, NC produced a high rate of formal paraphasias and a moderate rate of nonword phonological errors. Recall that there are two parameters in the IA model that regulate activation processes and word retrieval: Connection weight and decay rate. FL's error pattern was modelled with a connection weight lesion (slowing down the spread of activation). Martin et al. (1994) hypothesized that NC's error pattern resulted from impairment to the decay rate parameter manifested as too rapid decay of activated representations in the semantic-lexical-phonological network. As noted, formal paraphasias are presumed to occur at the lexical level and happen because connection strength is strong enough to feed back activation from phonological nodes to the lexical level over the course of lexical activation. Figure 4.2 illustrates the time course of feedforward-feedback processes in word retrieval in production.

As the feedforward-feedback cycles of activation begin in the word retrieval process, the target node (cat) and semantically related competitors (dog and rat) are the first nodes to be activated. Phonologically related lexical nodes (can) are primed later by feedback activation from primed phonological nodes. As the feedforward-feedback cycles occur, nodes that are primed increase in activation and then decay at a certain rate until the next cycle of activation occurs. This is to keep activation levels in check until word retrieval occurs. The target receives the most activation because it is the target. But, with respect to competitors that are activated during this process, semantically related lexical nodes (dog, rat) become more activated than competitors that are only phonologically related (can). This is because they are primed earlier than phonological competitors and accumulate more activation over the time course of lexical selection. Competitors that are similar both semantically and phonologically (rat) receive both feedforward and feedback activation. When all connections are subjected to an increase in the rate of activation decay, the activation advantage of semantically related competitors becomes a disadvantage, because earlier primed representations (target and semantic competitors) suffer more from the cumulative effects of too fast decay than the representations primed later (phonologically related word nodes). Thus, as decay rate is increased beyond the "normal" setting, the probability increases that these late-activated competitors (phonologically related words) will be selected in error.

Figure 4.3 illustrates the time course of feedforward-feedback processes in single word repetition. A decay rate lesion in this case would lead to an

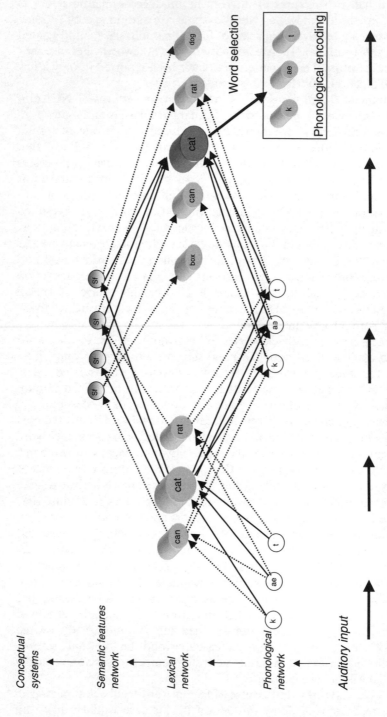

Figure 4.2 Temporal and spatial course of spreading activation during *repetition* of a single word in an interactive activation model.

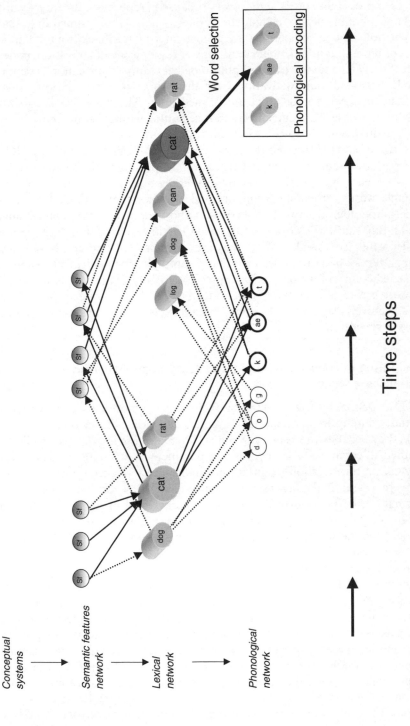

Figure 4.3 Temporal and spatial course of spreading activation during *production* of a single word in an interactive activation model.

increased probability of *semantic* errors because in repetition, the target word (cat) and phonologically related word nodes (cab, rat) are primed first, and semantically related competitors are primed later by feedback from semantic levels of representation. Under conditions of rapid decay of activation, nodes primed early (the target, cat, and phonological competitors, can, rat) cumulatively will lose more activation over the course of word retrieval than semantically related nodes that are primed later. The net effect is to shift probabilities of error in such a way that semantic errors become more likely (see Martin & Saffran, 1992 for further discussion).

Martin et al. (1994) tested the rapid-decay hypothesis by simulating NC's error pattern in both naming and repetition. Importantly, the same lesion (a global increase in decay rate) was used to model both naming and repetition of single words, providing computational evidence that a single semantic-lexical-phonological network could subserve both input and output processing. The finding that NC's error pattern could be simulated with a decay lesion further validated the idea of "processing" impairment and confirmed that error patterns could vary based on the type of processing impairment. Whereas weakened connection strength accounted for FL's high rate of phonological nonword errors and perseverations, abnormally fast decay rate accounted for NC's relatively high rate of formal paraphasias in naming and semantic errors in repetition.

Exploration of connection weight and decay impairments in a multiple case study

In 1997, Dell, Schwartz, Martin, Saffran, and Gagnon used the IA model to study naming impairments of 21 aphasic subjects. As in their previous work, they began with the assumptions (1) that aphasic impairment could be captured in cognitive terms by altering parameters of the model that affect information transmission (connection weight) and representational integrity (decay rate) and (2) that aphasic error patterns fell on a continuum between a "normal" error pattern and a random pattern. Dell et al. (1997) showed that by varying these two parameters globally within the semantic-lexical-phonological network, the model could simulate the distribution of correct and erroneous responses across error categories (e.g., semantic, formal paraphasias, and mixed errors).

Additionally, Dell et al. (1997) explored impairments of connection weight and decay rate as predictors of other error phenomena. First, they demonstrated what is called the "noun" effect. This prediction concerns formal paraphasias (word errors that are phonologically related to the target). In Dell's model, these errors can be true word selection errors (arising at lemma access) or phonological errors that by chance form real words. In a picture-naming task in which the target words are nouns, formal paraphasias that arise at lemma access should also be nouns at rates greater than chance because they are true word level errors. Moreover, these errors should be observed more often in subjects with impaired decay rate and strong connection strength, because the latter is needed support spread of feedback activation to the lexical network where these errors occur. Phonological errors that by chance form words should be nouns only at chance rates, and this pattern of error should occur in subjects whose naming impairment is due to weakened connection weights. Dell et al. (1997) divided their subject group into those with strong connection weights and those with weak connection weights. As predicted, formal paraphasias were nouns at rates greater than chance in the strong connection weight group and were nouns only at chance rates in the weak connection weight group.

The occurrence of mixed errors, word errors that are both semantically and phonologically related to the target word, also depends on strong feedback. Therefore, these errors should be more prevalent in subjects whose naming error pattern is fit with strong connection weights. Dell et al. (1997) found that whereas subjects with strong connection weights showed a substantial mixed error effect, subjects, with weak connection weights did not.

Using computational models to test theories of language

Ruml and Caramazza (2000) raised several of questions concerning the modelling study of Dell et al. (1997) and the validity of using computational models to evaluate theories of lexical processing. They claimed that the fits of patient-naming data to the model were poor in absolute terms, and therefore, did not support their theory of lexical access. Ruml and Caramazza (2000) produced a mathematical model that provided closer fits to the data but could not predict other aspects of error patterns (e.g., recovery patterns, lexical retrieval in other tasks such as repetition, the mixed-error effect, the noun effect) because the model is not based on a theory. Dell et al. (1997, 2000) make the important point (see also Popper, 1935, 1959) that the success of a model is marked by its ability to make predictions based on its fit to the data. Ruml and Caramazza (2000) argued that the predictions made by the model of Dell et al. (1997) did not substantiate their claims about the nature of lexical access and aphasic impairment. In reply, Dell et al. (2000) note that the role of computational modelling in developing theories of language involves systematic tests and refinement of those models. Using a computational model to develop a theory involves first fitting data to the model as closely as possible and then evaluating those fits with respect to the theory. Inadequate fits between data and the model could be due to the assumptions of the theory or to simplifying assumptions made to develop a computational instantiation of the theory. These factors need to be scrutinized and, perhaps, refined in light of those fits. Full discussion of the debate between Dell et al. (1997, 2000) and Ruml and Caramazza (2000) will take us too far from the main focus of this chapter. However, the reader is urged to refer to these papers for a thorough discussion of the role of computational modelling in cognitive research.

Scope of error patterns accounted for by the interactive activation model

An important criticism of the Dell et al. (1997) study is that it cannot account for all error patterns that have been observed in aphasia. When asked to name a picture, for example, a commonly observed error is the "no response", stating something like "I know it, but I can't say it". Versions of the IA model used by Dell et al. (1997; Foygel & Dell, 2000; Martin et al., 1994; Martin et al., 1996) do not include a mechanism for modelling "no response" errors, limiting its ability to account for those aphasic speakers who produce a high percentage of "no responses" on the picture-naming task. More recent versions of Dell's interactive activation model (Dell, Lawler, Harris & Gordon, in press) have incorporated a selection threshold parameter (e.g., Laine et al., 1998; Roelofs, 1992 and this volume, Chapter 3) to account for omission errors.

Another error pattern that is sometimes observed in aphasia is a high rate of semantic errors with few instances of other error types except "no responses". None of the patients reported by Dell et al. (1997) demonstrated this pattern, but, as discussed later, individuals with this pattern of error have been reported elsewhere and present a challenge to the IA model.

Rapp and Goldrick (2000) tested the abilities of several models to account for some less typical aphasic error patterns. They explored five different lexical access models that differed with respect to whether they included cascading, interactive spreading activation, no interaction or partial interaction. The models were evaluated with respect to normal speech errors patterns and error patterns of three brain damaged individuals with naming deficits. Rapp and Goldrick (2000) found that two of their patients, KE and PW, produced only semantic errors and no responses in naming, while a third patient, CSS, produced a variety of errors. Putting aside the issue of how to model "no responses", Rapp and Goldrick focused on identifying and modelling the locus of the lesion that gave rise to semantic errors produced by KE and PW. They determined that KE had a central semantic deficit because he produced semantic errors on a variety of input and output tasks that presumably tap into semantic processes. In contrast, PW's semantic errors in naming were determined to have a post-lexical origin, because he performed well on picture-word matching tests (a measure of single word comprehension), which Rapp and Goldrick interpreted as evidence of good semantic processing.

Rapp and Goldrick (2000) simulated these error patterns by adding noise to different levels of representation within the network. With this localized form of damage, they showed that only a model with interaction occurring between lexical and phonological levels could account for all three patterns (called the "restricted interactive activation model). Like the other modelling studies discussed thus far, Rapp and Goldrick's (2000) study illustrates that data from individual patients can place important constraints on our models of word-processing. Unlike the previous studies, Rapp and Goldrick provide independent evidence to localize the deficits of their patients within the word-processing model. Following this, they lesioned each of the five models by increasing noise at specific levels of representation. Their focus on site of lesion differed from that of Dell et al. (1997), who globally altered parameters that affect information transmission (connection weight) and integrity of activation (decay rate). Thus, whereas Rapp and Goldrick's study focused more on the effects of lesion site on error patterns, Dell et al. (1997) explored effects of different kinds of processing impairments.

Rapp and Goldrick's (2000) modelling study supported the long-held belief that lesions giving rise to aphasic symptoms can be localized within specific stages of lexical processing (e.g., semantic, phonological). When case studies are used to constrain a model, it is important to thoroughly document the empirical evidence that localizes the impairment within the lexical system. Although Rapp and Goldrick follow this approach, they provide somewhat sparse empirical evidence to localize the deficits of each patient compared to typical neuropsychological studies. In particular, evidence that PW does not have any semantic damage is fairly weak: He performs well on a word-to-picture matching task and can provide imprecise descriptions of words he cannot name (e.g., a picture of a zebra was named "a horse in the jungle"). The word-to-picture matching task measures the mapping of an auditorily activated lexical form onto one of four semantic representations (primed by visual input of the pictures) and is not equivalent to the mapping in picture naming between a conceptually activated semantic representation and one of all lexical forms in the lexicon. The competitive fields in which access takes place are obviously quite different in the two tasks, and it is likely that the naming task with a larger field of primed competitors is more difficult.

When identifying the locus of a naming impairment based on measures of input processing, severity is an important factor to consider. This variable should interact with task factors (input versus output processing) and locus of impairment (semantic or phonological lesion). It is noteworthy that PW's naming impairment was considerably milder than KE's (.72 versus .56 correct). It is conceivable that this difference in magnitude could affect the input and output mappings such that only the more difficult mapping used in naming suffers in milder cases and the easier mapping involved in a word-to-picture matching task suffers in more severe cases (Martin & Saffran, 2001).

The computational/empirical studies of Dell et al. (1997) and Rapp and Goldrick (2000) have each contributed important insights to our understanding of word processing and its impairment. Whereas Dell et al. (1997) introduced the idea that processing impairments could systematically affect word processing, Rapp and Goldrick (2000) demonstrate the importance of considering the effects of locus of impairment as well. The next study makes an attempt to consider both of these factors when modelling aphasic impairment.

Exploration of local lesions in the interaction activation model

Foygel and Dell (2000) compared two models derived from a two-step theory of lexical access with respect to their ability to account for aphasic speech error patterns in a picture-naming task: the weight-decay model (Dell et al., 1997, 2000) and the semantic-phonological model. As described earlier, the weight-decay model accounted for the different patterns of speech error by altering two parameters of the model, connection weight (affecting the amount of activation spread through the network) and decay rate (the speed at which activation is lost) globally; that is, they affected all connections in the semantic-lexical-phonological network. Dell et al. (1997) found that patients whose error patterns reflected good interaction were best modelled with decay rate lesions (an increase in decay rate), and patients whose error patterns reflected diminished interaction were best modelled with reduced connection weights. In the semantic-phonological model, Foygel and Dell (2000) attempted to capture these same differences in error patterns by holding constant the kind of processing impairment that could occur (weakened connection weights only) and varying the locus of damage within the model to affect semantic or phonological connections. This categorization was more in keeping with aphasiologists' long-standing characterization of word-processing impairments. Foygel and Dell (2000) found that error patterns reflecting good interaction (such as the decay rate lesions) were more likely to have reduced semantic weights and normal or near normal phonological weights. In contrast, error patterns reflecting reduced interaction (as in the global weight lesions) were best captured with normal or near normal semantic weights and reduced phonological weights.

Although the semantic-phonological model fared well in modelling the data that were fit to the weight-decay model, it failed to provide an account for patients with post-semantic damage whose error patterns include mostly semantic errors and few of any other error type. PW, whom we discussed earlier (Rapp & Goldrick, 2000), was this type of patient (72 per cent correct responses, 19 per cent mixed errors and 3 per cent unrelated errors and 0 per cent formal paraphasias). Using a pure lexical-semantic lesion, Foygel and Dell (2000) were able to model most of PW's error pattern except, importantly, the absence of formal paraphasias.

What do the modelling studies discussed thus far indicate about the relation between normal and pathological speech errors? Each effort began with a model of normal speech production, which, in all cases, produced mostly correct responses and a small number of errors distributed over a range of error types. Although theories do not fully agree on the architecture of the word-processing system or the mechanisms by which damage affects word processing, the evidence reviewed here suggests that quantitative and qualitative differences between aphasic and normal speech error patterns could result from converging influences of the locus, severity and type of processing impairment (affecting activation strength or integrity).

How do speech error patterns in aphasia change with partial recovery?

The idea that variation in aphasic speech error patterns could be attributed to type and severity of processing impairment led to further studies of error patterns as a function of severity. The model of Dell et al. (1997) predicts that in production, a decay rate lesion at milder levels results in errors that have some semantic component (semantic and mixed errors) while at more severe levels, rates of formal paraphasias and nonword errors increase relative to rates of semantic and mixed errors. A useful means of testing this prediction of the model is to look at the severity variable in reverse, that is, to examine changing error patterns that accompany recovery.

In an earlier section, I discussed the 1994 study by Martin et al. of patient NC who produced a high rate of formal paraphasias in naming and a high rate of semantic paraphasias in repetition. Both of these error patterns were qualitatively different from the normal speech error pattern. They modelled this error pattern by increasing decay rate to very high levels and keeping the connection weight at the setting used to simulate normal speech. In that study, Martin et al. (1994) also examined NC's error pattern after some recovery. The model used by Martin et al. (1994) predicted that with recovery NC's error pattern should shift towards the normal pattern. That is, there should be a reduction in formal paraphasias in naming with the rate of semantic errors staying about the same and in repetition, semantic errors should decline while formal paraphasias and nonwords should prevail. This pattern of recovery was simulated by gradually reducing the decay rate towards the normal settings. NC's recovery pattern followed this prediction precisely. After some partial recovery, he made few, if any, semantic errors in repetition of single words and fewer formal paraphasias in naming. In a follow-up study, Martin, Saffran, and Dell (1996) used the same model of repetition to predict that semantic errors would re-emerge in NC's repetition error pattern if he repeated two words rather than one. This was postulated because the occurrence of semantic errors in repetition is related to decay rate as well as the temporal interval between the time a stimulus is heard and the time it is repeated. Semantic errors should be more likely as time passes. In fact, semantic errors did re-emerge in NC's error pattern when he repeated two words rather than just one.

Dell et al. also investigated the recovery patterns of a subset of the 21 subjects whom they reported in 1997. They showed that changes in subjects' error patterns could be simulated in the model by gradually shifting the impaired parameters back toward their normal levels (i.e., lowered decay rate, increased connection weight). An important implication of these three studies of recovery (Dell et al., 1997; Martin et al., 1994) is that recovery of impaired cognitive mechanisms underlying speech production appears to follow a path the returns the word-processing system to its pre-morbid state.

A recent study by Schwartz and Brecher (2000) investigated a prediction of the Dell et al. (1997) model that phonological errors are sensitive to severity of impairment and semantic errors are not. They examined naming error patterns of 15 subjects in and observed, as the model predicted, that the rates of phonological errors increased with overall severity, but rates of semantic errors showed no such increase. Schwartz and Brecher then predicted that with partial recovery, error patterns would show a greater decrease in the rate of phonological errors than in the rate of semantic errors. This prediction was confirmed in a study of the partial recovery of naming impairments in 7 subjects. In this study, Schwartz and Brecher made no distinction between subjects whose semantic errors arise from central semantic deficits or from phonological output deficits (see Caramazza & Hillis, 1990), and thus, we cannot be certain that rtes of semantic errors in such patients would not change with recovery. Nonetheless, the finding that recovery leads to a drop in phonological errors sooner than semantic errors is an interesting one.

Concluding remarks

I have reviewed some recent studies that use some version of an interactive activation model to account for several aspects of aphasic speech errors including qualitative differences from normal speech errors and changes in error patterns that accompany recovery. Interactive activation theories make predictions about dynamic questions such as these that can be tested in computational models. Although the practice of using computer models to test a theory's predictions is in its early stages, the enterprise shows great promise. In several instances, these models have been able to demonstrate what is not intuitively obvious. Aphasic errors appear to differ qualitatively from normal speech error patterns, but it was shown in Martin et al. (1994) and Dell et al. (1997) that that this apparent difference can be captured in a model by varying parameters used to model normal speech errors. Comparison of empirical and computational data in recovery studies confirmed this conclusion. In Martin et al. (1996) and Schwartz and Brecher (2000), the IA model predicted that qualitatively different error patterns would resolve to resemble the normal error pattern more closely, and empirically, this was found to be the case.

The studies discussed here, as well as others using distributed connectionist models (e.g., Plaut, 1996; see Dell and Kim, this volume, Chapter 2, for a discussion of local and distributed connectionist models), have stimulated debate about dynamic issues of word processing and forced us to think about how empirical data can be interpreted in a dynamic system. A common denominator of the studies discussed in this chapter is the use of speech error data as evidence to investigate the architecture and behaviour of the word processing system. Historically, speech errors have proved invaluable in shaping our models of word retrieval. Virtually every model of word production holds that there are stages at which semantic and phonological representations of words are realized in some form. This revelation first appeared in early studies of speech errors (Fromkin, 1971; Garrett, 1975). The use of speech errors produced by both normal and aphasic speakers, and now by computational models, should continue to be useful data to investigate many aspects of word processing.

Acknowledgements

This work was supported by NIH grant number DC-01924–10 granted to Temple University (PI: N. Martin). Thanks go to Ulrich Schade and Zenzi Griffin for helpful comments on this chapter and to my colleagues, Gary Dell, Myrna Schwartz, Eleanor Saffran and Deb Gagnon for many helpful discussions that influenced the ideas expressed here.

Note

1 Martin, Roach, Brecher and Lowery (1998) note two possible accounts of whole word perseverations within an interactive activation model, one which involves only reduced connection weights and another which results from reduced connection weight in combination with a damaged post-selection inhibition mechanism.

References

Blanken, G. (1990). Formal paraphasias: A single case study. *Brain and Language, 38,* 534–54.

Bloch, D. E. (1986). *Defining the speech production impairment in a case of Wernicke's neologistic jargonaphasia:* A Speech Error Analysis. University of Pennsylvania unpublished doctoral dissertation.

Caramazza, A., & Hillis, A. E. (1990). Where do semantic errors come from? *Cortex, 26,* 95–122.

Dell, G. S. (1986) A spreading activation theory of retrieval in language production. *Psychological Review, 93,* 283–21.

Dell, G. S. & Kim, A. (2004). Speech errors and word-form encoding. In R. J. Hartsuiker, R. Bastiaanse, A. Postma, & F. N. K. Wijnen (Eds.), *Phonological encoding and monitoring in normal and pathological speech.* Hove, UK: Psychology Press.

Dell, G. S., Lawler, E. N., Harris, H. D., & Gordon, J. K. (in press). Models of errors of omission in aphasic naming. *Cognitive Neuropsychology.*

Dell, G. S., & O'Seaghdha, P. G. (1992). Stages in lexical access in language production. *Cognition, 42,* 287–314.

Dell, G. S., Schwartz M. F., Martin N., Saffran E. M., & Gagnon, D. A. (1997) Lexical access in aphasic and non-aphasic speakers. *Psychological Review, 104,* 801–38.

Dell, G. S., Schwartz, M. F., Martin, N., Saffran, E. M., & Gagnon, D. A. (2000). The role of computational models in neuropsychological investigations of language: Reply to Ruml and Caramazza. *Psychological Review, 107,* 635–45.

Foygel, D., & Dell, G. S. (2000). Models of impaired lexical access in speech production. *Journal of Memory and Language, 43,* 182–216.

Fromkin, V. A. (1971). The non-anomalous nature of anomalous utterances. *Language, 47,* 27–52.

Garnham, A., Shillcock, R. C., Brown, G. D. A., Mill A. I. D., & Cutler, A. (1982).

Slips of the tongue in the London-Lund corpus of spontaneous conversation. In A. Cutler (Ed.), *Slips of the tongue and language production*. Amsterdam: Mouton.

Garrett, M. F. (1975). The analysis of sentence production. In G. H. Bower (Ed.), *The psychology of learning and motivation*, Vol. 9. New York: Academic Press.

Garrett, M. F. (1982). Production of speech: Observations from normal and pathological language use. In A. W. Ellis (Ed), *Normality and pathology in cognitive functions*. London: Academic Press.

Harley, T. A. (1984). A critique of top-down independent levels models of speech production: Evidence from non-plan internal speech errors. *Cognitive Science, 8*, 191–219.

Howard, D., & Franklin, S. (1988). *Missing the meaning? A cognitive neuropsychological study of processing words by an aphasic patient*. Cambridge, MA: MIT Press.

Laine, M., Tikkala, A., & Juhola, M. (1998). Modelling anomia by the discrete two-stage word production architecture. *Journal of Neurolinguistics, 10*, 139–58.

Martin, N., Dell, G. S., Saffran, E. M., & Schwartz, M. F. (1994). Origins of paraphasias in deep dysphasia: testing the consequences of a decay impairment to an interactive spreading activation model of language. *Brain and Language, 47*, 609–60.

Martin, N., Roach, A., Brecher, A., & Lowery, J. (1998) Lexical retrieval mechanisms underlying whole-word perseveration errors in anomic aphasia. *Aphasiology, 12*, 319–33.

Martin, N., & Saffran, E. M. (1992) A computational account of deep dysphasia: Evidence from a single case study. *Brain and Language, 43*, 240–74.

Martin, N., & Saffran, E. M. (1997) Language and auditory-verbal short-term memory impairments: Evidence for common underlying processes. *Cognitive Neuropsychology, 14*, 641–82.

Martin, N., & Saffran, E. M. (2001). The relationship of input and output phonology in single word processing: Evidence from aphasia. *Aphasia, 16*, 107–50.

Martin, N., Saffran, E. M., & Dell, G. S. (1996). Recovery in deep dysphasia: Evidence for a relation between auditory-verbal STM and lexical errors in repetition. *Brain and Language, 52*, 83–113.

Plaut, D. (1996). Relearning after damage in connectionist networks: Toward a theory of rehabilitation. *Brain and Language, 52*, 25–82.

Popper, K. R. (1935) *Logic der Forschung*. Wien. English ed. (1959) *The logic of scientific discovery*. New York: Basic Books.

Rapp, B., & Goldrick, M. (2000). Discreteness and interactivity in spoken word production. *Psychological Review, 107*, 406–99.

Roelofs, A. (1992) A spreading activation theory of lemma retrieval in speaking. *Cognition, 42*, 107–142.

Ruml, W., & Caramazza, A. (2000). An evaluation of a computational model of lexical access: Comment on Dell et al. (1997). *Psychological Review, 107*, 609–34.

Schriefers, H. Meyer, A. S., & Levelt, W. J. M. (1990). Exploring the time course of lexical access in production: Picture-word interference studies. *Journal of Memory and Language, 29*, 86–102.

Schwartz, M. F. (1987). Patterns of speech production deficit within and across aphasia syndromes: Application of a psycholinguistic model. In M. Coltheart, G. Sartori and R. Job (Eds.), *The cognitive neuropsychology of language*. Hove, UK: Lawrence Erlbaum Associates Ltd.

Schwartz, M. F., & Brecher, A. (2000). A model-driven analysis of severity, response characteristics, and partial recovery in aphasic's picture naming. *Brain and Language, 73,* 62–91.

Schwartz, M. F., Saffran, E. M., Bloch, D. E., & Dell, G. S. (1994). Disordered speech production in aphasic and normal speakers. *Brain and language, 47,* 52–88.

Stemberger, J. P. (1985). An interactive model of language production. In A. W. Ellis (Ed.). *Progress in the psychology of language,* Vol. 1. (pp. 143–86). Hillsdale, NJ: Lawrence Erlbaum Associates, Inc.

5   Phonological encoding and conduction aphasia

Dirk-Bart den Ouden and
Roelien Bastiaanse

Abstract

This chapter discusses phonological encoding from an aphasiological perspective. It is argued that deficits of phonological encoding provide insight into the regular workings of the process. Such a deficit is the syndrome of conduction aphasia, which is claimed to consist of two types, one a deficit in the building of the phonological plan, at the level of individual segments, the other a verbal working memory deficit in the maintenance of this plan. Particular attention is paid to the input to phonological encoding, as well as to the time course of the process. Aphasic speech data indicate that the input consists of metrical frames, hierarchically organized as syllables, and autonomous segments or bundles of phonological features. These segments appear to be mapped onto the frames in a parallel fashion, as opposed to sequentially from left to right, while serial (length) effects may be generated by the maintenance process, which is a function of verbal working memory.

Introduction

In this chapter, we present a discussion of aphasiological work that has related aphasic symptoms to deficient phonological encoding. In particular, we focus on the syndrome of conduction aphasia, in which problems with sequential ordering of speech sounds have been widely noted. We argue that aphasic deficits at different levels of processing allow insight into the amount and type of phonological structure present at those specific levels. We also argue that conduction aphasia can either be related to a deficit in the building of the phonological speech plan or to a deficit in its maintenance (in working memory). Both types may provide insight into the nature of the phonological encoding process.

Phonological encoding is the building of the sound shape and structure of phonological words; in a sequential model (e.g., Levelt, Roelofs, & Meyer, 1999), it is the stage *after* lemma retrieval and *before* the execution of articulatory gestures. This definition yields a number of questions to be investigated, two of which receive special attention in this chapter:

1   Which (types of) elements form the *input* to phonological encoding?
2   What is the *time course* of phonological encoding, i.e., does the encoding of elements within words or even larger domains proceed in a parallel fashion, or is there a specific order in the encoding of separate elements?

After two general sections on speech errors and conduction aphasia, these two topics in phonological encoding research will be discussed in relation to findings and developments in aphasiology, mainly against the background of the model for single word production proposed by Levelt et al. (1999). The specific topic addressed is what conduction aphasia may tell us about the level of phonological encoding, particularly with regard to questions 1 and 2. This necessitates the investigation of what conduction aphasia itself constitutes exactly. We also relate the observations to developments in formal linguistic theory.

Genesis of speech errors in aphasia

For normal speech, it is generally held that segmental speech errors, i.e. substitution, transposition, deletion and addition of phonemes, are generated during phonological encoding. Therefore, all such speech errors have been interpreted as reflections of the type and amount of phonological structure involved in phonological encoding (Stemberger, 1990). Applying this approach to the interpretation of speech errors in aphasiology, however, may be too simple.

Different forms of aphasia are not regarded as communally stemming from the same deficient level of processing. Although individual patients may differ greatly in their patterns of aphasic symptoms and brain lesions are not constrained by functional modules, it is possible to distinguish clusters of symptoms in aphasia, for efficiency's sake regarded here as "syndromes". These syndromes are hypothesized to result from different functional loci of impairment and treated as such in research as well as in speech therapy programmes. Nevertheless, the particular clusterings of symptoms into a syndrome may well be more the result of anatomical factors than of functional associations (Poeck, 1983).

As the focus in this work is on phonological encoding, we will limit the following discussion to aphasic patients who exhibit so-called *literal paraphasias* in production. This term covers word-form errors, excluding neologisms and semantic paraphasias. We prefer it to the also commonly used term *phonemic paraphasia*, because it is by no means always likely that the erroneous units in such paraphasias are "phonemes", rather than the phonological, perceptual or articulatory features these phonemes are supposed to consist of.

Three major aphasic syndromes generally show large proportions of literal paraphasias in speech output: Wernicke's aphasia, Broca's aphasia and conduction aphasia. Wernicke's aphasia is a fluent lexical-semantic deficit, with impaired comprehension. Production is marked by many semantic para-phasias, as well as literal paraphasias. For conduction aphasia, the literal paraphasias and the laborious attempts at error correction are central charac-teristics. Patients are generally fluent, but speech may become hesitant and disfluent in the face of phonological errors, of which the patient is well aware. Comprehension is not impaired. Broca's aphasia is a nonfluent output deficit, marked by problems with functional syntactic items and sentence building.

The literal paraphasias produced by individuals with Broca's aphasia, whose syndrome often coincides with apraxia of speech, are considered to be generated at a more peripheral, phonetic level than the paraphasias of the other two syndromes (Blumstein, 1991). In a modular representation of the speech production process, distinguishing the lexicon from phonological encoding and articulatory planning, the functional deficit of individuals with conduction aphasia is often located in between, at the level of phonological encoding (e.g., Kohn, 1988).

Although some studies show that the literal paraphasias that are often part of these syndromes differ in type, structure and regularity (e.g., Bastiaanse, Gilbers, & Van der Linde, 1994; Nespoulous, Joanette, Béland, Caplan, & Lecours, 1984), there have also been claims that phonological structure is so pervasive throughout the system that all literal paraphasias should bear the same characteristics, formed under the influence of universal constraints of (un)markedness (Blumstein, 1973; Christman, 1992).

To the extent that aphasic symptoms can be associated with deficits at specific psycholinguistic levels, they can provide an even better mirror on underlying structure and processes than normal speech errors. This is the approach adopted here. Of course, if all error characteristics are ultimately shown to be alike, this argues in favour of a more holistic viewpoint, viz the view that all literal paraphasias are generated at the same functional level, or that phonological constraints are pervasive throughout the speech processing system, hard-wired from the abstract to the concrete.

As mentioned earlier, the aphasic syndrome that has typically been associ-ated with an impairment at the functional level of phonological encoding is conduction aphasia. The following section gives a brief overview of the symptoms and characteristics of this type of aphasia. After this, these char-acteristics will be discussed in greater detail, when they are related to the process of phonological encoding.

Conduction aphasia

First described by Carl Wernicke (1874), conduction aphasia is distinguished by the characteristic symptoms of literal paraphasias in the absence of articu-latory or comprehension deficits, coupled with repeated attempts at error correction, known as *conduites d'approche*. Contemporary aphasiologists use the term *reproduction conduction aphasia* for this type, as opposed to *rep-etition conduction aphasia*, which is typically characterized by an excessive proportion of phonological errors on repetition tasks, in combination with relatively unimpaired spontaneous speech (Caplan & Waters, 1992; Croot, Patterson, & Hodges, 1998; Shallice & Warrington, 1977). In what follows, we will use the term conduction aphasia to mean the "reproduction" type. Individuals with reproduction conduction aphasia do show impairment in spontaneous speech and on naming tasks, as well as on repetition tasks. It is reproduction conduction aphasia which is most adequately captured under the description of "breakdown at the level of organising phonemic strings" (Kohn, 1988, p. 103), i.e., the level of phonological encoding. Nespoulous et al. (1984) speak more specifically of "disruption of a serial-ordering mechanism" (p. 212), which they claim is also the origin of normal speech errors.

Despite these generally used definitions, conduction aphasia is far from a homogeneous syndrome. In fact, its apparent heterogeneity is notorious (Canter, Trost, & Burns, 1985; Feinberg, Rothi, & Heilman, 1986). Even though it is generally held that the functional locus of deficit lies in between lexical access and articulatory planning, the exact nature of conduction aphasia is still a matter of debate. This has much to do with the variable results of studies into the syndrome. For one, it is exceptional to find cases of "pure" conduction aphasia. This may be for anatomical reasons, as lesions are obviously not constrained by functional boundaries. However, even if apparently pure cases are considered, results of different studies with respect to the structural systematicity in error forms and the different variables that seem to affect the form of paraphasias are quite divergent. After Wernicke, conduction aphasia has been presented as a disturbance of "inner speech" (Goldstein, 1948), a type of oral apraxia (Luria, 1964), and as a short-term memory deficit (Warrington & Shallice, 1969). It seems that the definition and status of conduction aphasia have depended to a great extent on the different psycholinguistic models in which researchers have tried to fit this type of aphasia in the past century (Henderson, 1992; Köhler, Bartels, Herrmann, Dittmann, & Wallesch, 1998; Prins, 1987).

Length effects observed on the paraphasias in conduction aphasia have led to accounts of the syndrome as a verbal working memory deficit. According to Baddeley (1986, 1990; see also Baddeley & Wilson, 1985), working memory retains a generated phonological representation, which is then checked via a "phonological loop". If the working memory capacity is deficient, this leads to inadequate checking and thus to literal paraphasias of the type found in conduction aphasia (Hough, De Marco, & Farler, 1994; Miller, 2000). Brain imaging studies have yielded evidence that brain activity patterns related to phonological processing are quite compatible with and thus support the model of a checking loop as proposed by Baddeley and colleages (Démonet, Price, Wise, & Frackowiak, 1994; Démonet, Fiez, Paulesu, Petersen, & Zatorre, 1996; Miller, 2000; Poeppel, 1996; Price et al. 1996). We argue later that there may well be two types of "reproduction conduction aphasia" here: one in the building of phonological plans, the actual phonological encoding deficit, and one in the retention and checking of these plans, possibly in a phonological output buffer. Repetition conduction aphasia may fall within the latter category.

Conduction aphasia as a window on phonological encoding

In this section, we discuss the phonological encoding process in greater detail. The discussion is organized into two components: *input* and *time course*. Of course, the organizational division between input and time course is notwithstanding the fact that these two aspects of the process are strongly related and interdependent.

Input

To gain insight into the process of phonological encoding, it is important to establish what exactly the input to this process is, i.e., what representations are moulded into the end result of the process. With respect to the Levelt et al. (1999) model, the specific question is: What units does the form lexicon contain and what happens to these units during phonological encoding? We will investigate these questions by looking at conduction aphasia, in the course of which we will also spend time on observations about the syndrome itself.

In the adopted speech production model, lemmas contain the syntactic information that is associated with words, for example, their grammatical status. Lemmas, then, activate entries in the form lexicon. In the form lexicon, which provides the input to the phonological encoding process, speech sound specifications are stored separately from the metrical frames onto which they are mapped during encoding (e.g., Shattuck-Hufnagel, 1979). One of the reasons for such a distinction is that these pieces of information may be available independently, without the availability of the whole word form (e.g., Brown & McNeill, 1966). Phonological encoding consists of the association of the two types of information, which results in the full phonological structure that is needed by following functional levels to make sure that the correct form is articulated. The relatively large amounts of sequential errors observed in conduction aphasia have led to the hypothesis that these patients encounter problems in the mapping of sound specifications to the appropriate slots in metrical frames.

There is ongoing debate over the nature and structure of the metrical frame. In a study on speech errors in normal speech, Stemberger (1990) found contextual effects of syllable structure on additions, indicating a distinction between syllable structure (or word shape) and content (segments). Priming and reaction time experiments have yielded a diffuse pattern of results, so far. According to Meijer (1996), CV structure (the difference between consonants and vowels and the grouping of these categories into syllables) is stored in the mental lexicon and retrieved during phonological encoding. Sevald, Dell, & Cole (1995) also argue that segments are separable from syllable structure and that the latter is indeed an abstract *structure*, as opposed to a mere opaque chunk of grouped sounds. Hartsuiker (2000) shows that a computational speech-processing model that incorporates CV structure adequately simulates normal processing data. Others, however, conclude that the syllable does not play any functional role in phonological encoding (Schiller, 1997), and that the lexicon only contains information about the serial position of segments within morphemes, as opposed to syllables (Roelofs, 1996). Shattuck-Hufnagel (1992) stresses the special status of word-onset consonants in serial ordering, arguing against models which only rely on syllable structure in the analysis of speech errors. Wheeler and Touretzky (1997) argue that syllables or syllable frames are not stored in the lexicon, but that segments specified solely for their serial position are syllabified during phonological encoding. Levelt (1992) similarly refers to syllabification as a "late process in phonological encoding" (p. 16).

Basically, these authors agree on the fact that phonological encoding yields a syllabified string of segments, but there is disagreement over whether these segments are syllabified in a bottom-up fashion, or top down. Bottom up, the segmental content determines the eventual syllabic organisation, so syllable structure does not exist without segmental content. Top down, segments are mapped onto stored syllable templates. The bottom-up/top-down syllabification problem has been extensively discussed by phonological theorists (e.g., Cairns & Feinstein, 1982; Hayes, 1989; see Gilbers & Den Ouden, 1994 for a brief overview). Here, evidence for structurally strong or weak syllable positions is often taken to support hierarchical syllable structure and thus templates.

One approach that is currently quite popular, optimality theory, has done away with direction of syllabification entirely (Prince & Smolensky, 1993). The focus is on well-formed output and to establish this, different output candidates (for example, different syllabifications) are evaluated. The optimal candidate wins. This amounts to a compromise in that candidates are evaluated in terms of constraints that refer to segmental content as well as constraints that refer to positional, prosodic structure. In terms of a psycholinguistic processing model, the OT representation would be equivalent to an interactive determination of phonological structure, instead of a purely feedforward building of phonological plans.

If the literal paraphasias produced by aphasic speakers show the effects of constraints on output well-formedness that are induced by syllable structure preferences, as in the systematic deletion of structurally weak segment positions, this indicates a presence of such (hierarchical) structures at the level of deficit, for example phonological encoding (cf. Valdois, 1990).

Whereas especially individuals with Broca's aphasia have often been reported as systematically simplifying syllable structure (showing a preference for phonologically less marked forms), the errors in conduction aphasia do not seem to show such an obvious preference for, for example, consonant cluster reduction (Kohn, 1988; Nespoulous et al., 1984). Relative to other disorders, individuals with conduction aphasia produce a large proportion of transpositions of phonemes. Nespoulous, Joanette, Ska, Caplan, and Lecours (1987) noted this in repetition tasks, although on oral reading tasks they found significantly fewer "displacements" than additions and substitutions, indicating "more variability in the behavior of the conduction aphasics and . . . more stability in that of Broca's aphasics" (p. 58).

The form of paraphasias in conduction aphasia is not completely random with respect to linguistic structure. It has been widely noted that they do not, or only very rarely, violate language specific constraints on phonotaxis, or well-formedness (e.g., Buckingham 1992). Burns and Canter (1977) found that individuals with conduction aphasia do show a significant increase in segmental errors as the motor complexity of the targets increases. Specific phonological features may also pose problems in conduction aphasia, as shown in a case study by Béland and Lecours (1989) for the vowel feature advanced tongue root (ATR). These authors also observed difficulty with branching (complex) syllable constituents in their patient. Lecours and Lhermitte (1969) as well as Hough et al. (1994) show that many phoneme substitutions involve substitutions of only one or two features, which the latter authors ascribe to rapid decay of memory traces, leading to partial access of intended phonemes. Together, these facts show that mainly segmental restrictions influence the paraphasias in conduction aphasia.

This may mean that hierarchical syllable structure, in the form of templates onto which segments are mapped, is not functional at the level of phonological encoding. Only the type of segments retrieved from the lexicon will constrain the errors generated at this processing level. Contrariwise, it may also indicate that the functional deficit of conduction aphasia does not lie in the segment-to-frame mapping during phonological encoding at all and that the metrical frames do not constrain the form of conduction aphasic paraphasias for this reason.

In an alternative analysis of the literal paraphasias in Broca's aphasia, den Ouden (2002a, 2002b) argues that the form of their errors is really due to dominant factors of *segmental* markedness, as opposed to syllable markedness. In tautosyllabic consonant clusters, these patients quite systematically delete the sonorant (more vowel-like) consonants, whereas optimal syllables rather prefer to end in a sonorant than in a non-sonorant consonant.

Den Ouden (2002a, 2002b) looked specifically at patterns of segment deletion in fluent and nonfluent aphasic speech. The deficit in fluent aphasia (Wernicke's and conduction aphasia), whether lexical or postlexical in nature, is considered to lie in the building of the phonological plan. The form of their paraphasias is ascribed to abstract phonological factors, i.e., the constraints that play a role up to and including the stage of phonological encoding. The errors of nonfluent patients (Broca's aphasia with apraxia of speech), who display halting speech, are interpreted as more articulatorily constrained. Individuals with conduction aphasia are generally fluent.

The comparison between fluent and nonfluent patients' structural reductions (segment deletions) on a monosyllabic repetition task revealed that both groups of patients reduced tautosyllabic clusters of consonants to single segments. For fluent patients, there was an effect of preferred syllable shape as well as of segmental markedness. The nonfluent patients' paraphasias could be ascribed to segmental markedness alone. The interpretation of these data was that syllable structure, together with segmental structure, plays a role up to and including the stage of phonological encoding, whereas after that stage, only segmental structure remains functional.

Among the 10 fluent patients tested with the monosyllabic repetition task were 4 patients who had been diagnosed as conduction aphasic. Their deletion patterns are shown in Figure 5.1. The bars show the percentages of deletions in specific syllable positions, clarified with the example word *sprints*, which, being bimorphemic, was not part of the list of items to be repeated.

Patients CA 1 and CA 2 show the patterns of deletions that may be expected from the perspective of segmental markedness, with relatively more deletions of sonorant consonants, regardless of their position within the syllable. Patients CA 3 and CA 4 rather appear to show a length effect, with more deletions towards the end of (even) these monosyllabic stimuli.

Within four patients, this counts as a completely normal pattern of variation and we may leave it at that. It is also possible that these data reveal only a quantitative effect, in that they reflect a more severe disturbance in CA 1 and CA 2, than in CA 3 and CA 4. However, I will speculate on an alternative account for the division between these four patients.

It seems that there is at least a subgroup of patients diagnosed as suffering from conduction aphasia whose literal paraphasias are similar to those of patients with a peripheral articulatorily constrained deficit. They are sensitive mostly to linguistic structure at the level of individual segments. The fact that this is not what is found for conduction aphasia in general, indicates that a subclass of individuals with conduction aphasia have a type of deficit that is insensitive to these abstract (linguistic) constraints. A verbal working memory deficit, roughly equal in its effects to a deficit in phonological output buffer storage capacity, would be an alternative candidate for these patients (Goodglass, 1992; Hough et al., 1994; Kohn & Smith, 1992).

What remains is that syllable structure does play a role at or before the stage of phonological encoding, as indicated by the results of the fluent patients as a group, but apparently not in the process that is disturbed in conduction aphasia. During phonological encoding, segments are thus autonomous from syllable structure. If patients with an earlier deficit than that in conduction aphasia do show effects of syllable structure, this may indicate that the metrical frames onto which the segments are later mapped have the form of hierarchically organized syllable templates. A deficit at the level of metrical frames is hypothesized to result in literal paraphasias that show effects of syllable markedness.

It is our position, then, that the surface characteristics of the conduction aphasic syndrome, viz preserved comprehension, fluent production of literal paraphasias and *conduites d'approche*, cover two different but related types

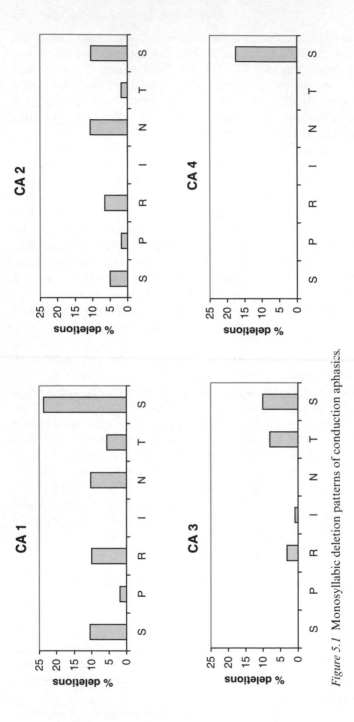

Figure 5.1 Monosyllabic deletion patterns of conduction aphasics.

of functional deficit. One is in the building of the phonological plan, specifically at the level of individual segments, while the other is in maintaining the activation of the phonological plan. The latter process may form the link between phonological encoding and the specification of articulatory gestures for speech output. It is the difference between these two types of deficit that is responsible for the wide range of accounts of this aphasic "syndrome".

It is quite possible that a subgroup of conduction aphasia with a verbal working memory deficit will display relatively great difficulty with repetition, in particular of nonwords. If activation from the lexicon is lacking, it may be even more difficult to retain a phonological plan. This subgroup of patients is probably the group labelled repetition conduction aphasic by Shallice and Warrington (1977). Note, however, that repetition will not necessarily be particularly problematic for *all* individuals with conduction aphasia with a working memory deficit.

The input to the process of phonological encoding, then, consists of segments, or bundles of phonological features, and metrical frames in the form of syllable templates. These are mapped onto one another, during which problems can arise with the assignment of segments to their proper slots in the frame, as well as with the individual markedness of segments.

Time course

Another set of questions concerns the time course of the mapping of segments to their metrical slots. In parallel models of speech production, segments within words or morphemes are selected simultaneously (Dell, 1986, 1988), whereas in serial models, they "are released in a linear [(left-to-right)] fashion for assignment to the frame" (Wheeldon & Levelt, 1995, p. 312; also Levelt, 1989, 1992; Levelt et al., 1999; Shattuck-Hufnagel, 1992). Note, by the way, that although Dell's original model is indifferent to serial order, he does suggest that it must be changed in order to accommodate effects that point to a sensitivity to serial order in speech errors. In particular, he mentions the apparent special status of syllable and word-initial segments, which are more prone to error than others and which provide better cues than other segments in word retrieval (Dell, 1988, p. 140).

Wheeldon and Levelt (1995) used phoneme detection times to establish the time course of phonological encoding. Subjects had to silently translate words (English–Dutch) while self-monitoring for specific phonemes. The results of this study showed a syllable-by-syllable effect, indicating incremental, left-to-right activation. However, it is unclear to what extent these results were influenced by the fact that Wheeldon and Levelt used not only bisyllabic, but also bimorphemic test items. Also, there may well be language-particular variation, as some languages appear to be more sensitive to syllable structure than others, which typically allow ambisyllabicity (Cutler 1993; Cutler, Mehler, Norris, & Segui, 1986).

Possible effects of the time course of phonological encoding on aphasic output are hard to predict. A deficit in working memory capacity is more likely to produce a length effect if segments are serially mapped to their slots, than if the process is parallel. Crucially, what is meant here with "word length effect" is not only the phenomenon that more errors are produced on longer words, something that has been observed in conduction aphasia (Köhler et al., 1998) as well as in most other types of aphasia, but rather the effect of more errors towards the *ends* of words. If segments are selected in a left-to-right fashion, one might expect a metrical frame-internal length effect anyway. However, such an effect could also be due to the relative strength of structural edge positions, especially if the metrical frames are small. If the frames are large, the effects might be due to processing capacity overload at a stage earlier or later than phonological processing, or at an entirely independent level. In the Levelt et al. (1999) model, phonetic encoding of prosodic words only starts after completion of their full phonological code.

Hough et al. (1994) have suggested that the working memory deficit in conduction aphasia, "rapid decay of a memory trace" (p. 244), may present itself in the form of substitutions with changes of only a few (i.e. one or two) features. They hypothesize this decay to occur in the phonological buffer, which in the Levelt et al. (1999) model serves as input to phonetic encoding (although Hough et al. use a different model, based on the phonological loop proposed by Baddeley, 1986). Nevertheless, one might argue that the memory traces of feature combinations (segments) must also be maintained during phonological encoding itself. In this case, an absence of word length effects in the presence of many single feature changes seems easiest to account for when segment-to-frame mapping is a parallel process.

Romani and Calabrese (1998) studied the deficit of Broca's aphasic patient DB and their interpretation of his impairment is very well compatible with the suggestion in Hough et al. (1994). They relate DB's articulatory difficulties to his limited digit span by claiming that a deficit at the level of articulatory planning leads to simplification of the representations that form the input to this level. If the articulatory programme is too complex for the patient, simplification of the phonological representation will take place in the buffer. Although this account requires backtracking between processing levels, which is highly unpopular in the Levelt et al. (1999) model, it does address the similarity of errors due to simplification of phonological structure in nonfluent patients and a subgroup of fluent patients, as discussed already. It also means that phonological (segmental) structure, and not only more general cognitive factors such as item length, must still be visible and functional in this output buffer.

In the previous section, we interpreted the divergent results of studies into conduction aphasia as indicating that there are in fact two deficits with broadly similar surface characteristics. The paraphasias of patients with a deficit in the building of the phonological plan show effects of segmental markedness, whereas the paraphasias of patients with a deficit in the maintenance of this plan show length effects. With respect to the time course of the encoding process, this suggests that phonological encoding of segments within metrical (syllabic) frames is parallel, but that serial (length) effects may be generated by the maintenance process, a function of verbal working memory.

Again, the picture emerging from aphasiological studies is of working memory interacting with the process of phonological encoding, in which phonological structure plays a functional role. It will be interesting to see whether there are (conduction or other) aphasic patients who can be shown to have no working memory difficulties *at all*, while still producing more errors towards word ends. Such an observation would indicate that segment-to-frame mapping proceeds in a serial fashion, as opposed to parallel.

Conclusion

Conduction aphasia as a syndrome has been presented as a phonological encoding deficit, but we maintain here that only a subgroup of individuals with conduction aphasia have specific problems with the encoding process. Other patients with conduction aphasia suffer from a verbal working memory deficit and have problems retaining the activation of the phonological plan. The first group of patients provides direct insight into the characteristics of the phonological encoding process, showing, for example, that individual segments function independently from hierarchically organized syllables as functional units at this processing level. The second group, however, shows the close link that exists between processing capacity (working memory) and the building of speech surface structure.

It is even possible that these differences in type of deficit are merely gradual, and that working memory performs an essential function in phonological encoding. If the articulatory rehearsal and checking of phonological content, as proposed by Baddeley (1986), are essential to the phonological encoding process, the memory deficit may not be so different from the linguistic deficit after all.

In our discussion of phonological encoding, we have split the process into two components: *input* and *time course*. With regard to the input, we claim that sound specifications are mapped onto hierarchically organized metrical frames, in the form of syllables. The syllabification itself is a late process in phonological encoding, but the metrical frames are already hierarchically organized in the form lexicon. Because of the interaction with working memory deficits, it is not straightforward to gain insight into the time course of phonological encoding through aphasiological studies. Our interpretation of the data suggests that phonological encoding within metrical frames is parallel, yielding structural effects rather than length effects on impairment. Serial (length) effects are due to a verbal working memory deficit. It may be the interaction of segment-to-frame mapping and working memory itself that provides insight into the nature of the process.

It will be clear from this chapter that different approaches to the process of phonological encoding, even within the domains of formal phonological theory, psycholinguistics and neurolinguistics, are not always easy to distinguish and compare. This is because of definitions and terminology, but also because these domains do not always intend to address the same issues. Nevertheless, we feel that these different domains of research will all benefit from attempts at communication between them.

Acknowledgements

This chapter was written as part of the first author's project "Phonological encoding deficiencies in aphasia", funded by the Dutch Organization for Scientific Research (NWO) under grant #575–21–001. We are grateful to Albert Postma, Frank Wijnen and Ulrich Schade for their reviews of earlier versions of this paper, from which it has benefited greatly. Needless to say, any errors remain our own.

References

Baddeley, A. (1986). *Working memory*. Oxford: Clarendon Press.
Baddeley, A. (1990). *Human memory: Theory and practice*. Needham Heights, MA: Allyn & Bacon.
Baddeley, A., & Wilson, B. (1985). Phonological coding and short-term memory in patients without speech. *Journal of Memory and Language, 24*, 490–502.
Bastiaanse, R., Gilbers, D. G., & van der Linde, K. (1994). Sonority substitutions in Broca's and conduction aphasia. *Journal of Neurolinguistics, 8*, 247–55.
Béland, R., & Lecours, A. R. (1989). Analyse phonologique de séquences d'approximations. *Revue Québécoise de Linguistique Théorique et Appliquée, 8*, 267–85.
Blumstein, S. E. (1973). Some phonological implications of aphasic speech. In H. Goodglass & S. Blumstein (Eds.), *Psycholinguistics and aphasia*. Baltimore, MA: Johns Hopkins University Press.
Blumstein, S. E. (1991). Phonological aspects of aphasia. In M. T. Sarno (Ed.), *Acquired aphasia*. San Diego, CA: Academic Press.
Brown, R., & McNeill, D. (1966). The 'tip of the tongue' phenomenon. *Journal of Verbal Learning and Verbal Behavior, 5*, 325–37.
Buckingham, H. W. (1992). Phonological production deficits in conduction aphasia. In S. E. Kohn (Ed.), *Conduction aphasia*. Hillsdale, NJ: Lawrence Erlbaum Associates, Inc.
Burns, M. S., & Canter, G. J. (1977). Phonemic behavior of aphasic patients with posterior cerebral lesions. *Brain & Language, 4*, 492–507.
Cairns, C. & Feinstein, M. (1982). Markedness and the theory of syllable structure. *Linguistic Inquiry, 13*, 193–226.
Canter, G. J., Trost, J. E., & Burns, M. S. (1985). Contrasting speech patterns in apraxia of speech and phonemic paraphasia. *Brain & Language, 24*, 204–22.
Caplan, D., & Waters, G. (1992). Issues arising regarding the nature and consequences of reproduction conduction aphasia. In S. E. Kohn (Ed.), *Conduction aphasia*. Hillsdale, NJ: Lawrence Erlbaum Associates, Inc.

Christman, S. S. (1992). Uncovering phonological regularity in neologisms: Contributions of sonority theory. *Clinical Linguistics & Phonetics, 6*, 3, 219–47.

Croot, K., Patterson, K., & Hodges, J. R. (1998). Single word production in nonfluent progressive aphasia. *Brain and Language, 61*, 226–73.

Cutler, A. (1993). Language-specific processing: Does the evidence converge? In G. T. M. Altmann & R. Shillcock (Eds.), *Cognitive models of speech processing: The second Sperlonga meeting.* Hillsdale, NJ: Lawrence Erlbaum Associates, Inc.

Cutler, A., Mehler, J., Norris, D., & Segui, J. (1986). The syllable's differing role in the segmentation of French and English. *Journal of Memory and Language, 25*, 385–400.

Dell, G. S. (1986). A spreading activation theory of retrieval in sentence production. *Psychological Review, 93*, 283–321.

Dell, G. S. (1988). The retrieval of phonological forms in production: Tests of predictions from a connectionist model. *Journal of Memory and Language, 27*, 124–42.

Démonet, J. F., Price, C., Wise, R., & Frackowiak, R. S. J. (1994). A PET study of cognitive strategies in normal subjects during language tasks: Influence of phonetic ambiguity and sequence processing on phoneme monitoring. *Brain, 117*, 671–82.

Démonet, J. F., Fiez, J. A., Paulesu, E., Petersen, S. E., & Zatorre, R. J. (1996). PET studies of phonological processing: a critical reply to Poeppel. *Brain and Language, 55*, 352–79.

Feinberg, T., Rothi, L., & Heilman, K. (1986). Inner speech in conduction aphasia. *Archives of Neurology 43*, 591–3.

Gilbers, D. G., & Den Ouden, D. B. (1994). Compensatory lengthening and cluster reduction in first language acquisition: A comparison of different analyses. In A. de Boer, H. de Hoop & H. de Swart (Eds.), *Language and cognition 4: Yearbook 1994 of the research group for theoretical and experimental linguistics of the University of Groningen,* 69–82.

Goldstein, K. (1948). *Language and language disturbances.* New York: Grune & Stratton.

Goodglass, H. (1992). Diagnosis of Conduction Aphasia. In S. E. Kohn (Ed.), *Conduction aphasia.* Hillsdale, NJ: Lawrence Erlbaum Associates, Inc.

Hartsuiker, R. J. (2000). *The addition bias in Dutch and Spanish phonological speech errors: The role of structural context.* University of Nijmegen manuscript.

Hayes, B. (1989). Compensatory lengthening in moraic phonology. *Linguistic Inquiry, 20*, 253–306.

Henderson, V. W. (1992). Early concepts of conduction aphasia. In S. E. Kohn (Ed.), *Conduction aphasia.* Hillsdale, NJ: Lawrence Erlbaum Associates, Inc.

Hough, M. S., DeMarco, S., & Farler, D. (1994). Phonemic retrieval in conduction aphasia and Broca's aphasia with apraxia of speech: underlying processes. *Journal of Neurolinguistics, 8*, 235–46.

Köhler, K., Bartels, C., Herrmann, M., Dittmann, J., & Wallesch, C.-W. (1998). Conduction aphasia – 11 classic cases. *Aphasiology, 12*, 865–84.

Kohn, S. E. (1988). Phonological production deficits in aphasia. In H. A. Whitaker (Ed.), *Phonological processes and brain mechanisms.* New York: Springer Verlag.

Kohn, S. E., & Smith, K. L. (1992). Introduction: On the notion of 'aphasia syndrome'. In S. E. Kohn (Ed.), *Conduction aphasia.* Hillsdale, NJ: Lawrence Erlbaum Associates, Inc.

Lecours, A. R., & Lhermitte, F. (1969). Phonemic paraphasias: Linguistic structures and tentative hypotheses. *Cortex, 5*, 193–228.

Levelt, W. J. M. (1989). *Speaking: From intention to articulation*. Cambridge, MA: MIT Press.

Levelt, W. J. M. (1992). Accessing words in speech production: Stages, processes and representations. *Cognition, 42*, 1–22.

Levelt, W. J. M., Roelofs, A., & Meyer, A. S. (1999). A theory of lexical access in speech production. *Behavioral and Brain Sciences, 22*, 1–38.

Luria, A. R. (1964) Factors and forms of aphasia. In A.V. S. de Reuck, & M. O'Connor (Eds.), *Disorders of language*. London: Churchill, 143–61.

Meijer, P. J. A. (1996). Suprasegmental structures in phonological encoding: The CV structure. *Journal of Memory and Language, 35*, 840–53.

Miller, N. (2000). Changing ideas in apraxia of speech. In I. Papathanasiou (Ed.), *Acquired neurogenic communication disorders: A clinical perspective*. London and Philadelphia: Whurr.

Nespoulous, J.-L., Joanette, Y., Béland, R., Caplan, D., & Lecours, A. R. (1984). Phonological disturbances in aphasia: Is there a "markedness effect" in aphasic phonemic errors? In F. C. Rose (Ed.), *Advances in aphasiology, Vol. 42: Progress in aphasiology*. London: Raven Press.

Nespoulous, J.-L., Joanette, Y., Ska, B., Caplan, D., & Lecours, A. R. (1987). Production deficits in Broca's and conduction aphasia: Repetition vs. reading. In E. Keller & M. Gopnik (Eds.), *Motor and sensory processes in language*. Hillsdale, NJ: Lawrence Erlbaum Associates, Inc.

Ouden, D. B. den (2002a). *Phonology in aphasia: Syllables and segments in level-specific deficits*. Groningen: Groningen Dissertations in Linguistics (GRODIL).

Ouden, D. B. den (2002b). Segmental vs syllable markedness: Deletion errors in the paraphasias of fluent and nonfluent aphasics. In E. Fava (Ed.), *Clinical linguistics: Language pathology, speech therapy, and linguistic theory*. CILT series. Amsterdam/Philadelphia: John Benjamins.

Poeck, K. (1983). What do we mean by "aphasic syndromes"? A neurologist's view. *Brain and Language, 20*, 79–89.

Poeppel, D. (1996). A critial review of PET studies of phonological processing. *Brain and Language, 55*, 317–51.

Price, C. J., Wise, R. J. S., Warburton, E. A., Moore, C. J., Howard, D., Patterson, K, Frackowiak, R. S. J., & Friston, K. J. (1996). Hearing and saying: The functional neuro-anatomy of auditory word processing. *Brain, 119*, 919–31.

Prince, A., & Smolensky, P. (1993). *Optimality theory: Constraint interaction in generative grammar*. Rutgers University Center for Cognitive Science Technical Report 2.

Prins, R. S. (1987). *Afasie: Classificatie, behandeling en herstelverloop*. Unpublished dissertation, University of Amsterdam.

Roelofs, A. (1996). Serial order in planning the production of successive morphemes of a word. *Journal of Memory and Language, 35*, 854–76.

Romani, C., & Calabrese, A. (1998). Syllabic constraints in the phonological errors of an aphasic patient. *Brain & Language, 64*, 83–121.

Schiller, N. O. (1997). *The role of the syllable in speech production*. Nijmegen University PhD thesis.

Sevald, C. A., Dell, G. S., & Cole, J. S. (1995). Syllable structure in speech production: Are syllables chuncks or schemas? *Journal of Memory and Language, 34*, 807–20.

Shallice, T., & Warrington, E. (1977). Auditory-verbal short-term memory and conduction aphasia. *Brain and Language, 4*, 479–91.

Shattuck-Hufnagel, S. (1979). Speech errors as evidence for a serial order mechanism in sentence production. In W. E. Cooper & E. C. T. Walker (Eds.), *Sentence process-ing: Psycholinguistic studies presented to Merrill Garrett*. Hillsdale, NJ: Lawrence Erlbaum Associates, Inc.

Shattuck-Hufnagel, S. (1992). The role of word structure in segmental serial ordering. *Cognition, 42*, 213–59.

Stemberger, J. P. (1990). Wordshape errors in language production. *Cognition, 35*, 123–57.

Valdois, S. (1990). Internal structure of two consonant clusters. In J.-L. Nespoulous & P. Villiard (Eds.), *Morphology, phonology and aphasia*. New York: Springer Verlag.

Warrington, E. K., & Shallice, T. (1969). The selective impairment of auditory verbal short-term memory. *Brain, 92*, 885–96.

Wernicke, C. (1874). *Der Aphasische Symptomencomplex: Eine psychologische Studie auf anatomischer Basis* [The aphasia symptom complex. A psychological study on an anatomic basis]. Breslau: Cohn & Weigert. Translated in G. H. Eggert (1977) *Wernicke's works on aphasia: A sourcebook and review*. New York: Mouton.

Wheeldon, L. R., & Levelt, W. J. M. (1995). Monitoring the time course of phono-logical encoding. *Journal of Memory and Language, 34*, 311–34.

Wheeler, D. W., & Touretzky, D. S. (1997). A parallel licensing model of normal slips and phonemic paraphasias. *Brain & Language, 59*, 147–201.

6   Phonological encoding in young children who stutter

Kenneth S. Melnick, Edward G. Conture, and Ralph N. Ohde

Abstract

Recently, a growing body of research and theory has suggested that linguistic factors such as phonological, semantic and syntactic encoding play just as much of a role in the development of stuttering in children as motoric variables. One prominent theory of stuttering that has received considerable attention is the Covert Repair Hypothesis (CRH) (e.g., Kolk & Postma, 1997), which suggests that stuttering is a by-product of a slower than normal ability to phonologically encode. Although empirical studies have been performed to evaluate the process of phonological encoding, few have systematically assessed or manipulated pertinent variables such as speech reaction time of people who stutter in response to a picture-naming task. To date, those studies of these variables have typically involved adults who stutter, with only two focusing on young children who stutter (CWS). For the latter, preliminary results indicate that both CWS and children who do not stutter (CWNS) benefit from manipulation of phonological segments. However, CWNS demonstrate a significant negative correlation between scores on a standardized test of articulation and speech reaction time while CWS show little to no relationship between these variables. Such findings suggest continued study of the speech-language planning and production abilities of CWS and seem supportive of commonly made clinical suggestions to parents of CWS, for example, to minimize interrupting and to allow more planning time for children's speech-language production.

Introduction

Theoretical accounts of stuttering take two general forms: those that try to explain stuttering from the perspective of onset and development versus those that try to explain the nature and/or occurrence of instances or "moments" of stuttering (Bloodstein, 1995, pp. 60–67). Among the latter, some have explained stuttering as a difficulty with speech motor control or, more specifically, as a motor execution deficit resulting in disturbances in spatial/temporal coordination of the peripheral speech mechanism.

While motoric aspects (e.g., speech motor control of articulation, phonation, and respiration) of stuttering have received considerable attention in the past 20 years, developing lines of evidence suggest that linguistic (e.g., phonological, semantic and syntactic) variables also contribute a good deal to childhood stuttering. For example, CWS more frequently exhibit phonological problems than CWNS (for an overview of the possible relationship between phonological disorders and stuttering, see, e.g., Howell & Au-Yeung, 1995; Louko, Conture & Edwards, 1999; Louko, Edwards & Conture, 1990; Nippold, 1990; Paden & Yairi, 1996; Paden, Yairi & Ambrose, 1999; Pellowski, Conture & Anderson, 2000; Throneburg, Yairi, & Paden, 1994). There is also evidence that CWS, when compared to CWNS, demonstrate greater disparity between scores on standardized tests of receptive vocabulary and receptive and expressive language (i.e., semantics, syntax, and morphology) (Anderson & Conture, 2000). Furthermore, Yairi, Ambrose, Paden and Throneberg (1996), have shown that children close to the onset of stuttering exhibiting lower scores on a standardized test of language abilities are more apt to exhibit persistent stuttering than children with higher language performance scores. In addition, others (Bernstein Ratner & Sih, 1987; Howell, Au-Yeung, & Sackin, 1999; Logan & Conture, 1995; 1997; Melnick & Conture, 2000; Yaruss, 1999; Zackheim & Conture, 2003) have repeatedly shown that increases in utterance length and grammatical complexity, as well as certain word types (i.e., function versus content), are associated with increases in frequency of stuttering.

These results, based on over 12 empirical studies, would not seem easily explained by purely motoric accounts of stuttering (e.g., the notion that stuttering is caused by discoordination among articulatory, laryngeal and respiratory events). What is needed, therefore, are theoretical accounts for those linguistic processes (e.g., phonology) occurring *prior to* motor execution of speech that appear to appreciably influence instances of stuttering. In general, a better understanding of these processes and their relationship to stuttering should broaden our perspective on stuttering beyond that of considering it to be chiefly resulting from motoric difficulties. In specific, such an approach should provide meaningful insights into the role that linguistic processes play in the initiation and/or cause of instances of stuttering in children.

Theoretical background

In attempts to develop a theoretical account for how disruptions in linguistic processes lead to instances of stuttering, we have employed essential elements of the theoretical and empirical work of Levelt and his colleagues in terms of normal speech and language production (e.g., Levelt, Roelofs & Meyer, 1999; Levelt & Wheeldon, 1994), as well as constructs from a Levelt-influenced model of stuttering, the CRH (e.g., Kolk & Postma, 1997; Postma & Kolk, 1993). Greatly simplifying the stipulation of Levelt et al., the process of speech-language production is partitioned into three components: (1) conceptualizer, where the speaker's "intention" is created, (2) the formulator, where the speaker's linguistic plan to be spoken is created; and (3) the articulator, where the speaker's phonetic plan is realized in the form of overt communication. Although each component has relevance to speech-language production, we will focus on the formulator component (whose sub-components consist of such processes as phonological encoding) as a result of our own research (e.g., Anderson & Conture, 2000; Logan & Conture, 1997; Logan & LaSalle, 1999; Melnick, Conture, & Ohde, 2003), as well as that of others.

Starting from the position that linguistic processes contribute to the cause and/or initiation of instances of stuttering, it is our basic assumption that instances of stuttering, at least in part, are related to the process of *planning for* speech and language production. Based on this assumption, our model leads us to suggest that the most common instances of childhood stuttering (e.g., sound/syllable repetitions, sound prolongations and single-syllable whole-word repetitions) reflect relatively slower (when compared to normal) planning (formulation) of linguistic speech and language processes, particularly those processes that must interface rapidly, smoothly and accurately to communicate the speaker's intent.

Stuttering: A temporal disruption in planning

This slower than normal planning may be viewed, at least in part, as a temporal disruption. As Kent (1984) suggested, given the definition of stuttering as a disruption in rhythm or fluency of speech, whatever causes such a disruption is more than likely temporal in nature. In fact, according to Hall, Amir and Yairi (1999), phone rates (phones per second) differ between CWS and CWNS, indicating that CWS, at the segmental/subsegmental level of speech production, appear to have difficulties regulating the temporal aspects of speaking, a finding consistent with Kent's (1984) notion that stuttering is associated with a disruption in the temporal structure of processing. Chang, Ohde, and Conture (2002) found a greater differentiation in formant transition rate for place of articulation in CWNS compared to CWS, suggesting a subtle difficulty in the speed of speech-language production in the latter than former group. It is reasonable to suggest that these temporal disruptions can take many forms, including: (1) overall slowness during encoding (e.g., selecting sounds); (2) slowness in "mapping" one process (e.g., the *meaning* of a word, to another; the *form* of a word); and (3) encoding elements correctly but not in their sequence. According to Woodworth (1938, p. 238): "Time as a dimension of every mental or behavioural process ... can be used as an indicator of the complexity of the performance or the participant's readiness to perform." In our own work to date, in this area (Melnick, Conture, & Ohde, 2003), we have tried to answer questions about the structure and function of a covert system, that is, linguistic/information processing, by measuring overt behavior, for example, how long it takes participants to name objects.

While phonological encoding contributions to stuttering have, to date, received the greatest amount of theoretical attention (Kolk & Postma, 1997), it is just as possible that other aspects of linguistic planning also contribute to instances of stuttering. For example, (1) retrieving the lemma (i.e., syntactic/ meaning aspects of word) from the mental lexicon; (2) morphological-syntactic construction of surface structure; and (3) mapping the lemma onto the lexeme (i.e., phonological aspects of the word) and/or being able to appropriately select speech targets at a rate commensurate with the phonological encoder's ability to activate the same.

Differences in frequency due to differences in capability

As shown in Figure 6.1, it is our general assumption that similar linguistic variables (e.g., utterance complexity) influence the production of speech (dis)fluency for both CWS and CWNS; however, the difference in absolute frequency of disfluency, between CWS and CWNS, relates to between-group differences in linguistic capability. Whether these difficulties arise because of genetic, environmental or combined genetic-environmental factors is not the focus of the present discussion. Rather, it is our contention that if results of empirical studies suggest that such difficulties are present, they deserve further empirical investigation as well as theoretical explanation. The current chapter will address whether relatively brief, subtle disruptions at the level of phonological encoding are associated with childhood stuttering (i.e., phonological encoding *capabilities* of CWS are slower than those of CWNS). In this discussion, we have employed the model just discussed, and some of its testable assumptions/hypotheses, to help address specific questions outlined in this chapter.

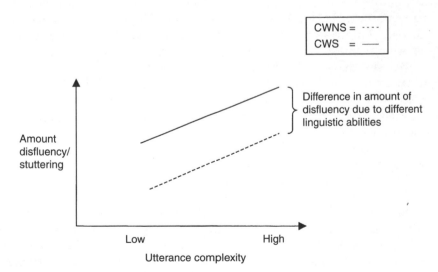

Figure 6.1 Difference in amount of disfluency due to different linguistic abilities for both children who stutter (CWS) and children who do not stutter (CWNS).

As already indicated, we assume that phonological encoding/processing (and related aspects of planning for speech-language production) contributes to, at least in part, the cause(s) of stuttering. Given that assumption, it appears quite appropriate that our empirical investigations of childhood stuttering have focused on linguistic processes (i.e., phonological encoding/processing) that CWS use to plan their intended messages prior to overt communication. The following is a brief discussion of phonological encoding.

Phonological encoding

According to Levelt's (1989) model, phonological encoding takes place within the formulator (which is also where grammatical and semantic encoding take place). Theoretically, the input into the formulator consists of fragments of messages (and, in particular, the surface structure from the grammatical encoder), and the output is the phonetic or articulatory plan (Levelt, 1989). According to Meyer and Schriefers (1991), phonological encoding can be defined as, "the retrieval of the phonological form of a word (i.e., information about the word's morphology, phonology and prosody), given its meaning" (p. 1146). In most phonological encoding models, syllables are often viewed as "frames" or "slots", and the units encoded, in succession, are syllable *constituents* (i.e., onset, nucleus and coda; Shattuck-Hufnagel, 1979, 1983) rather than complete syllables (Meyer & Schriefers, 1991). More specifically then, phonological encoding is usually assumed to involve the retrieval of phonological segments, the creation of a "frame", and then the insertion of the segments into the slots of the frame (Meyer & Schriefers, 1991).

According to Levelt (1989, p. 12), the function of the phonological encoder is to retrieve or build a phonetic or articulatory plan for each lemma (i.e., syntactic word) and for the utterance as a whole. It should be mentioned that the output of the formulator (which includes the phonological encoder) is a phonetic representation of an utterance, which Levelt (1989) identified as *internal* speech (as opposed to overt speech) in which the speaker has only a certain, parsed, awareness of the entire message (Levelt, 1989). The stage in which the message is overtly produced occurs at the final, articulatory phase.

Levelt's (1989) psycholinguistic model of spoken language (speech) production has lead to numerous experiments attempting to assess its constructs (e.g., Dell & O'Seaghdha, 1991; Meyer, 1991; Roelofs, 1997). As Meyer and Schriefers (1991) point out, however, the time required to access the meaning and form of a word is highly speculative.

Until fairly recently (e.g., Levelt & Wheeldon, 1994; Van Turennout, Hagoort, & Brown, 1997), empirical experiments on the time course of phonological encoding have been limited. As suggested earlier, we still have mainly a theoretical understanding of the form in which the sounds are accessed, as well as the manner (i.e., order) in which they are made available for production. For instance, in Dell's (1986) model, all segments of a given syllable become highly activated at the same time and can be inserted into the slots of a syllable frame in any order. This model differs from Shattuck-Hufnagel's (1979, 1983) model in which all slots of a word must be filled in a particular order (Meyer & Schriefers, 1991). In fact, according to Van Turennout et al. (1997), not only does phonological encoding proceed in a left-to-right manner, but the initial phase of semantic activation proceeds phonological encoding.

One method of carefully controlling the nature and time course of phonological encoding is through picture-naming tasks. What follows, therefore, is a brief discussion of the process of picture naming, particularly as it relates to measuring the time course of phonological encoding.

Picture naming

In general, picture recognition requires only the relationship between noun and corresponding object (Glaser, 1992). From a technical perspective, however, picture naming involves four stages, including: (1) the perception of the picture (i.e., conceptual identification); (2) lemma retrieval; (3) word-form encoding; and (4) articulation (Roelofs, 1992).

Until recently (Meyer, 1990, 1991; Meyer & Schriefers, 1991), phonological studies in picture naming have been limited, especially as they relate to young children (Brooks & MacWhinney, 2000). One method that has been frequently used with adults (Meyer, 1990, 1991; Meyer & Schriefers, 1991) is based on a Stroop paradigm[1] (Stroop, 1935) in which a distracter (either visual or auditory) stimulus prior to picture presentation must be suppressed. Therefore, in a typical picture-naming task using this design, a preceding stimulus ("prime"), followed by a picture (i.e., target) stimulus, must be suppressed before the target is articulated. Thus, in a "priming" (i.e., phonological facilitation) experiment, the independent variable is the instruction concerning the prime and the semantic or associative relatedness between the prime and the target (e.g., the participant can be instructed to ignore the prime or use it to aid in a more efficient response), and the dependent variable is usually the response latency between onset of target presentation and onset of target naming (Glaser, 1992). According to Glaser (1992), results of these types of experiments generally show that response latencies are gradually *reduced* (i.e., made faster) depending on the prime-target similarity (e.g., an auditory prime that presents the same-first versus a different-first sound of the name of the target that follows).

Experimental studies of phonological priming

For some time (i.e., since at least the 1970s), priming has been extensively used in cognitive psychology (Collins & Ellis, 1992). Although many of these studies have involved semantic (or lexical) priming (McNamara & Holbrook, 2002; see Neely, 1991 for a review of this area), fewer have been conducted in phonological priming. One of the first influential studies involving lexical priming, conducted by Meyer and Schvaneveldt (1971), demonstrated that lexical decisions for written word pairs were identified faster when the words were related in meaning than when they were unrelated (Collins & Ellis, 1992), findings consistent with Glaser's (1992) theory regarding prime-target similarity.

According to Radeau, Morais, and Dewier (1989), phonological priming is the "effect on word target recognition that arises from some phonological relationship between a prime and the target" (p. 525). Although several studies in *phonological* priming have been conducted since the 1970s (for an overview, see Collins & Ellis, 1992), findings are somewhat mixed on the consequence of the phonological relationship between stimuli for processing of the target item. That is, some studies show facilitation (i.e., faster speech reaction time during a priming versus no prime condition), others show inhibition, and still others show a mixture of effects (Collins & Ellis, 1992). Central to most of these studies are theoretical constructs such as those proposed by Dell's (1986) theory of spreading activation and Stemberger's (1982, 1985) theory, which implies that more highly activated items are executed first. In their study, Collins and Ellis (1992) conducted a series of experiments designed to test the strength of these theories and reported the following: (1) facilatory effects for words and non-words when primes were related (similar) and unrelated (nonsimilar) to targets and (2) priming is more of an automatic than strategic process, that is, the longest stimulus onset asynchrony (SOA) (1000 ms) was no more helpful than the shortest (0 ms). Overall, these results seem to support Dell's (1986) theory (Collins & Ellis, 1992).

One common criticism of both lexical and phonological priming involves the question of automatic versus strategic processes (Martin & Jensen, 1988). In other words, do participants strategically exploit the time between prime and target to reduce response latency? In a series of studies conducted by Rouibah, Tiberghien, and Lupker (1999), a masking procedure[2] was introduced in an attempt to discourage participants from using such strategies. In their experiments, Rouibah et al. (1999) used various designs, ranging from colour matching, where participants were required to use a button press, to experiments that included a verbal response to primes that were either homophonic or rhyming. Results support not only the theory that priming phonological segments can be achieved, but also that processing effects appear to be automatically rather than strategically based (Rouibah et al., 1999).

In certain experimental paradigms, "primes" (whether sharing elements or not in common with the target), are considered to be "interfering stimuli" (IS). That is, trials containing an IS are expected to result in longer naming latencies than trials without an IS. Thus, the salient dependent variable is the difference in average naming latency between trials that contain IS that share common segments, meaning, etc. (i.e., related IS) and trials that contain IS that do not share common segments, meaning, etc. (i.e., unrelated IS). As with most such paradigms, many procedural variables will influence findings, for example, Meyers and Schriefers (1991) suggest that if the activation of segments occur too rapidly such that an IS is too far ahead of the target or picture presentation, then the facilatory effect will be lost (i.e., the activation decays prior to picture or target naming). Thus, activation must occur at an optimum time (relative to picture naming) for one to observe a facilatory effect (i.e., lessening of the interference effect) to be observed (Meyer & Schriefers, 1991); however, whether optimal times are similar for children and adults is presently unclear.

In the Meyer and Schriefers (1991) experiments, adult participants were presented with begin-related, begin-unrelated, end-related and end-unrelated ISs. During these experiments, "primes" were presented at 4 different SOAs which included −300 (minus indicates onset of prime prior to onset of target), −150, 0 and +150 ms. Results indicated facilatory effects of both begin- and end-related "primes", but that end-related (facilatory) effects began to appear at *later* SOAs. This suggests that phonological encoding of the first syllable begins *before* the encoding of the second syllable and that the encoding within a syllable also proceeds in a left to right manner (Meyer & Schriefers, 1991). Other, more general findings indicated that reaction times tended to be shorter on trials with related ISs than on trials with unrelated ISs, but that both related and unrelated conditions revealed longer reaction times than the silent condition. Finally, another finding was that the longest (negative) SOA did not produce any significant facilatory effects (between related and unrelated primes). This suggests that the prime had *decayed* before the target was presented (Meyer & Schriefers, 1991).

Although findings from these word- and picture-naming studies do not irrefutably demonstrate the time-course sequence of phonological encoding, they do provide evidence for how phonological encoding proceeds. Of most importance, it appears that phonological encoding proceeds in a left-to-right manner, and that the unit of encoding may indeed consist of syllable constituents rather than whole syllables or words.

Although picture-interference experiments, such as those conducted by Meyers and Schriefers (1991), were originally intended to assess the rate of activation or time-course sequence of phonological encoding in people *without* any speech and language impairments, a similar procedure has been used to examine the speech and language abilities of adults and CWS. In particular, it has been used to test at least one prominent theory of stuttering, the Covert Repair Hypothesis (CRH) (Kolk & Postma, 1997; Postma & Kolk, 1993). The following is a brief description of the CRH (for a more detailed description of this and related theories, see Conture, 2001, pp. 30–45), followed by a more in-depth discussion of several experiments that have used picture-interference studies to examine this theory.

The Covert Repair Hypothesis (CRH)

Wingate (1988) set the stage for current psycholinguistic approaches to stuttering by suggesting that: "There is ample evidence to indicate that the defect is not simply one of motor control or coordination, but that it involves more central functions of the language production system" (p. 238). Since that time, Postma and Kolk's CRH (e.g., Kolk, 1991; Kolk & Postma, 1997; Postma & Kolk, 1993) has become one of the more comprehensive, psycholinguistically driven explanations of stuttering. This theory explicitly attempts to account for the occurrence of sound/syllable repetitions and sound prolongations (i.e., instances of stuttering) by using an overarching model of speech communication (e.g., Levelt, 1989; Levelt et al., 1999) as well as empirical studies of speech disfluencies and errors (e.g., Blackmer & Mitton, 1991; Bredart, 1991; Clark & Wasow, 1998; Dell & Juliano, 1991; Levelt, 1983).

The basic premise of the CRH is that the speech sound units of young CWS are slow to activate, a fact that means their intended units are more apt to remain in competition (for being selected) with unintended units for a longer period of time. The possibility that CWS experience a lengthened period of competition – due to the slowness of their speech target activation – is speculated to increase chances for misselecting during the process of phonological encoding. This is thought to be particularly problematic if these children attempt to initiate speech and/or make speech sound selections at an inappropriately fast rate. If they do, they are believed to be more apt to produce speech sound selection errors, because the child's rate of selection has exceeded his/her rate of speech unit activation. Because internal speech allows one to detect "trouble" before the speaker has fully articulated the utterance (Levelt, 1989, p. 13), it seems plausible that the speaker can revise their phonetic plan in the event a "troublesome element" arises (p. 13). As the frequency of their misselections increase, these children are hypothesized to more frequently revise their "articulatory program", a revision that often entails tracing back to the beginning of the sound, syllable or word. That is, the speaker self-repairs an "unintended message" or speech error having either (a) just occurred, (b) is in the process of occurring or (c) is about to occur, with an instance of stuttering (e.g., sound/syllable repetition) resulting as a by-product. The CRH suggests that many self-repairs exhibited by people who stutter reflect their attempts to accommodate for or adapt to an impaired (i.e., slower than normal) ability to "phonologically encode", with instances of stuttering resulting as a by-product of these self-repairs.

By itself, slowness in phonological encoding would not be a problem as long as the child made his or her phonological selections at a rate commensurate with his or her system's rate of activation for this variable. If, however, for whatever the reason, the child initiates or selects too soon (e.g., the child's internal or external environment encourages him to rush the planning of speech-language production), chances increase that inappropriate sounds, words and/or surface structure elements get placed into the phonetic plan (see Conture, 2001, Figures 1.3 and 1.4, for analogies to such temporal mismatches for people who stutter). Such occurrences, when they are detected by the speaker, would lead to disruptions in the forward flow of speech (i.e., "cutoff"), resulting in self-repairs and speech disfluencies.

It is important to note that even though the CRH provides a framework with which to explain how stuttering occurs, relatively few studies in phonological priming have been conducted to evaluate the CRH with adults who stutter, and an even fewer number with CWS. The following is a brief description of some of these studies.

Experiments in phonological encoding with children and adults who stutter

One of the earliest studies was conducted by Wijnen and Boers (1994) who presented both adults who do and do not stutter (i.e., "primed") with the initial C or CV of a word prior to saying the target word. Although both groups responded more quickly during the CV than in the C-alone condition, the adults who did not stutter benefited more than those that did stutter in the C-alone condition. Results showed that, for the adults who stuttered, a significant priming effect occurred, but only if both the consonant *and* following vowel were preactivated (i.e., preactivation of the initial C alone did not show any significant priming effect). Wijnen and Boers (1994) took their results to suggest that, if adults who stutter were having phonological encoding difficulties, the problem was with the syllable rime (a speculation seemingly related to Wingate's (1988) "Fault-Line Hypothesis").

In an attempt to replicate this study, Burger and Wijnen (1999) conducted a similar study with adults who do and do not stutter. In their study, both groups of adults responded similarly during the C and CV conditions. Although similar in procedure to the Wijnen and Boers (1994) study, results of the more recent study do not support the hypothesis that stuttering is specifically related to a difficulty in the phonological encoding of the stress-bearing part of the syllable (Burger & Wijnen, 1999).

Although results of these priming studies with adults seem to provide equivocal support for the CRH, research with CWS may be more supportive of the CRH. One such study was conducted by LaSalle and Carpenter (1994) who had CWS and CWNS participate in an experimental story-telling situation where the complexity of phonological encoding was reduced relative to a control story-telling situation (i.e., in the "less complex", experimental condition, all words ended in "ing", while in the control condition, word endings were allowed to normally vary). In their study, LaSalle and Carpenter (1994) reported significantly fewer overall speech disfluencies and sound prolongations during the experimental story-telling situation than during the control story-telling situation.

Although LaSalle and Carpenter (1994) investigated phonological facilitation with young children, they did not control for several pertinent variables, for example, the reaction time between the onset of the target and utterance response. In fact, in all of the phonological priming studies with adults and children discussed thus far, only one (i.e., Meyer & Schriefers, 1991) experimentally controlled for not only the aforementioned reaction time, but also time latency from the onset of the prime to the onset of the target. Further-more, all these studies did not always measure both the frequency of stutter-ing and phonological difficulties (both articulatory errors and slips of the tongue) of the experimental and control groups. A study similar in design to Meyer and Schriefers (1991), which quantitatively measures speech reaction time stuttering frequency, and phonological errors for CWS, would be most appropriate to test the CRH model.

Picture naming and phonological priming of children: Preliminary results

In attempts to adapt the picture-naming task (e.g., Meyer & Schriefers, 1991) to young CWS, the authors presented 18 CWS and 18 CWNS between the ages of 36 and 72 months old with three priming conditions (Melnick, Conture, & Ohde, 2003): (1) *silent* (i.e., no auditory stimulus was presented prior to picture presentation); (2) *related-primed* (i.e., the initial CV or CCV of the picture ("prime") was presented auditorily from a speaker just prior (i.e., 500 ms) to picture presentation); and (3) *unrelated-primed* (i.e., an initial CV or CCV not related to the picture was presented auditorily just prior (i.e., 500 ms) to picture presentation). This research indicated that all children benefited from the related-primed condition more so than either the silent or unrelated-primed condition. More importantly, however, CWNS, but not CWS, demonstrated a significant relationship between the speech reaction times in all priming conditions and their percentile scores on a test of articulatory mastery (Goldman–Fristoe Test of Articulation – Goldman & Fristoe, 1986). CWNS demonstrated, for each of the three priming conditions (no prime, related and unrelated) a significant negative correlation between articulation scores and speech reaction time while CWS demonstrated little or no re-lationship between these variables. Interestingly, Lahey, Edwards, and Munson (2001) report similar results for 4- to 9-year-old children with language problems, that is, no relationship between measures of naming latencies and scores on standardized tests of language abilities. Thus, less than well-organized relationships between speed and accuracy of various aspects of speech-language production characterize CWS as well as children with language problems.

It should be noted, however, that because this study (i.e., Melnick, Conture, & Ohde, 2003) appears to be the first, or one of the first, studies of its kind conducted with young children, several procedural issues make it difficult to achieve unambiguous results and interpretation. The following, therefore, is a brief discussion of some of these issues.

Picture naming and phonological priming of children: Procedural issues

One of the first procedural issues, when using the picture-naming task, involves comprehension of the task itself by young children. For example, although adults are be able to easily comprehend the nature of a picture-interference task and thus, readily name pictures shown to them on a face of a computer, young children have a much more difficult time. That is, young children's attention can easily wander resulting in an artificially large reaction time. Or, children grasp, at one moment, the concept that they are only to name the picture target rather than repeat the auditory prime, only to "forget" the concept part-way through the experimental condition.

Another procedural issue that had to be addressed, particularly as it related to young children was the SOA. In Meyer and Schriefers (1991), several SOAs were used (e.g., −300 ms to +150 ms). Initially, we attempted to manipulate the SOA for the young children. However, it quickly became apparent that presentation of the auditory prime in too close proximity to the onset of the picture target was confusing – so much so that children were not able to complete the task with any reasonable level of accuracy. Consequently, it was discovered that using a SOA of −500 ms permitted most children to complete the task, however, the "ideal" SOA for use with young children is still an empirical question.

One might argue, of course, that setting an SOA at −500 ms might create too long a gap between prime and target. In other words, such a gap may not truly permit a priming effect to occur (i.e., if too much time has elapsed since the onset of the prime, it may have decayed, thus, eliminating any possible facilitation/inhibition from occurring). Without question, this is a legitimate concern and one that we have been trying to rectify in more recent experiments. For instance, by allowing children to "practise" the task with a non-test or practice set of pictures beforehand (i.e., acclimate them better to the procedure ahead of time), we may be able to manipulate the SOA without confusing the children.

Third, there may be difficulties using the aforementioned paradigm to measure accuracy rather than speed of production. That is, when measuring speed or response latency during a picture-naming task, the experimenter must know, a priori, that the pictures employed in the task are named by participants with a relatively high degree of accuracy (for example, 8 per cent or greater). However, if an experimenter were interested in and wanted to measure accuracy (rather than latency) of picture-naming responses and uses pictures that were already identified with 80 per cent accuracy, there would be little opportunity to measure this parameter of the participant's response.

Finally, at the conclusion of each experimental condition, decisions needed to be made as to how to deal with those target productions where a reaction time was recorded but did not appear to accurately represent the child's naming of the picture target (see Ratcliff, 1992, for review of methods for dealing with reaction time outliers). Thus, various "decision rules" were created, for example, one decision rule dealt with the issue of an extraneous noise (e.g., the child's mother trying to encourage her son/daughter, despite experimenter instructions not to) inadvertently triggering the computer's voice key. Another dealt with the child accidentally repeating the prime rather than naming the picture target. Although Meyer and Schriefers (1991) provide some explanation for how they dealt with artifact "errors" in data, it was obvious that working with young children required a quantitatively as well as qualitatively different set of guidelines. In the end, statistical analysis was performed on *only* those data that seemingly represented "true" reaction time values, based on accurate, correctly articulated, fluent picture-naming responses.

Conclusion

Our studies to date of young CWS make clear that we have only begun to explore the nature of childhood phonological encoding in general and specifically, and how this process may contribute to instances of stuttering produced by young children. From our studies as well as others, it appears as if some CWS demonstrate an impaired ability to quickly and accurately phonologically encode relative to their non-stuttering peers. However, in addition to problems exhibited within the phonological encoder, there may be additional linguistic processes (e.g., semantic and syntactic) that are problematic for CWS.

For instance, other linguistic (e.g., semantic and syntactic) variables involved in the planning or formulation of the utterance have been shown to be associated with stuttering. For example, increases in utterance length and grammatical complexity have been shown to be significantly associated with instances of stuttering (e.g., Bernstein Ratner & Sih, 1987; Logan & Conture, 1995, 1997; Logan & LaSalle, 1999; Melnick & Conture, 2000; Yaruss, 1999). In fact, Zackheim and Conture, (2003), recently found that it is not only utterance characteristics that influence stuttering, but the relationship of these properties to the child's mean length of utterance that are highly associated to childhood stutterings. Importantly, these utterance characteristics (e.g., utterance length and complexity), seemingly change at a speed at least as rapid if not more rapid than the act of stuttering itself (the latter being a necessary aspect of any variable thought to be associated with instances of stuttering). Indeed, the predictability of what grammatical units and/or lexical items in the utterance are associated with instances of stuttering (Bloodstein, 1995, pp. 246–8) strongly suggests the need to consider *covert* processes that typically occur prior to *overt* motoric execution of articulation, phonation and respiration. Consequently, we have begun to examine differences in speech reaction time between CWNS and CWS during semantic and syntactic priming tasks (work similar to that recently reported by Smith and Wheeldon, 2001, with adults with typical speech and language abilities).

Implications for such findings include a number of suggestions to parents or caregivers of young CWS. For instance, if children cannot quickly and accurately encode phonological (or semantic or syntactic) units, then perhaps allowing such children additional planning time during conversational speech may help them. Similarly, not interrupting children may, likewise, enable them more time in which to plan or construct utterances, retrieve words, and/ or develop a phonetic plan.

Whether CWS experience, as a group, subtle to more gross difficulties with linguistic planning is, of course, an empirical question. Thus, suggesting intervention strategies, based on findings from such study, is still premature. However, a growing body of evidence suggests that linguistic variables/ planning for CWS contribute to their speaking difficulties and if future research findings proves this to be the case, intervention suggestions such as those mentioned here should be consistent with as well as receive support from empirical evidence.

Notes

1 For example, a person is presented with and has to name the word "green" that is superimposed on a red background. Because the word "green" conflicts with the different coloured background, the background colour must be suppressed before the word is named.
2 For example, the order of presentation might be: (1) mask, then (2) prime, then (3) mask, and then (4) target.

References

Anderson, J. D., & Conture, E. G. (2000). Language abilities of children who stutter. *Journal of Fluency Disorders, 25*, 283–304.

Bernstein Ratner, N., & Sih, C. (1987). Effects of gradual increases in sentence length and complexity on children's disfluency. *Journal of Speech and Hearing Disorders, 52*, 278–87.

Blackmer, E. R., & Mitton, J. L. (1991). Theories of monitoring and the timing of repairs in spontaneous speech. *Cognition, 39*, 173–94.

Bloodstein, O. (1995). *A Handbook on Stuttering*. San Diego, CA: Singular Publishing Group, Inc.

Bredart, S. (1991). Word interruption in self-repairing. *Journal of Psycholinguistic Research, 20*, 123–38.

Brooks, P. J., & MacWhinney, B. (1997). Phonological priming in children's picture naming. *Journal of Child Language, 27*, 335–66.

Burger, R., & Wijnen, F. (1999). Phonological encoding and word stress in stuttering and nonstuttering participants. *Journal of Fluency Disorders, 24*, 91–106.

Chang, S., Ohde, R., & Conture, E. (2002). Coarticulation and formant transition rate in young children who stutter. *Journal of Speech, Language, and Hearing Research, 45*, 676–88.

Clark, H., & Wasow, T. (1998). Repeating words in spontaneous speech. *Cognitive Psychology, 37*, 201–42.

Collins, A. F., & Ellis, A. W. (1992). Phonological priming of lexical retrieval in speech production. *British Journal of Psychology, 83*, 375–88.

Conture, E. G. (2001). *Stuttering: Its nature, diagnosis, and treatment*. Needham Heights, MA: Allyn & Bacon.

Dell, G. S. (1986). A spreading activation theory of retrieval in language production. *Psychological Review, 93*, 283–321.

Dell, G., & Juliano, C. (1991). Connectionist approaches to the production of words. In H. F. M. Peters, W. Hulstijn and C. W. Starkweather (Eds.), *Speech motor control and stuttering* (pp. 11–36). Amsterdam: Elsevier Science Publishers, BV.

Dell, G. S., & O'Seaghdha, P. G. (1991). Stages of lexical access in language production. In W. J. M. Levelt (Ed.), *Lexical access in speech production*. Amsterdam: Elsevier Science Publishers, BV.

Glaser, W. R. (1992). Picture-naming. *Cognition, 42*, 61–105.

Goldman, R., & Fristoe, M. (1986). *Goldman-Fristoe test of articulation* (GFTA). Circle Pines, MN: American Guidance Service, Inc.

Hall, K., Amir, O., & Yairi, E. (1999). A longitudinal investigation of speaking rate in preschool children who stutter. *Journal of Speech, Language, and Hearing Research, 42*, 1367–77.

Howell, P., & Au-Yeung, J. (1995). The association between stuttering, Brown's factors, and phonological categories in child stutterers ranging in age between 2 and 12 years. *Journal of Fluency Disorders, 30*, 331–44.

Howell, P., Au-Yeung, J., & Sackin, S. (1999). Exchange of stuttering from function to content words with age. *Journal of Speech, Language, and Hearing Research, 42*, 345–54.

Kent, R. (1984). Stuttering as a temporal programming disorder. In R. Curlee, & I. W. Perkins (Eds.), *Nature and treatment of stuttering: New directions* (pp. 283–302). Boston: College-Hill.

Kolk, H. (1991). Is stuttering a symptom of adaptation or of impairment? In H. F. M. Peters, W. Hulstijn, & C. W. Starkweather (Eds.), *Speech motor control and stuttering* (pp. 131–40). Amsterdam: Elsevier/Excerpta Medica.

Kolk, H. & Postma, A. (1997). Stuttering as a covert repair phenomenon. In R. Curlee, & G. Siegel (Eds.), *Nature and treatment of stuttering: New directions* (2nd ed., pp. 182–203). Needham Heights, MA: Allyn & Bacon.

Lahey, M., Edwards, J., & Munson, B. (2001). Is processing speed related to severity of language impairment? *Journal of Speech, Language, and Hearing Research, 44*, 1354–61.

LaSalle, L., & Carpenter, L. (1994). *The effect of phonological simplification of children's speech fluency*. Paper presented at the Annual Conference of the American Speech, Hearing and Language Association, New Orleans, November.

Levelt, W. J. M. (1983). Monitoring and self-repair in speech. *Cognition, 14*, 41–104.

Levelt, W. J. M. (1989). *Speaking: From intention to articulation*. Cambridge, MA: MIT Press.

Levelt, W. J. M., Roelofs, A., & Meyer, A.S. (1999). A theory of lexical access in speech production. *Behavioral and Brain Sciences, 22*, 1–75.

Levelt, W. J. M., & Wheeldon, L. (1994). Do speakers have access to a mental syllabary? *Cognition, 50*, 239–269.

Logan, K. & Conture, E. (1995). Relationship between length, grammatical complexity, rate, and fluency of conversational utterances. *Journal of Fluency Disorders, 20*, 35–61.

Logan, K. & Conture, E. (1997). Selected temporal, grammatical and phonological characteristics of conversational utterances produced by children who stutter. *Journal of Speech, Language, and Hearing Research, 40*, 107–120.

Logan, K., & LaSalle, L. (1999). Grammatical characteristics of children's conversational utterances that contain dislfuency clusters. *Journal of Speech, Language, and Hearing Research, 42*, 80–91.

Louko, L., Conture, E., & Edwards, M.L. (1999). Treating children who exhibit co-occurring stuttering and disordered phonology. In R. Curlee (Ed.), *Stuttering and related disorders of fluency* (2nd ed.). New York: Thieme Medical Publishers.

Louko, L. J., Edwards, M. L., & Conture, E. G. (1990). Phonological characteristics of young stutterers and their normally fluent peers: Preliminary observations. *Journal of Fluency Disorders, 15,* 191–210.

Martin, R. C., & Jensen, C.R. (1988). Phonological priming in the lexical decision task: A failure to replicate. *Memory and Cognition, 16,* 505–21.

McNamara, T. P., & Holbrook, J. B. (2002). Semantic memory and priming. In I. B. Weiner (Series Ed.), A. F. Healy, & R. Proctor (Vol. Eds.), *Comprehensive handbook of psychology: Vol. 4. Experimental psychology.* Chichester Wiley.

Melnick, K. & Conture, E. (2000). Relationship of length and grammatical complexity to the systematic and nonsystematic errors and stuttering of children who stutter. *Journal of Fluency Disorders, 25,* 21–45.

Melnick, K., Conture, E., & Ohde, R. (2003). Phonological priming in picture naming of young children who do and do not stutter. *Journal of Speech, Language, and Hearing Research, 46,* 1428–32.

Meyer, A. S. (1990). The time course of phonological encoding in language production: The encoding of successive syllables of a word. *Journal of Memory and Language, 29,* 524–45.

Meyer, A. S. (1991). Investigation of phonological encoding through speech error analysis: Achievements, limitations, and alternatives. In W. J. M. Levelt (Ed.), *Lexical access in speech production.* Amsterdam: Elsevier Science Publishers, BV.

Meyer, A.S., & Schriefers, H. (1991). Phonological facilitation in picture-word interference experiments: Effects of stimulus onset asynchrony and types of interfering stimuli. *Journal of Experimental Psychology: Learning, Memory, and Cognition, 17,* 1146–60.

Meyer, D. E., & Schvaneveldt, R. W. (1971). Facilitation in recognizing pairs of words: Evidence of a dependence in retrieval operations. *Journal of Experimental Psychology, 90,* 227–34.

Neely, J. (1991). Semantic priming effects in visual word recognition: A selective review of current findings and theories. In D. Benser and G. Humphreys (Eds.), *Basic processes in reading: Visual word recognition* (pp. 264–336). Hillsdale, NJ: Lawrence Erlbaum Associates, Inc.

Nippold, M. (1990). Concomitant speech and language disorders in stuttering children: A critique of the literature. *Journal of Speech and Hearing Disorders, 55,* 51–60.

Paden, E., & Yairi, E. (1996). Phonological characteristics of children whose stuttering persisted or recovered. *Journal of Speech and Hearing Research, 39,* 981–90.

Paden, E., Yairi, E., and Ambrose, N. (1999). Early childhood stuttering II: Initial status of phonological abilities. *Journal of Speech, Language and Hearing Research, 42,* 1113–24.

Pellowski, M., Conture, E., & Anderson, J. (2000). *Articulatory and phonological abilities of children who stutter.* Poster presentation presented at the Third Conference of the International Fluency Association, Nyborg, Denmark.

Postma, A., & Kolk, H. (1993). The covert repair hypothesis: prearticulatory repair processes in normal and stuttered disfluencies. *Journal of Speech and Hearing Research, 36,* 472–87.

Radeau, M., Morais, J., & Dewier, A. (1989). Phonological priming in spoken word recognition: Task effects. *Memory and Cognition, 17,* 525–35.

Ratcliff, R. (1992). Methods for dealing with reaction time outliers. *Psychological Bulletin, 11*, 3, 510–32.

Roelofs, A. (1992). A spreading-activation of lemma retrieval in speaking. *Cognition, 42*, 107–42.

Roelofs, A. (1997). The WEAVER model of word-form encoding in speech production. *Cognition, 64*, 249–84.

Rouibah, A., Tiberghien, G., & Lupker, S. J. (1999). Phonological and semantic priming: Evidence for task-independent effects. *Memory and Cognition, 27*, 3, 422–37.

Shattuck-Hufnagel, S. (1979). Speech errors as evidence for a serial-order mechanism in sentence production. In W. E. Cooper & E. C. T. Walker (Eds.), *Sentence processing: Psycholinguistic studies presented to Merrill Garrett*. Hillsdale, NJ: Lawrence Erlbaum Associates, Inc.

Shattuck-Hufnagel, S. (1983). Sublexical units and suprasegmental structure in speech production planning. In P. F. MacNeilage (Ed.), *The production of speech* (pp. 109–136). New York: Springer Verlag.

Smith, M., & Wheeldon, L. (2001). Syntactic priming in spoken sentence production – an online study. *Cognition, 78*, 123–64.

Stemberger, J. P. (1982). The nature of segments in the lexicon: Evidence from speech errors. *Lingua, 56*, 43–65.

Stemberger, J. P. (1985). An interactive activation model of language production. In A.W. Ellis (Ed.), *Progress in the psychology of language*, Vol. 1 (pp. 143–186). Hillsdale, NJ: Lawrence Erlbaum Associates, Inc.

Stroop, J. R. (1935). Studies of interference in serial verbal reactions. *Journal of Experimental Psychology, 18*, 643–61.

Throneburg, R., Yairi, E., & Paden, E. (1994). Relation between phonologic difficulty and the occurrence of disfluencies in the early stage of stuttering. *Journal of Speech and Hearing Research, 37*, 504–509.

Van Turennout, M., Hagoort, P., & Brown, C. M. (1997). Electrophysiological evidence on the time course of semantic and phonological processes in speech production. *Journal of Experimental Psychology: Learning, Memory, and Cognition, 23*, 4, 787–806.

Wijnen, F., & Boers, I. (1994). Phonological priming effects in stutterers. *Journal of Fluency Disorders, 19*, 1–20.

Wingate, M. (1988). *The structure of stuttering*. New York: Springer Verlag.

Woodworth, R.S. (1938). *Experimental psychology*. New York: H. Holt and Company.

Yairi, E., Ambrose, N., Paden, E. & Throneberg, R. (1996). Pathways of chronicity and recovery: Longitudinal studies of early childhood stuttering. *Journal of Communication Disorders, 29*, 51–77.

Yaruss, J. S. (1999). Utterance length, syntactic complexity, and childhood stuttering. *Journal of Speech, Language and Hearing Research, 42*, 329–44.

Zackheim, C., & Conture, E. (2003). Childhood stuttering and speech disfluencies in relation to children's mean length of utterance: A preliminary study. *Journal of Fluency Disorders, 28*, 115–42.

7 Syllables in the brain: Evidence from brain damage

Chris Code

Abstract

Syllabification appears to play a significant organizational role in speech production, and it has been suggested that it is hard-wired in the brain. In this chapter, psycholinguistic and bio-evolutionary models of syllable production form the basis for an examination of evidence from a range of studies of retained and impaired syllabification in brain-damaged individuals. Some aspects of syllabification survive significant brain damage very well, which raises the question of the status of the mental representation of syllabification. The review concludes that while some more automatic and overused aspects of syllabification involve diffuse and bilateral processing, less automatic, more online, syllable production involves a network of structures in the left inferior frontal and temporal lobes.

Introduction

Syllabification appears to enjoy a significant organizational role in speech production. The ways in which consonants and vowels cluster together to form patterns we call syllables is a prominent feature of the sound structure of language. Is it therefore reasonable to expect that syllabification should be well represented neurally and there should be evidence to show this? Most aspects of syllabification appear to survive brain damage well and Sussman (1984) hypothesized that this is because syllabification is hard-wired in the brain, specifically in the left hemisphere.

The cognitive neuroscientific approach to neuropsychology seeks convergence of evidence from the psycholinguistics laboratory, the speech science laboratory, the imaging suite and the clinic. In this chapter, we focus on the effects of brain damage on syllable production to see what light it can throw on our understanding of the theoretical status of the syllable and the neural representation of syllable production. Some people with left hemisphere brain damage appear to show impairments of syllable production, while others do not. Some lesions, while having a significant impact on speech and language processing, appear to leave unimpaired some features of syllable production. Studies range from those that have examined the effects of small discreet lesions to studies of the remaining speech of people who have had the complete left cerebral hemisphere removed through surgery.

We conduct this examination with reference to psycholinguistic and neurobiological models: the psycholinguistic model of syllable production proposed by Levelt and colleagues (Levelt, 1989; Levelt & Wheeldon, 1994) and the frame/content theory of the evolutionary origins and neural representation of syllable production developed by MacNeilage (1998a), where syllabification is seen as central to the very origins of human speech. The reader is also referred to Chapter 1 of the current volume, where Hartsuiker et al. present the continuity thesis, which holds that pathological deviations in speech can be explained similarly to 'normal' deviations as the result of impairments to specific components of the speech formulation mechanism and of interactions between these components.

We do not consciously guide all of our mental and motor activity. There is a great deal that is automatic and routine in speech production and much of speech processing is not under moment-to-moment control, with each segment being individually planned and sequentially executed online. This principle appears to apply to all levels of language processing, including syllable production. Syllables are formed from a combining of consonant and vowel speech gestures: the basic or simplest form being the CV syllable. The syllable organizational concept of sonority has been used by phonologists in the description of sonority hierarchies and in the description of sequencing of syllables, and in the ordering of segments within syllables. Sound segments can be ordered along a "sonority" hierarchy or scale from most to least sonorous with obstruents (stops, fricatives and affricates) at the least sonorant end, followed by nasals, liquids, glides to vowels at the most sonorant end. The sonority sequencing principle (SSP) (Clements, 1990) aims to account for segment ordering within syllables, by positing a syntagmatic relationship between the segments that is defined by relative sonority.

This approach sees the syllable peak (normally a vowel) as being highlighted by there being an increase of sonority from the syllable onset to the peak, and then a decrease of sonority from the syllable peak to the coda. Syllables are divided into demisyllables. The onset and peak of a syllable make up the initial demisyllable, and the peak and coda make up the final demisyllable. The ideal expression would be for obstruents to take the onset and coda positions, resulting in a maximum difference in sonority between those outlying positions and the peak.

Some syllables are used by speakers more than others. With something like the 80 most frequently used syllables, a speaker can generate about 50 percent of their speech, even though over 12,000 syllabic combinations can occur in English (Levelt, 1989). This fact has prompted researchers to postulate that more often used high frequency syllable combinations are produced more automatically, and should have discrete cognitive processes underlying their organization and production. Levelt and colleagues (e.g., Levelt, 1989; Levelt

& Wheeldon, 1994) have investigated a two-route phonetic encoding model which proposes that syllables that are more frequently used are stored as pre-programmed units and less frequently used syllable sequences require online assembly each time they are used by a speaker. Levelt and Wheeldon's (1994) reaction time experiments suggested that normal speakers have at their disposal this dual route encoding for syllable production. Normal speech is therefore constructed from more automatically produced and more frequently used syllables via a direct encoding route and less frequently used syllables, requiring online assembly, from an indirect route. There have been recent attempts to explain some of the features of acquired apraxia of speech (AOS) with reference to the two-route model and we examine these here.

According to MacNeilage's theory, syllable "frames" evolved through natural selection from ingestive cycles basic to feeding: Speech production originally developed in humans from the combination of mandibular oscillations, first used only in chewing, and laryngeal sounds. (The original purpose of the larynx was to prevent food passing into the airway.) The "syllabification" produced by the coming together of articulators with the sound produced by the larynx formed a primitive proto-speech. Syllabification, according to the theory, is seen as the oldest and most fundamental organizational system for speech. Speech became overlaid on this basic frame. Independence from this basic frame emerges, giving rise to syllabic *content*, which is mainly shaped by the lips and tongue, accounting for segmental phonological features. Studies by MacNeilage and his colleagues (MacNeilage, 1998a; MacNeilage & Davis, 2000; MacNeilage, Davis, Kinney, & Matyear, 1999a, 1999b) on the development of babbling in infants suggests an early frame-without-content stage, before words emerge. Babbling, which emerges universally at about 7 months, is characterized by a fairly strict order of appearance of consonant/vowel (CV) combinations. This ontogeny mirrors the hypothesized phylogenic development of speech in evolution and MacNeilage (1998a) suggests separate neural representation for frames and content in adult brains. He has put forward the hypothesis that syllabic frames are generated by the supplementary motor area (SMA) and anterior cingulate in the left dorsomedial frontal cortex, while syllabic content is represented in and around Broca's area in lateral inferior frontal left hemisphere. Commentators on MacNeilage's theory question the role of these particular neural sites in frame and content control (Abbs & DePaul, 1998; Jürgens, 1998), the likelihood that frame and content enjoy separate neural representation (Lund, 1998), the idea that speech developed from the jaw movements of mastication (Jürgens, 1998), and whether syllables are anything more than epiphenomenal consequences of speech processing (Ohala, 1998).

Using the dual-route hypothesis and the frame/content theory we shall examine how syllabification is represented in the brain from the perspective of the evidence from studies of retention and impairment in syllable processing in individuals with brain damage.

Syllabification following left brain damage

Brain damage in adult life can result in a wide range of speech and language impairments, but in this section we shall be concerned solely with those studies with brain-damaged people that have focused on syllable production. Syllabification has been examined particularly in aphasic speech automatisms, jargon aphasia, apraxia of speech (AOS), supplementary motor area (SMA) damage and left hemispherectomy. Studies in aphasia and apraxia of speech support the idea that certain kinds of speech and language breakdown may involve loss of control over more complex syllable structures and in separate aspects of syllable production.

Syllabification in nonfluent and fluent aphasia

Two major types of aphasic speech automatism that can occur in nonfluent motor aphasia have been identified, and their essential features have been clarified in recent years (Code, 1982, 1996; Wallesch, 1990). *Speech automatism* is the general term used for stereotyped and involuntarily reiterative utterances that can commonly occur in "motor" aphasia, whether made up of real legal words (lexical) or concatenated CV syllables (non lexical). *Recurring utterance* (RU) is also used to refer to the non-lexical variety of speech automatism made up of concatenated CV syllables. Examples of both types appear in Table 7.1.

An important feature of NLSAs is that, for the most severely affected, the utterance is perceptually indistinguishable from previous productions each time it is produced, although meaningful and communicatively functional intonation is relatively unimpaired. Among other aphasic and possibly apraxic impairments, there appears to be a failure of retrieval of new syllabic constituent structure.

Lexical speech automatisms are made up of recognizable words and are syntactically correct structures in the overwhelming majority of cases (Code, 1982). The utterances do not break the syntactic rules of the language. Analysis has shown that NLSAs are mainly made up of reiterated and concatenated CV syllables (although CVC and VCV occur too), and do not break the phonotactic constraints of the native language of the speaker.

Where the frequency of phones used in the lexical variety correlates highly

Table 7.1 Selected lexical speech automatisms (LSAs) and non-lexical speech automatisms (NLSAs) (from Code, 1982)

Lexical speech automatisms		Non-lexical recurring utterances	
I can't	I can talk	/tu tu tu uuuu/	/wi wi wi/
I can try	I said	/bi bi/	/di di/
I want	I want to	/ta ta/	/du du du/
bloody hell	fucking hell		

with normal English phoneme counts, for NLSAs the frequency of occurrence does not correlate with normal usage. There is a marked increase in vowel articulations in NLSAs: The ratio of consonants to vowels was found to be 47 percent to 53 percent (normal English = 62.54 percent to 37.46 percent) and only 21 of the available 24 phonemes of British English were used (data from Code, 1982).

The distribution of consonants in terms of the articulatory features voice and place in non-lexical recurring utterances is similar to conversational English. However, the manner of articulation – stop, fricative, nasal, etc. – shows that stops account for over 62 percent of consonant productions (normal English = 29.21 percent), fricatives for over 22 percent (normal English = 28.01 percent) (these both making the phonological feature obstruent), and sonorants for 7.5 percent (normal English = 19.42 percent); nasal sonorants were examined separately, and accounted for 7.5 percent (normal English = 18.46 percent) (Code, 1982). So there is a distinct increase in the use of the motorically simpler and unmarked articulations with a corresponding reduction in motorically more complex and more marked articulation.

An aphasic non-lexical speech automatism represents perhaps one of the most primitive utterances a human being can produce, paralleling perhaps the development of babbling in infant speech. Unlike infant babbling, however, they are invariant and unchanging. The speaker is unable, in the most severe cases, to vary the utterance (although they can in many cases vary suprasegmental features, and use this in compensatory ways to aid communication).

Code and Ball (1994) explored syllabification in aphasic non-lexical speech automatisms and the surviving speech of adult left hemispherectomees. We examined the syllable structure of the NLSAs of English and German aphasic speakers. We accessed two main collections of data on non-lexical speech automatisms, those reported for British English subjects in Code (1982), and those for German speakers described in Blanken, Wallesch, and Papagno (1990). This resulted in a total of 102 syllables for British English corpus, and 119 syllables for the German corpus.

We conducted a sonority analysis to see how far NLSAs adhere to normal syllabification patterns. We divided all syllables into demisyllables and all demisyllables were further divided into utterance peripheral (i.e., initial or final) and embedded (initial and final embedded). Demisyllables were constructed from the English and German data. All demisyllables were assigned to a demisyllable context, syllable shape (CV, CCV, V, VC), and demisyllable sonority profile (obstruent-vowel, nasal-vowel, vowel-obstruent, etc). Initial and embedded initial demisyllables were most frequently of the form CV. Of these CV types, obstruent-vowel was the most common demisyllable shape for both demisyllable types in both languages (over 50 percent in both English and German).

Only two initial consonant clusters occurred in the English data, both of the obstruent-liquid-vowel type (/pr/ and /br/), and both in embedded initial demisyllables. The vowel initial pattern occurred in 31 percent of the utterance initial demisyllables, and 15 percent of the utterance embedded. In German vowel initials were found in 11 percent of the utterance initial and 9 percent of the utterance embedded. Utterance final and embedded final demisyllables were both overwhelmingly of the vowel type in both languages. In syllable onset position (both utterance initial and embedded initial demisyllables) for both English and German aphasic speakers, by far the most common obstruent category was stop, agreeing with the notion of the maximal change from the onset to the syllable peak.

In short: (i) the syllable shapes used are generally of the simplest type phonotactically; (ii) the sonority patterns of the demisyllables adhere closely to those predicted in sonority theory; and (iii) no examples were found of language specific phonotactic ordering that supersede the sonority sequencing principle. Phonotactic constraints are rigidly adhered to and strict syllabification retained.

These facts may suggest that the initial production (the first time the utterance is produced following the brain injury) of a non lexical speech automatism is by a severely damaged left hemisphere encoding system. NLSAs represent frame without content, in the sense that, while they are CV in structure, they are unchanging; a sort of *frame aphasia*, as Abry, Stefanuto, Vilain, and Laboissière (2001) have termed it (although the term could just has well have been "content" aphasia, given that the impairment appears to be with content, rather than frame production). The syllabic content of the utterance is unchanging and invariant, suggesting damage to those areas directly responsible for syllabic content or for inhibitory control of repeated content of the syllable.

Blanken (1991) and Code (1994) proposed that an impairment to the articulatory buffer (Levelt, 1989), responsible for holding the syllable, can account for the unchanging nature of an individual NLSA – and therefore production of new "content". It may be damage to neural structure underlying the buffer that prevents the assembly of new articulatory programmes.

Kornhuber (1977) suggested that NLSAs result from damage to the left basal ganglia, a structure that he pioneered as a program generator. Brunner, Kornhuber, Seemuller, Suger, and Wallesch (1982) examined CT scans from 40 left hemisphere-damaged patients and concluded that as well as damage to the retrolanguage cortex, a lesion of the caudate and the lenticular nucleus of the basal ganglia was critical for the emergence of RUs. However, a further area that has been implicated in speakers with NLSAs is the posterior aspect of the arcuate fasciculus. Dronkers, Redfern, and Shapiro (1993) found that lesions severing this fibre bundle as it emerges out of the temporal lobe are common for speakers with NLSAs. Damage to the arcuate fasciculus is, of course, the classical site for the impairment of repetition, the core feature of conduction aphasia. The arcuate fasciculus is seen as the main route for the transmission of information from Wernicke's area to the anterior speech areas, hence the suggestion that a lesion here is essential for conduction aphasia, although there has been failure to confirm that damage to the arcuate fasciculus is required for repetition impairment, and there is evidence to suggest that the bisection of this fiber tract causes a global impairment of speech production (Dronkers, Redfern, & Knight, 1998; Dronkers, Redfern, & Shapiro, 1993).

An examination of sonority in a nonfluent and agrammatic Broca's aphasic speaker (Romani & Calabrese, 1998) produced similar findings of retained, but simplified, sonority leading the authors to suggest that as this speaker finds an articulatory programme too complex to deal with, then the phonological representation is simplified, resulting in deletions, substitutions and additions. Phonological segments become "syllabified", according to Romani and Carabrese, in the output buffer. The simplification typical of this speech occurs when articulatory planning transforms the abstract phonological features into muscle commands.

Christman (1992) analyzed syllable structure in three neologistic jargon-aphasic speakers. Neologistic jargon aphasia is characterized by apparently phonologically ordered, wordlike utterances, fluently produced but not forming recognizable words. Although they do not make recognizable words, neologisms do obey sonority constraints and they are not constructed with phonological abandon, but rather with a certain degree of phonological regularity. Christman found that initial demisyllable shapes are predominately CV and final demisyllables are most commonly VC. This is a normal, if limited, patterning and is in contrast to English words where other patterns feature relatively highly. The overwhelming majority of both CV and VC patterns in neologistic speech have an obstruent in the C position. In English words, obstruents were also the most common consonant in these patterns, although other types featured to a higher degree. The operation of sonority, then, is not significantly impaired and syllable construction is normal. This led Christman (1992) to support the view that sonority is a hard-wired component of the language system.

The three speakers in Christman's study had predominantly temporoparietal lesions, with one who had some inferior frontal damage. But, in all three jargon aphasia speakers, syllabic frame and content were intact. This may suggest that control for syllabification is more frontally based, and not diffusely represented throughout the brain.

Syllabification and damage to the supplementary motor area

The role of the supplementary motor area (SMA) in speech encoding has received close attention in recent years. In a seminal study, Jonas (1981) reviewed 53 published cases of speech disturbance involving the SMA. Patients had either paroxysmal speech disturbance involving neoplasmic invasion of the SMA (N = 19), speech disturbance with slowly developing neoplasmic SMA lesions (N = 23) or speech disturbance following sudden SMA lesions. A range of impairments were reported – aphonic mutism, uncontrollable involuntary utterances (in paroxysmal disturbances), per-severation, stuttering, dysarthria, and apraxia of speech (AOS). These led Jonas to propose that the SMA facilitates the initiation of propositional speech, has a role in the suppression of non-propositional speech and the pacing of speech, as well as the control of articulation and phonation.

Ziegler, Kilian, and Deger (1997) examined the effects of damage following haemorrhage to the SMA on the syllable production of a 48-year-old woman (SR) who showed an apparent dissociation between syllable frame and con-tent control. Magnetic resonance scanning showed a lesion where "the cortical region including the posterior part of the SMA and anterior cingular cortex was disconnected from the primary motor cortex" (Ziegler et al., 1997, p. 1198). Extensive testing showed that SR was not aphasic and did not have apraxia of speech. She had clear articulation without phonemic or phonetic distortions, although she was "moderately dysfluent, with frequent and pro-longed pausing, false starts and repetitions" (p. 1198). A series of careful experiments suggested that SR had no difficulties with segmental production. She was able to produce real words of length and complexity. However, when asked to produce pseudowords of more than two syllables she became disfluent.

SR's disfluency was related to utterance length rather than segmental content, features which appear to imply that processing associated with the syllabic frame was impaired but not the content, in contrast to the speaker with a NLSA: a suggestion supported by MacNeilage (1998b) and Abry et al. (2001). This evaluation of SR would appear to suggest that the SMA is not involved in the content of syllables, because it was syllable length rather than segmental complexity that was compromised in repetition for SR. The SMA, the authors conclude, must be particularly concerned in multiple segmental and sequential movements and may have "a critical role in the generation of short term memorized motor sequences" (Ziegler et al., 1997, p. 1201). This suggested for Ziegler et al. support for the view that the frames and the content of syllable production have separate neural representation. There appears to be a problem for SR in what Levelt (1989) calls the "unpacking" of the subprogrammes of an assembled programme. A function for the SMA is to apparently download the unpacked programme to Broca's area. The neural networks underlying the articulatory buffering may be represented in a network of structures, given that different kinds of impairments in speech production, resulting from lesions in different locations, may suggest prob-lems with buffering. Therefore, we would expect to find dissociations in syllable production impairments, as indeed we do.

Apraxia of speech

Acquired apraxia of speech (AOS) has been well researched since Broca's (1861) first patient, Leborgne, who was probably the first case of AOS described, as well as the first with a non-lexical speech automatism (*tan, tan*) to be described. AOS is a speech production problem that can be distinguished from aphasia and dysarthria and presents clinically as nonfluent speech. The following discussion is concerned with acquired AOS and the reader is referred to Chapter 8 in the current volume (Nijland & Maassen) for discussion of the impact of developmental apraxia of speech on syllable planning and programming. AOS is variously described as a planning, programming or execution impairment, but recent important discussions (Van der Merwe, 1997; McNeil, Doyle & Wambaugh, 2000) have made significant contributions to clarifying terminological, theoretical and clinical confusion in the field. For these authors pure AOS is clearly a speech *planning* disorder (and specifically *not* a speech *programming* or *execution* disorder, impairments here cause dysarthria), that has four kernel clinical features: (1) lengthened segment durations in vowels in multisyllabic words or words in sentences and in consonants in both phonemically "on target" and "off target" syllables, words, phrases and sentences; (2) lengthened intersegment durations; (3) spectrally distorted (in movement transitions) phonemically on target utterances; (4) distorted sound substitutions, (excluding anticipations, perseverations and exchanges).

This characterization specifically excludes such traditional features of AOS as inconsistency in error production, effortful articulatory searching and groping in the absence of significant motor impairments and problems with initiation of speech and voice as *differentially* diagnostic of AOS (i.e., as able to distinguish AOS from aphasic phonemic paraphasia), while accepting that they can occur *with* AOS. These impairments can arise from phonological specification, speech programming or execution deficits – outside speech planning. Many of these features are true for slips-of-the-tongue as well. (See Hartsuiker et al., Chapter 1 of the current volume, for discussion.) It also implies that the traditional "severity spectrum" of AOS, where AOS can present from mild to severe to mute, should be redefined in terms of other impairments in speech or non-speech motor production impairments that are not due to aphasia or dysarthria. The inconsistent utilization of a variety of terms used to describe non-dysarthric and non-aphasic speech production impairments, like *anarthria, aphemia/dysphemia, phonetic disintegration* may or may not all describe variants of speech planning, programming and/or execution impairments. It also emphasizes, importantly, that many, perhaps most, past studies have examined speakers who may or may not have AOS, according to this characterization. This characterization has a phonemic specification, received from the pre-motor planning phonological phase, as the fundamental unit for articulatory planning.

Workers have observed that a core feature of apraxia of speech seems to be an impairment at the level of syllabification. Keller (1987) suggested that normal speakers can either retrieve more frequently used syllables from a store or need to reassemble less frequently used syllables when they speak. Kent and Rosenbek (1982) have talked of an impairment of independent syllable generation and AOS has been characterized as resulting from some reduced articulatory buffer capacity where the buffer is unable to handle more than one syllable at a time (e.g., Rogers & Storkel, 1999).

The *articulatory buffer* (Levelt, 1989) is a temporary store for generated speech from the phonetic plan: it is the sub-component between the phonetic plan and overt articulation where some forms of apraxic impairment may arise. It deals with situations where generated speech is ahead of articulatory execution. "The Articulator retrieves successive chunks of internal speech from this buffer and unfolds them for execution" (Levelt, 1989, pp. 12–13). For some (e.g., Romani & Calabrese, 1998) syllabification and other parameters, such as pitch and tone, are actually set in the buffer. Errors arising from this executive retrieval and unfolding process can occur that, observed following brain damage, we might call apraxic. Speech errors that appear to be due to problems with programming on Van der Merwe's (1997) model may be most associated with the transition from buffer to execution. Errors that appear to rely on articulatory buffering and arising because of increased memory load would occur more frequently during imitation or repetition and would increase with increase utterance length.

There has been a recent attempt to explain some of the features of AOS with reference to Levelt's (Levelt, 1989; Levelt & Wheeldon, 1994) notion of a direct-indirect, dual-route phonetic-encoding model, which proposes that syllables that are more frequently used, and therefore more automatically produced, are stored as pre-programmed units and more infrequently used syllable sequences require online assembly each time they are used by a speaker. Whiteside and Varley (Varley & Whiteside, 2001; Whiteside & Varley, 1998) have invoked Levelt and Wheeldon's essential distinction and have claimed that many features of AOS suggest that speakers have lost access to stored syllables and have to construct all their speech online using the indirect route only. (Note that Whiteside and Varley's application of the model reverses Levelt's terminology and their direct route is Levelt's indirect route, and vice versa. The authors also deny phoneme selection.) Varley and Whiteside (2001) suggest that such a model would predict dissociations that should result in at least three broad types of AOS: Problems with direct access, problems with indirect access and problems with both kinds of access. A general feature, they suggest (Whiteside and Varley, 1998) is that the speech of an AOS speaker shares similarities with the speech of a non-AOS speaker who is carefully choosing each syllable during attempts to express ideas "online" during an interview or a presentation. For the AOS speaker, access to more frequent and automatic syllable structures is lost to various degrees.

McNeil et al. (2000) and Ziegler (2001) have questioned whether AOS is similar to a normal speaker carefully delivering a talk or in an interview, where most of their production will require less automatically accessed and pre-programmed syllables. Normal speakers have relatively few problems producing unfamiliar words, AOS speakers have major problems. Ziegler (2001) points out that one would expect AOS speakers to articulate all words normally, irrespective of their frequency, if only access to the high frequency store is the problem. Non-dysarthric speech production impairment can present as a continuum from mutism to a mild articulatory imprecision, implying more than damage only to a directly accessed high frequency syllabary.

While researchers still seek the syllabary, psycholinguistic evidence for its existence is shaky. A criticism of Levelt and Wheeldon's (1994) study is that it did not control sufficiently some crucial variables, and in a re-analysis of the Levelt and Wheeldon (1994) data, Levelt and Meyer (reported in Hendriks & McQueen, 1995) attempted to replicate the syllable frequency effect but while controlling for segment frequency, demisyllable frequency and word frequency. With these variables better controlled, the syllable frequency effect disappeared.

We would want to observe double dissociations between speakers with damage only to automatic syllabic access and only to low frequency online syllabic access. At the lexical level and above we can observe speakers with some retained use of automatic speech and at least one case of right basal ganglia damage has suggested that automatic and propositional speech can dissociate.

Speedie, Wertman, Ta'ir, and Heilman (1993) described a right-handed Hebrew–French bilingual whose automatic speech was disrupted following haemorrhage involving the right basal ganglia. The patient had normal language but had marked difficulties counting up to 20 and reciting the Hebrew prayers and blessings before eating. These prayers and blessing were so familiar to him that he had recited them daily throughout his life. He could not recite the intoned prayers or sing highly familiar songs, although he could hum some of them. His comprehension of emotional prosody was intact but he could not produce emotional prosody. He had an impaired ability to swear and curse also, although he had been but an occasional swearer. He was unable to provide the appropriate expletive for particular situations or complete a curse. Despite these impairments in production he was able to comprehend the automatic and nonpropositional speech he could not produce. At three years post-onset he had not recovered these automatic and nonpropositional speech abilities. This appears to be the first case to demonstrate a dissociation between nonpropositional and propositional speech and provide some evidence of right hemisphere dominance for automatic and nonpropositional aspects of speech. The authors suggest that the lesion may have disrupted limbic system input to automatic speech production while leaving comprehension intact.

Despite this dramatic case of impaired automatic and retained propositional speech at the word and phrase production level (although it is probable that nonpropositionally produced words and phrases are produced as holistic chunks; see Code, 1987, and Van Lancker, 1987, for arguments in favour of this hypothesis), it is less clear that such dissociations can be observed at the syllabic production level, although we might note that more automatically produced speech is made up mainly of high frequency syllable combinations, which confound attempts to tease apart the two parameters.

Since Broca's time, the area named after him has been the traditional lesion site for AOS and its central role is speech *planning* is not disputed (see Van der Merwe, 1997, for review). More recently Dronkers (1996) compared the CT or MRI scans of 25 speakers she classified as apraxic on traditional features, with 19 stroke survivors without AOS. For AOS speakers she found lesions that all included the precentral gyrus of the anterior insula of the left hemisphere, but the insula was spared in all 19 speakers without AOS. The anterior insula, she concludes, may be involved in articulatory planning. Others (McNeil et al., 2000) have questioned whether the selection criteria for speakers with AOS used by Dronkers could have included speakers with aphasic phonemic paraphasia.

McNeil, Weismer, Adams, and Mulligan (1990) used stricter criteria for participant selection (outlined further later) and found that in 4 participants with pure AOS the only shared lesion area was the postcentral facial area. However, there is fMRI evidence that for normal, non-aphasic, speakers the anterior insula is engaged during speech that is executed, and not only planned (Dogil et al., 2002). The insula has connections to most parts of the brain, including the cingulate (Flynn, Benson, & Ardila, 1999) and is implicated in a number of language-related processes including calculation (Cowell, Egan, Code, Harasty & Watson, 2000), phonological decision making (Rumsey, Horwitz, Donohue, Nace, Maisog & Andreason, 1997) and verbal affect (Ardila, 1999).

The insidious degeneration in speech production from mild to mute observed with progressive fronto atrophy (Ball, Code, Tree, Dawe, & Kay, 2004; Code, Tree, Dawe, Kay, Ball, & Edwards, 2002) appears to provide additional support for a wide neurally and phylogenically represented network underlying speech planning, programming and execution. It appears that damage to a number of left frontotemporal areas can disrupt syllable production in various ways, providing support for the existence of a network of structures engaged in the transformation of the products of phonological encoding into the input for phonetic encoding. These structures are the posterior SMA, anterior cingulate, Broca's area and the anterior insula. However, there is evidence that, at least for more automatic aspects of syllable production, a left hemisphere is not required at all. Adult left hemispherectomy patients have a range of retained, if very limited, speech production abilities (Code, 1996, 1997), and in the final section we consider the effects of complete removal of the left hemisphere on syllable production.

Left hemispherectomy

Sussman (1984) hypothesized that syllable structure survives the most severe left hemisphere damage and phonotactic constraints are not seen to be violated in even the most severely aphasic speakers, and this is because syllabification is hard-wired in the brain, specifically in the left hemisphere. He develops a neuronal model where each consonant and vowel position is associated with a specific cell assembly network.

For the adult patients E.C. and N.F. (Burklund & Smith, 1977; Smith & Burklund, 1966), the surgery was sufficiently radical to rule out the possibility of the involvement of remaining left subcortical structures and the standardized testing sufficiently detailed to allow the confident conclusion that only the right hemisphere could be responsible for the observed speech (see Code, 1996, for further discussion). Importantly, E.C and N.F. were adults in their middle years, with fully mature neural systems.

The remaining speech of E.C. and N.F. appears to be predominantly nonpropositional and formulaic, although there was some good object naming (with some paraphasia) and digit, word and sentence repetition. E.C. and N.F. produced novel speech in response to questions and other stimuli in the environment, much of this appears to be situation specific and reactive rather than novel and generative (e.g., "Got a match?"). Phonotactic constraints are not broken in the speech of these subjects and syllabification is organized according to normal sonority. That is to say, removal of the left hemisphere in these right-handed adults, although devastating for speech and language processing, does not appear to impede syllabification of remaining speech. While syllabification was not examined directly, there are no instances in the reported data where phonotactic and sonority rules are broken.

This seems to confirm that Sussman's hypothesis that syllabification is hard-wired specifically in the left hemisphere cannot be correct but, if hard-wired at all, syllabification is diffusely represented throughout the brain.

One further speculation is that the nonpropositional utterances of left hemispherectomy speakers and the lexical (but not the non-lexical) speech automatisms of aphasic speakers, were generated by a left hemisphere system in early development. The right hemisphere's processing of automatic and nonpropositional speech may be its part of a task-sharing metasystem between right and left hemispheres. This would allow the left hemisphere more processing space for the online generation of novel speech and language, presumably the most demanding and exacting of human activities. Syllabification of nonpropositional utterances may have been well established during earlier extended pre-surgery usage by the speaker without a left hemisphere. Automatic aspects of syllabification at least clearly survive global damage to the neurolinguistic system and even complete left hemispherectomy. It would therefore appear to be a most successful survivor of brain damage.

Conclusions

Figure 7.1 presents a summary of some conclusions we might draw from the brain damage evidence. This shows some implicated neural sites where syllable frame and content processing may occur as suggested by studies of syllable production in brain damaged individuals.

Results of damage	Neural structure	Cognitive process
Impairment of syllable frame processing (Case SR)	Posterior SMA anterior cingulate	Syllable frame generation

Impairment of syllable content processing (NLSAs)	Broca's area	Syllable content generation

Figure 7.1 Neural representation of aspects of syllable frame and constant processing as suggested from studies of syllable production following brain damage.

Separate internally generated and externally triggered action systems have been identified (Bradshaw, 2001; Jahanshahi & Frith, 1998). For actions that are internally generated, voluntary and self-initiated, the dorsolateral prefrontal cortex, anterior cingulate, SMA, putamen and thalamus in the basal ganglia are engaged. For actions that are externally triggered the lateral premotor and inferior parietal areas combine with anterior cingulate, but SMA is not involved. There would appear to be an SMA-anterior cingulate-basal system responsible for initiation and "moving on" for speech and voice and an inferior frontal-Broca's-operculum-premotor-basal system with parietal input responsible for syntax and sequential gestural communication (Arbib, in press; Corballis, 2002). NLSAs appear to arise from the left SMA deprived of basal ganglia inhibition (Abry et al., 2001; Code, 1994).

Ziegler's case SR would appear to suggest that the posterior SMA and anterior cingulate may constitute the structure where syllabic frames are generated. Extra articulatory buffering appears to be necessary for the processing of less familiar syllable combinations. If syllabic content is unimpaired by SMA damage, but is impaired with damage to Broca's area (the "frame" aphasia of the speaker with a NLSA) and the anterior insula (maybe the buffering problems of the AOS speaker), this may suggest that buffering relies on structures in and around Broca's area and the anterior insula in the left frontotemporal brain. Damage to these structures results in various kinds of distinct disruptions to speech production entailing syllabic control and they appear to be crucial for syllable generation and the holding of syllabic elements while combining into strings.

The survival of frame syllabification following brain damage, even left hemispherectomy, might simply mean that it enjoys no mental reality and is simply an inevitable by-product of speech production, supporting suggestions (Code & Ball, 1994; Ohala, 1998) that it may be a non-causal consequence of neurophysiology and the mechanico-inertial constraints of speech-motor mechanisms. The most robust aspect of "syllabification" then is the basic framing of syllable production, surviving massive brain damage, suggesting highly diffuse representation throughout the cortical and subcortical brain. Aspects of syllable "content" may survive quite well also. Sonority constraints, at least, are not violated in the surviving speech of such varied conditions as jargon aphasia from posterior left hemisphere damage, a variety of acquired and progressive speech production impairments arising from anterior left hemisphere damage, and even total left hemispherectomy. However, severe impairments of speech production accompany most of these conditions. Psycholinguistic research too has so far been unable to confirm the existence of the syllabary, a store for higher frequency syllables.

For Hughlings Jackson (1874) automatic language could come from both the left and right hemispheres, a hypothesis well supported by modern research. Perhaps this same principle underlies syllable production, as well as processing above the syllable. Frequently used syllables, or maybe frequently used syllable frames, may enjoy bilateral representation, and frequently used syllables make up frequently used words, but structures in the left dorsomedial and inferiofrontal brain alone can assemble online a less frequently required syllable. Perhaps beginning at around 7 months with babbling, highly familiar syllable templates get laid down in bilateral networks, and these are utilized in frequently used words and less propositional phrases and expressions. Following some kinds of left brain damage access to bilaterally represented highly familiar syllabic combinations, making up nonpropositional language above the syllable, may be possible; in other kinds they may not.

Acknowledgements

I am grateful to Christian Abry, Michael Arbib, Harvey Sussman and Wolfram Ziegler for comments on an earlier draft of this chapter. This chapter was completed while the author was a visiting fellow of the Hanse Institute for Advanced Study, Delmonhorst, Germany.

References

Abbs, J., & DePaul, R. (1998). Motor cortex fields and speech movements: simple dual control is implausible. *Behavioral and Brain Sciences, 21*, 511–12.

Abry, C., Stefanuto, M., Vilain, A., & Laboissière, R. (2001). What can the utterance "tan, tan" of Broca's patient Leborgne tell us about the hypothesis of an emergent "babble-syllable" downloaded by SMA? In J. Durand, & B. Laks (Eds.), *Phonetics, phonology and cognition* (pp. 226–43). Oxford: Oxford University Press.

Arbib, M. (in press). Beyond the mirror system: From monkey-like action recognition to human language. *Behavioral & Brain Sciences*.

Ardila, A. (1999). The role of insula in language: An unsettled question. *Aphasiology*, *13*, 79–87.

Ball, M. J., Code, C., Tree, J. Dawe, K. & Kay, J. (2004). Phonetic and phonological analysis of progressive speech degeneration: A case study. *Clinical Linguistics & Phonetics*, *18*, 447–62.

Blanken, G. (1991). The functional basis of speech automatisms (recurring utterances). *Aphasiology*, *5*, 103–27.

Blanken, G., Wallesch, C.-W., & Papagno, C. (1990). Dissociations of language functions in aphasics with speech automatisms (recurring utterances). *Cortex*, *26*, 41–63.

Bradshaw, J. L. (2001). *Developmental disorders of the frontostriatal system*. Hove, UK: Psychology Press.

Broca, P. (1861). Remarques sur le siège de la faculté du langage articulé suivi d'une observation d'aphemie (perte de la parole). *Bulletin de la Societé d'Anatomie de Paris*, *36*, 330–57.

Brunner, R. J., Kornhuber, H. H., Seemuller, E., Suger, G., & Wallesch, C.-W. (1982). Basal ganglia participation in language pathology. *Brain and Language*, *16*, 281–99.

Burklund, C. W., & Smith, A. (1977). Language and the cerebral hemispheres. *Neurology*, *27*, 627–33.

Christman, S. S. (1992). Uncovering phonological regularity in neologisms: contributions of sonority theory. *Clinical Linguistics & Phonetics*, *6*, 219–47.

Clements, G. N. (1990). The role of the sonority cycle in core syllabification. In Kingston, J., & Beckman, M. (Eds.), *Papers in laboratory phonology I: Between the grammar and the physics of speech*. Cambridge: Cambridge University Press.

Code, C. (1982). Neurolinguistic analysis of recurrent utterance in aphasia. *Cortex*, *18*, 141–52.

Code, C. (1987). *Language, aphasia, and the right hemisphere*. Chichester: Wiley.

Code, C. (1996) Speech from the right hemisphere? Left hemispherectomy cases E.C. and N.F. In C. Code, C.-W. Wallesch, Y. Joannette, & A.-R. Lecours (Eds.), *Classic cases in neuropsychology*. Hove, UK: Psychology Press.

Code, C. (1994). Speech automatism production in aphasia. *Journal of Neurolinguistics*, *8*, 135–148.

Code, C. (1997). Can the right hemisphere speak? *Brain & Language*, *57*, 38–59.

Code, C. (1998). Models, theories and heuristics in apraxia of speech. *Clinical Linguistics & Phonetics*, *12*, 47–66.

Code, C. & Ball, M. J. (1994). Syllabification in aphasic recurring utterances: contributions of sonority theory. *Journal of Neurolinguistics*, *8*, 257–65.

Code, C., Tree, J., Dawe, D., Kay, J., Ball, M., & Edwards, M. (2002). *A case of progressive speech deterioration with apraxias*. Paper presented to the Joint BAS-BNS Autumn Meeting, 3–4 October, University of York, UK.

Corballis, M. C. (2002). *From hand to mouth: The origins of language*. Princeton, NJ: Princeton University Press.

Cowell, S. F., Egan, G. F., Code, C., Harasty, J., & Watson, J. (2000). The functional neuroanatomy of simple calculation and number repetition: A parametric PET activation study. *NeuroImage, 12,* 565–73.

Dogil, G., Ackermann, H., Grodd, W., Haider, H., Kamp, H., Mayer, J., Rieckman, A., & Wildgruber, D. (2002). The speaking brain: A tutorial introduction to fMRI experiments in the production of speech, prosody and syntax. *Journal of Neurolinguistics, 15,* 59–90.

Dronkers, N. (1996). A new brain region for coordinating speech articulation. *Nature, 384,* 159–61.

Dronkers, N., Redfern, B. B., & Knight, R. (1998). The neural architecture of language disorders. In M. S. Gazzaniga (Ed.), *The new cognitive neurosciences.* Cambridge, MA: MIT Press.

Dronkers, N. F., Redfern, B. B., & Shapiro, J. K. (1993). Neuroanatomic correlates of production deficits in severe Broca's aphasia. *Journal of Clinical and Experimental Neuropsychology, 15,* 59–60.

Flynn, F. G., Benson, D. F., & Ardila, A. (1999). Anatomy of the insula-functional and clinical correlates. *Aphasiology, 13,* 55–78.

Hendriks, H., & McQueen, J. (1995). *Annual report of the Max-Planck-Institut für Psycholinguistik.* Nijmegen, The Netherlands.

Jackson, J. H. (1874). On the nature of the duality of the brain. In J. Taylor (Ed.), *Selected writings of John Hughlings Jackson,* Vol. II. London: Staples Press.

Jahanshari, M., & Frith, C. D. (1998). Willed action and its impairments. *Cognitive Neuropsychology, 15,* 483–533.

Jonas, S. (1981). The supplementary motor region and speech emission. *Journal of Communication Disorders, 14,* 349–73.

Jürgens, U. (1998). Speech evolved from vocalization, not mastication. *Behavioral and Brain Sciences, 21,* 519–20.

Keller, E. (1987). The cortical representations of motor processes of speech. In E. Keller & M. Gopnik (Eds.), *Motor and sensory processes of language.* Hillsdale, NJ: Lawrence Erlbaum Associates, Inc.

Kent, R. D. & Rosenbek, J. (1982). Prosodic disturbance and neurologic lesion. *Brain & Language, 15,* 259–91.

Kornhuber, H. H. (1977). A reconstruction of the cortical and subcortical mechanisms involved in speech and aphasia. In J. E. Desmedt (Ed.), *Language and hemispheric specialization in man: Cerebral ERPs.* Basel: Karger.

Levelt, W. J. M. (1989). *Speaking: From intention to articulation.* Cambridge, MA: MIT Press.

Levelt, W. J. M., & Wheeldon, L. (1994). Do speakers have access to a mental syllabary? *Cognition, 50,* 39–269.

Lund, J. P. (1998). Is speech just chewing the fat? *Behavioral and Brain Sciences, 21,* 522.

MacNeilage, P. (1998a). The frame/content theory of evolution of speech production. *Behavioral and Brain Sciences, 21,* 499–546.

MacNeilage, P. (1998b). Reply: The frame/content theory of evolution of speech production. *Behavioral and Brain Sciences, 21,* 499–546.

MacNeilage, P., & Davis, B. L. (2000), On the origin of internal structure of word forms. Serial-output complexity in speech. *Science, 288,* 527–31.

MacNeilage, P., Davis, B. L., Kinney, A., & Matyear, C. L. (1999a). The motor core of speech: a comparison of serial organization patterns in infants and languages. *Child Development, 71,* 153–63.

MacNeilage, P., Davis, B. L., Kinney, A., & Matyear, C. L. (1999b). Origin of serial-output complexity in speech. *Psychological Science, 10*, 450–59.

McNeil, M. R., Doyle, P. J., & Wambaugh, J. (2000). Apraxia of speech: A treatable disorder of motor planning and programming. In L. J. Gonzalez Rothi, B. Crosson, & S. E. Nadeau (Eds.), *Aphasia and language: Theory to practice*. New York: Guildford Publications.

McNeil, M. R., Weismer, G., Adams, S., & Mulligan, M. (1990). Oral structure non-speech motor control in normal, dysarthric, aphasic, and apraxic speakers: Isometric force and statis position control. *Journal of Speech & Hearing Research, 33*, 255–68.

Ohala, J. (1998). Content first, frame later. *Behavioral and Brain Sciences, 21*, 525–6.

Rogers, M. A., & Storkel, H. L. (1999). Planning speech one syllable at a time: the reduced buffer capacity hypothesis in apraxia of speech. *Aphasiology, 13*, 793–805.

Romani, C., & Calabrese, A. (1998). Syllabic constraints in the phonological errors of an aphasic patient. *Brain and Language, 64*, 121–2.

Rumsey, J. M., Horwitz, B., Donohue, B. C., Nace, K., Maisog, J. M., & Andreason, P. (1997). Phonological and orthographic components of word recognition: a PET-rCBF study. *Brain, 120*, 739–59.

Smith, A., & Burklund, C. W. (1966). Dominant hemispherectomy. *Science, 153*, 1280–82.

Sussman, H. M. (1984). A neuronal model for syllable representation. *Brain and Language, 22*, 167–77.

Speedie, L. J., Wertman, E., Ta'ir, J., & Heilman, K. M. (1993). Disruption of automatic speech following a right basal ganglia lesion. *Neurology, 43*, 1768–74.

Van der Merwe, A. (1997). A theoretical framework for the characterization of pathological speech sensorimotor control. In M. R. McNeil, (Ed.), *Clinical management of sensorimotor speech disorders* (pp. 1–25). New York: Thieme.

Van Lancker, D. (1987). Nonpropositional speech: Neurolinguistic studies. In A. W. Ellis (Ed.), *Progress in the psychology of language*, Vol. II. Hove, UK: Lawrence Erlbaum Associates Ltd.

Varley, R. A., & Whiteside, S. P. (2001). What is the underlying impairment in apraxia of speech? *Aphasiology, 15*, 39–49.

Wallesch, C.-W. (1990). Repetitive verbal behaviour: functional and neurological considerations. *Aphasiology, 4*, 133–54.

Whiteside, S. P., & Varley, R. A. (1998). A reconceptualisation of apraxia of speech: A synthesis of evidence. *Cortex, 34*, 221–31.

Ziegler, W. (2001). Apraxia of speech is not a lexical disorder. *Aphasiology, 15*, 74–7.

Ziegler, W., Kilian, B., & Deger, K. (1997) The role of the left mesial frontal cortex in fluent speech: evidence from a case of left supplementary motor area hemmorrhage. *Neuropsychologia, 35*, 1197–208.

8 Syllable planning and motor programming deficits in developmental apraxia of speech

Lian Nijland and Ben Maassen

Abstract

This chapter gives an overview of research aiming to determine at which levels of speech production the deficits of children with developmental apraxia of speech might be located. We conclude that two levels might be involved in developmental apraxia of speech, namely syllable planning (including the syllabary) and motor programming. Next, the results of two experiments are discussed, each focussing on one of these two levels. The first experiment, in which the syllable structure was manipulated, demonstrated no systematic durational patterns in children with developmental apraxia of speech, a result that is interpreted as signifying a deficit in syllable planning, specifically in using prosodic parameters in articulation. The second experiment showed a deviant effect of a bite-block in children with developmental apraxia of speech as compared to normally speaking children, which supported the interpretation of a motor programming deficit in developmental apraxia of speech. Our conclusion is that in developmental apraxia of speech both syllable planning and motor programming are involved. Insufficient durational control plays a central role at both of these levels.

Introduction

Developmental apraxia of speech is a speech disorder that is characterized by low intelligibility due to the large number of consonantal errors, especially (contextual) substitutions and omissions. Inconsistency of errors and groping (searching articulatory behavior) are typical for developmental apraxia of speech (McNeil, Robin, & Schmidt, 1997). Errors and distortions in vowel productions have also been reported (Pollock & Hall, 1991; Walton & Pollock, 1993), as well as inappropriate stress patterns (Shriberg, Aram, & Kwiatkowski, 1997). Vegetative movements (like coughing, chewing, and swallowing) and non-speech *oral-motor* actions, such as licking an ice cream, or blowing do not necessarily cause difficulties as in oral apraxia.

Describing developmental apraxia of speech as a speech disorder does not preclude the possibility that children with developmental apraxia of speech may demonstrate additional problems, for instance, language or language-related problems (Groenen, Maassen, Crul, & Thoonen, 1996; Guyette & Diedrich, 1981; Hodge, 1994; Hoit-Dalgaard, Murry, & Kopp, 1983; Marion, Sussman, & Marquardt, 1993; McCabe, Rosenthal, & McLeod, 1998). Various studies reported production as well as perception errors. A study of Hoit-Dalgaard et al. (1983), for example, shows that apraxic subjects demonstrate problems in both production and perception of the voicing feature of phonemes. A similar relation between production and perception problems was found in children with developmental apraxia of speech with respect to the feature 'place-of-articulation' (Groenen et al., 1996) in rhyming abilities (Marion et al., 1993). Children with developmental apraxia of speech also often demonstrate 'soft' neurological signs, such as clumsiness and motor coordination problems (Guyette & Diedrich, 1981; Ozanne, 1995; Pollock & Hall, 1991; Robin, 1992).

There is debate among researchers on the exact speech symptoms of developmental apraxia of speech as well as the accompanying non-speech characteristics. Guyette and Diedrich (1981) noted that there are no pathognomic (i.e., differential diagnostic) features to diagnose developmental apraxia of speech and to differentiate developmental apraxia of speech from other speech output disorders. More recent discussions focus on finding the "diagnostic marker" for developmental apraxia of speech. Shriberg et al. (1997) suggested inappropriate stress as a diagnostic marker, which might be applicable to a subtype in approximately 50 per cent of the children diagnosed as developmental apraxia of speech. Some researchers discussed the possibility of a more general inability underlying developmental apraxia of speech (Davis, Jakielski, & Marquardt, 1998; Velleman & Strand, 1994). A study by Thoonen, Maassen, Gabreëls, and Schreuder (1994) yielded a measure for degree of involvement of developmental apraxia of speech based on the maximum repetition rate (MRR), especially in repetitions of trisyllabic utterances (e.g., /pataka/). In contrast, involvement of dysarthria can be assessed on the basis of monosyllabic repetition rate (e.g., /papapa/). This underlined the importance of both monosyllabic and trisyllabic MRR as a diagnostic criterion.

Despite the dispute about pathognomic features, there is more or less agreement about a set of more central or core diagnostic symptoms of developmental apraxia of speech. These comprise a high number of consonant errors, especially substitution in place of articulation, inconsistency in repeated productions, difficulty in sequencing phonemes, especially in diadochokinetic tasks (/pataka/), groping, and resistance to therapy (also see Davis et al., 1998; Hall, Jordan, & Robin, 1993; Thoonen, 1998). Setting aside the ongoing debate, we adopted the selection criteria as proposed by Thoonen, Maassen, Wit, Gabreëls, and Schreuder, 1996.

Besides the dispute on the operational definition of developmental apraxia of speech, also in neuropsychological or neurolinguistic approaches a diversity of views exists with regard to the underlying deficit. Explanations for developmental apraxia of speech range from a disturbance localized at the level of phonological representation, the phonological encoding process, the generation of a phonetic program, to the motor planning, programming and execution levels (Ballard, Granier, & Robin, 2000; Dodd & McCormack, 1995; Hall et al., 1993; McNeil et al., 1997; Ozanne, 1995; Shriberg & Kwiatkowski, 1982; Van der Merwe, 1997). In this chapter we first give an overview of the levels of speech production at which deficits might occur in children with developmental apraxia of speech, and describe speech symptoms that might arise from a deficit at each level. As will be discussed, the specificity of these symptoms for the differentiation of developmental apraxia of speech from other speech disorders in children is low. Subsequently, two experiments are described, that were conducted to test in a more explicit manner the involvement of deficits in syllable planning and motor programming. Finally, we discuss the results and provide answers about the location of the underlying deficit in the speech production process in children with developmental apraxia of speech.

Speech production model

Phonological encoding

According to Levelt (1989), phonological encoding starts with retrieval of the word-form ("lexeme"). Phonological encoding comprises the spelling out of the word's metrical and segmental properties and inserting the segments in the metrical template, resulting in a phonological plan (Levelt, Roelofs, & Meyer, 1999). Deficits at this level may range from underspecified or incorrect lexemes, to an inadequate or delayed phonological rule system that is different from both the target adult form and the age-appropriate developmental level form. In clinical linguistic descriptions an error pattern that remains the same over different events, for example the consistent use of non-developmental (atypical) rules, is often interpreted as referring to these underlying deficits. In addition, one might find phonotactic errors and phoneme sequencing errors, such as true sound substitutions (not distortions perceived as substitutions) and transpositions, including metathesis. For example, 'bath' pronounced as 'path' results from an error at the level of phonological encoding when the wrong (first) phoneme is selected. However, this error might also concern a distortion (rather than a substitution) that emerges at a later stage in speech production (see motor programming), namely when voicing in the first phoneme (differentiating /b/ from /p/) is initiated too late and the /b/ is consequently perceived as /p/. Since phonological planning includes planning of suprasegmental features, prosodic disturbances may also result from this level (Ozanne, 1995; Van der Merwe, 1997).

Mental syllabary

The mental syllabary, as proposed by Crompton (1982 in Levelt et al., 1999, p. 32) and followed by Levelt et al. (1989; Levelt & Wheeldon, 1994), is a repository of gestural programs of frequently used syllables that are collected during phonetic planning (which will be discussed later). Making use of the syllabary has the advantage that the motor plan of a frequently uttered syllable needs not to be computed time and again, but is stored and can be retrieved on demand. Thus conceived, the syllabary can be interpreted as a mechanism for automaticity to ensure fast and effortless production (Varley & Whiteside, 2001;[1] Ziegler, 2001). In addition, it is suggested that there is more coherence of spatial and temporal aspects of articulatory gestures within the syllables than between syllables (Browman & Goldstein, 1997). Syllables that are stored in a syllabary are likely to show more cohesion. A problem in accessing the mental syllabary or restoring a (precompiled) gestural program might thus lead to prolongation and less cohesion of the sounds within the syllable.

Phonetic planning

During phonetic planning a phonological plan is translated into a phonetic plan (McNeil et al., 1997; Ozanne, 1995; Velleman & Strand, 1994). For this, the spatial and temporal goals of the articulatory movements for speech sound productions (the phonetic plan) are collected from a sensorimotor memory and adapted to the surrounding phonemes, or precompiled gestural syllabic programs are collected from the syllabary. A breakdown at this level could cause difficulty in recalling or restoring the correct phonetic plans of specific phonemes resulting in groping behavior on verbal tasks. Also, enhanced differences in performance on voluntary speech versus more automatic, standardized utterances could occur, because the former, being produced "on the fly", requires more contextual adaptation than the latter, which are overlearned. Children with a speech disorder at this level might be able to utter words spontaneously but unable to imitate them, or to produce a sound but unable to do so in the appropriate context. This is due to specific inability in adapting phonemes to the phonetic context arising from a disorder at this processing level (e.g., a child aged 6 who produced "car" as [da], but "dog" as [pɒk]; Ozanne, 1995, p. 108). Thus, investigation of the articulatory cohesion within the syllable (within syllabic coarticulation) could provide information about a possible problem in phonetic planning (Van der Merwe, 1997).

Motor programming

Unlike Levelt & Wheeldon (1994), who suggested an articulatory network as the last stage of speech production in which the exact movement trajectories of the articulators are calculated, others (e.g., Ozanne, 1995; Van der Merwe, 1997) subdivided this last level in two stages: motor programming and motor execution. During motor programming the (more abstract) phonetic plans, that is the articulatory "gestures", are translated into precise articulatory instructions (in a so-called "task dynamical system"; see Browman & Goldstein, 1997; Fowler & Saltzman, 1993). This means that the gesture (defined during phonetic planning) only defines the task of the articulators in an abstract way and does not delineate the exact means to accomplish this task. For example, one of the tasks in producing the consonant /p/ is "lip closure." The execution can consist of movements of the mandibular, the lower lip, both lips, or combinations of these articulators. The information required to reach the set goal is not specified until the motor programming stage.

The motor programming stage also allows compensation, for example, it permits speakers to still produce intelligible speech while clenching a bite-block between the teeth. A malfunction in motor programming affects the process of specifying muscle tone, rate, direction, and range of movements (Van der Merwe, 1997), resulting in problems such as sound distortions, voicing errors, resonance inconsistencies, or phonetic variability of production. Furthermore, a fine motor incoordination might result in slow diadochokinetic rates and the inability to maintain syllable structure, by producing perseverative responses (Ozanne, 1995). The two deficits of poor compensation (in, for example, a bite-block speech condition) and dyscoordination (slow diadochokinetic rates) could interact resulting in complex context-dependent speech patterns (see also Towne, 1994).

Motor execution

In the final stage of motor execution the motor program is transformed into automatic (reflex) motor adjustments, that is, it is implemented by the muscles involved in articulation. Problems at this stage might be due to anatomical anomaly, such as cleft palate, or due to neurological damage affecting muscle strength and coordination (dysarthric qualities).

Modeling developmental apraxia of speech

How do possible underlying deficits in developmental apraxia of speech fit into the model we have just sketched? Diverse explanations for the frequently noted unintelligible speech of children with developmental apraxia of speech range from an impairment in storing and retrieving word-forms, in producing the correct sequence of speech sounds in syllables and words (phonological encoding), in automating speech patterns such as syllables, to deficient phonetic planning and motor programming. Most authors agree that developmental apraxia of speech is not caused by an oral-motor deficit such as dysarthria, although a concomitant dysarthria is possible. Although one might be tempted to interpret speech symptoms in developmental apraxia of speech as a manifestation of one specific processing deficit, which in itself can be a seminal heuristic exercise leading to interesting predictions of possible combinations of symptoms or contexts in which they can occur, one should be very cautious and wait for firm experimental evidence to construct the definite model of developmental apraxia of speech.

One core feature of developmental apraxia of speech is *inconsistency*. Inconsistency of articulatory errors suggests a processing rather than a representational deficit; no consistent use of atypical phonological behavior (i.e. non-developmental rules) has been reported for developmental apraxia of speech that would indicate a common underlying phonological representation problem. Also the fact that most children with developmental apraxia of speech (from age 5 onward) do not demonstrate consistent problems in producing phonemic contrasts on request, suggests that developmental apraxia of speech can occur with a complete and intact *phonological repertoire*.

Furthermore, there is evidence that the origin of the speech symptoms in children with developmental apraxia of speech is to be found in a stage following word-form retrieval, and is a processing rather than (phonological) representation problem (Thoonen, 1998). The evidence consists of studies that reported small differences in number of errors produced by children with developmental apraxia of speech when imitating meaningful as compared to nonsense words, which was in contrast to normally speaking children who produced considerably more errors in nonsense words (Thoonen, Maassen, Gabreëls, & Schreuder, 1994). Following Ozanne (1995) we would argue that developmental apraxia of speech arises from an impairment somewhere in the transition from word-form retrieval into the final articulo-motor output.

Phonetic transcriptions of utterances by children with developmental apraxia of speech have revealed information about the type and amount of speech errors that these children produce in spontaneous speech as well as in repeated utterances. Although large quantitative differences between developmental apraxia of speech and normally speaking children have been reported, namely higher substitution and omission rates, very few qualitative differences in error patterns have been found between children with developmental apraxia of speech, children diagnosed with a phonological speech output disorder and normally speaking children[2] (Forrest & Morrisette, 1999; Thoonen et al., 1994). Thus, both the specificity of the phonological error patterns in children with developmental apraxia of speech and the suggestion of the phonological encoding as *the* underlying deficit can be seriously questioned.

Given the fact that so few specific symptoms are found at the level of phonological encoding and their origin is presumed to lie after the word-form retrieval process, we hypothesize the following. Although children with developmental apraxia of speech produce many phonemic errors, in phonemically *correct* productions in which it can be assumed that the phonological plan was correct, we argue that these children will have problems in the transformation of the phonological plan into a phonetic plan and/or a motor program. This could then become manifest in qualitative differences in the speech productions of children with developmental apraxia of speech as compared to trouble-free productions in normally speaking children.

These qualitative differences in phonemically correct utterances cannot be perceived auditorily, and therefore require a different methodology; acoustical measurements do allow these differences in articulation to be established. For example, prolongation of transitions, steady states, and inter-syllabic pauses, all characteristic of developmental apraxia of speech, can easily be assessed acoustically, but are difficult to recognize perceptually. Acoustic analysis of the speech may, thus, provide further indications with respect to the location of the underlying deficit in developmental apraxia of speech (from phonological encoding onward) and may allow a distinction to be made between a deficient phonetic or syllable plan, a problem in the mental syllabary, or a deficit in motor programming.

The articulatory realization of a segment is highly dependent on the phonetic environment, leading to coarticulation due to preplanning (i.e., anticipatory coarticulation) or carry-over (i.e., perseveratory coarticulation) effects. This means that before a phoneme is actually uttered features of this phoneme (e.g., spectral quality and duration) can influence the preceding phonemes (Whalen, 1990). Problems in planning or in programming of speech movements could influence the syllabic coherence and thus leave their traces in anticipatory coarticulation patterns. The influence of an upcoming vowel in preceding phonemes can be determined by measuring the formant frequencies (especially first and second formant) through the utterance, which is assessed in the present study. For example, the high second formant frequency of an upcoming /i/ versus the low second formant frequency of an /o/ can be found earlier in an utterance (for instance, the Dutch utterance 'ze schiet' /zə#sxit/ ['she shoots'] versus 'ze schoot' /zə#sxot/ ['she shot'] as described later, in experiment 1), reflecting anticipatory coarticulation. Thus, investigating the coarticulation pattern and contextual interdependency in utterances might provide us valuable information about possible problems in planning or programming speech.

In short, children with developmental apraxia of speech seem to have problems in the planning or in the programming of speech movements. In this study, results of two experiments, each focussing on one of these two levels of the speech production process, are discussed (detailed descriptions of the experiments and the results can be found in Nijland, Maassen, & Van der Meulen, 2003, and Nijland, Maassen, Van der Meulen, Gabreëls, Kraaijmaat, & Schreuder, 2003). In the first experiment, we investigated phonetic planning and the mental syllabary. The second experiment focussed on the level of motor programming and execution.

Developmental apraxia of speech: A problem in phonetic planning?

In order to find evidence of deviant phonetic *planning*, a study of the articulatory cohesion within the syllable was conducted (Nijland et al., 2002; Nijland, et al., 2003). Based on the findings that cohesion of articulatory movements within syllables is stronger than between syllables (Byrd, 1995; Levelt et al.,

1999; Nittrouer, Studdert-Kennedy, & Neely, 1996; Whalen, 1990) we argue that articulation is organized on the basis of a stored repository of syllabic gesture scores. As a consequence, the syllable structure of a particular utterance is determinative of the amount of segmental coarticulation. Therefore, we manipulated the syllable structure in an otherwise unchanging sequence of sounds. An example in English is 'I scream' versus 'ice cream' in which the phonemic sequence is identical in both phrases. If the syllable structure is indeed relevant to the amount of coarticulation, then, in this example, the anticipatory coarticulation of the vowel on the preceding /s/ is expected to be stronger in the first phrase (within syllabic coarticulation) than in the second phrase (between syllabic coarticulation). In the first experiment similar manipulations were applied. On the basis of the assumption that developmental apraxia of speech is a problem of phonetic planning, we expected to find different effects of the syllable structure manipulation in children with developmental apraxia of speech as compared to normally speaking children.

Developmental apraxia of speech: A problem in accessing or storing the mental syllabary?

In addition to syllable structure, the first experiment looked at the contrast between highly frequent syllables and syllables with an extremely low (zero) frequency. The assumption is, that a necessary (but not sufficient) condition for storage of syllables in the syllabary is their frequent use in speech. Syllables that are used frequently in the ambient language are therefore more likely to be stored in the syllabary than low frequency syllables. Even if a child is in the process of building a syllabary, we may expect an effect of syllable frequency. If a child is unable to store syllables or to access the syllabary, no difference in coarticulation is expected between high and low frequency syllables.

Developmental apraxia of speech: Deviant motor programming or motor execution?

In order to explore whether in developmental apraxia of speech a deviance might occur during the final stages of speech production we compared the ability of normally speaking children and children with developmental apraxia of speech to compensate their articulatory movements for perturbations (Nijland, Maassen, & Van der Meulen, 2003). Such a compensation is possible from the level of motor programming onward (Van der Merwe, 1997). In the second experiment, children were asked to produce utterances in the condition in which the mandible was fixed by a bite-block clenched between the teeth, such that vertical articulatory movements were blocked. These utterances were compared to a condition without bite-block. It was our premise that problems in compensating articulatory movements in such a bite-block condition might reveal an underlying disruption in motor programming. We expected the children with developmental apraxia of speech to show more problems in adapting to the bite-block condition than the normally speaking children.

Developmental apraxia of speech: A problem in using stress?

An alternative hypothesis was put forward by Shriberg, et al. 1997, who reported that children with developmental apraxia of speech especially have problems in using stress in that unstressed syllables are also stressed. These authors interpreted the deviating durational patterns in the utterances of children with developmental apraxia of speech as resulting from problems in rhythm and prosody, which, rather than reflection differences in movement durations (or "prearticulatory sequencing"), correspond to deficiencies in durational control. These findings are in line with Manuel (1999) who concluded: "Prosody clearly has to do with timing, so it seems likely that prosody and temporal coordination of articulatory gestures are strongly linked" (p. 196).

Experiment 1: Evidence concerning phonetic planning and the mental syllabary deficits

In this first experiment the hypothesis that children with developmental apraxia of speech show a specific deficit of phonetic planning (including the syllabary) was evaluated by manipulating syllable structure and syllable frequency (see Table 8.1).

Coarticulatory cohesion, using second formant measures throughout the

Table 8.1 List of stimuli items (with translations), together with syllable frequency of first and second syllable

Syllable structure	*Meaningful utterance*	*Syllable frequency*		*Nonsense utterance*	*Syllable frequency*	
		First	*Second*		*First*	*Second*
ʉs#xV	zus giet (*'sister pours'*)	1413	394	fus giek	13	8
	zus goot (*'sister poured'*)	1413	427	fus gook	13	0
	zus gaat (*'sister goes'*)	1413	30067	fus gaak	13	0
ə#sxV	ze schiet (*'she shoots'*)	392675	1946	de schiek	3471753	0
	ze schoot (*'she shot'*)	392675	3474	de schook	3471753	0
	ze schaat-sen (*'they skate'*)	392675	143	de scha-tel	3471753	11343

Note: The syllable frequencies were based on the Dutch database CELEX (Baayen, Piepenbroek, & Gulikers, 1995) consisting of 42 million lexical word forms.

utterance, and durational pattern were determined in the utterances produced by six children with developmental apraxia of speech and six normally speaking children. The children with developmental apraxia of speech were selected according to the clinical criteria described by Hall et al. (1993) and Thoonen et al. (1996) (for a detailed description see Nijland et al., 2002, 2003). All children were native speakers of Dutch, between the ages of 5 and 10 years, with normal sense of hearing and language comprehension. Furthermore the children with developmental apraxia of speech did not exhibit organic disorders in the orofacial area, gross motor disturbances, dysarthria, or below normal intelligence.

As a first result, it was found that although the children with developmental apraxia of speech were able to repeat the utterances correctly, they also produced erroneous utterances, especially in the [sx] sequence. The normally speaking children were all able to produce the utterances without difficulties. The error data on the [sx] sequence indicated more problems in producing the onset-cluster [sx] sequence than in producing the tautosyllabic consonant string (in which syllable boundary occurs between the two consonants). These results suggest that syllable structure plays an important role during speech production in children with developmental apraxia of speech, just as in normally speaking children. Some children with developmental apraxia of speech, contrariwise, produced deviations from syllabic organization by producing pauses within the /sx/ cluster, which did not occur in normally speaking children.

Second, the coarticulation pattern in the utterances showed a significant within-syllable coarticulation effect of the vowel on the preceding consonant [x] in both groups. The crucial test was whether an effect of syllable structure on coarticulatory cohesion would occur on the consonant [s] that changed syllable position due to syllable structure manipulation (either belonging to the same syllable as the vowel or belonging to the preceding syllable). Such an effect was not found, that is coarticulation strength and extent were not affected by syllable structure. The absence of a syllable structure effect on coarticulatory cohesion, being a negative result, could mean that the spectral measure was either not affected at all by syllable structure, or not sensitive enough to demonstrate subtle planning differences. However, a significant difference in coarticulatory cohesion due to syllable structure was found in the first vowel in both groups (stronger coarticulation in the [#sx] utterance than in the [s#x] utterance). This might be interpreted as an effect due to phonological specification of the first vowel, that is the /ʉ/ is more specified than /ə/, and therefore less vulnerable for coarticulation.

The durational structure, by way of contrast, revealed a difference in syllabic planning between children with developmental apraxia of speech and normally speaking children more strongly than the spectral data. Normally speaking children showed clear effects of syllable structure on segment durations, in which two different effects seemed to be operative: A metric and a prosodic effect. First, a shortening of the [x] and of the second vowel in the [#sx] utterances as compared to [s#x] was interpreted as an adjustment to the change in metrical structure of the second syllable due to the extra segment /s/. In children with developmental apraxia of speech adjustment to the change in metrical structure was only found in the second vowel, which was shorter in the [#sx] utterances than in the [s#x] utterances (see also Code, this volume, Chapter 7). Second, the shortening of the first vowel in the [#sx] condition as compared to the [s#x] condition could not be explained by a change in metrical structure (after all, the effect is the other way around). Yet, the first syllables differed prosodically, that is the closed syllable /CV$_1$s#/ was stressed whereas the open syllable /CV$_1$#/ is not. Significant differences in duration between spondaic (both syllables are stressed, as in CV$_1$s#xV$_2$C) and iambic utterances (only the second syllable is stressed, as in CV$_1$#sxV$_2$C) found in the first vowel in the normally speaking children corresponded with reports of shorter durations in prosodically weak positions (Lehiste, 1976). This effect was not found in children with developmental apraxia of speech. This result is an indication for a deviant effect of prosodic parameters on articulation in children with developmental apraxia of speech confirming the finding of Shriberg et al. (1997) and Velleman and Shriberg (1999).

Third, under the assumption that the articulatory gestures of frequently used syllables are stored and therefore will show more cohesion, we expected to find stronger coarticulation in high frequency as compared to low frequency syllables.

Results showed that syllable frequency did not affect the strength or extent of the coarticulation, neither did it account for differences in duration. From the absence of a syllable frequency effect in both groups we must conclude that the existence of a syllabary, including a possible deficient syllabary in children with developmental apraxia of speech, could not be substantiated (see also Code, this volume, Chapter 7). This could mean that either the theoretical construct of a syllabary is false or the effect of the syllable frequency manipulation was not strong enough in our data. Note that in the construction of the speech material only the frequency of the second syllable was strongly manipulated.

Finally, the variability among speakers was not significantly different between the two groups, neither on spectral measures nor on durational measures. This indicates that the group of children with developmental apraxia of speech was not more heterogeneous on the measurements than the normally speaking children. In contrast to this finding, significantly higher variability in repeated utterances (within speaker variability) was found in children with developmental apraxia of speech as compared to normally speaking children, which is interpreted as an indication of poor automatisation of production processes.

Experiment 2: Evidence concerning a motor programming deficit

A second experiment investigated a disturbance at the motor programming and execution level of speech production in children with developmental apraxia of speech, by comparing the compensatory abilities to a bite-block manipulation in normally speaking children to those of children with developmental apraxia of speech. For this, simple bisyllabic utterances ([dəCV] (C=/b,d,x,s/ and V=/a,i,u/) were uttered in a condition with a bite-block clenched between the teeth (bite-block condition) and without it (normal speech condition), by five children with developmental apraxia of speech and five normally speaking children (the five normally speaking children and one child with developmental apraxia of speech also participated in experiment 1).

The results showed a differential effect of the bite-block manipulation between the two groups of children on spectral measures as well as durational measures. The spectral measures showed that during normal speech, normally speaking children produced significantly stronger distinctions between the different vowels (/a,i,u/), and slightly stronger intra-syllabic coarticulation than the children with developmental apraxia of speech did. In the bite-block condition, however, the difference in vowel distinctiveness between the two groups decreased, and the difference in inter-syllabic coarticulation strength increased. The former effect was particularly due to an increase in distinction between vowels found in children with developmental apraxia of speech and the latter effect was a result of the weaker coarticulation in children with developmental apraxia of speech in the bite-block condition as compared to the normal speech condition.

Although normally speaking children could not completely compensate for the bite-block, it hardly affected the extent of anticipatory coarticulation. In contrast, in children with developmental apraxia of speech the distinction between the vowels /a,i,u/ increased in the bite-block condition, which resulted in more "normal" patterns. Nevertheless, the groups still differed highly in coarticulatory pattern: Children with developmental apraxia of speech showed less anticipatory coarticulation (within as well as between syllables) compared to normally speaking children.

The finding that children with developmental apraxia of speech made more distinction between the vowels due to the bite-block was quite remarkable. It turns out that children with developmental apraxia of speech were actually helped by the bite-block. A similar pattern was described by Netsell (1985) in an example of a subject with Parkinson's disease. He speculated that the bite-block both slows the speaking rate and requires the subject to increase the range of lip and tongue movements. Furthermore, the reduction of degrees of freedom (jaw movement is fixed) might also result in an improvement of the lip and tongue movements. Nevertheless, in the present study the articulatory patterns still showed aberrance in children with developmental apraxia of speech as compared to normally speaking children. In conclusion, children with developmental apraxia of speech showed differential effects to the bite-block manipulation compared to normally speaking children, which suggests a deviance in the final stages of speech production (motor programming and/ or motor execution).

Results of the durational pattern showed a stable pattern in the normally speaking children, despite the increase of consonant and second vowel durations in the bite-block condition. Thus, apparently these children use a compensatory strategy by slowing down the process of speech production while controlling for the intrinsic durational differences and contextual interdependency. The children with developmental apraxia of speech reacted differently to the bite-block as compared to normally speaking children. Although, also an increase of consonant duration was found, the duration of the second vowel decreased. Apparently, these children do not use a similar compensatory strategy of equally slowing down as the normally speaking children do. The aberrant durational pattern in children with developmental apraxia of speech as compared to the normally speaking children due to the bite-block were assumed to result from differences in movement durations that are not controlled for. That is, some movements are slowed down more than others without evidence of a "higher" control mechanism. These conclusions corroborate the findings of Shriberg et al. (1997) who suggested that the problems that children with developmental apraxia of speech exhibit in using stress (all syllables are stressed) result from a higher level of rhythm and prosody, rather than reflecting compensatory effects.

Furthermore, the results on the variability analyses of spectral and durational measures revealed that within-speaker variability of the spectral measures in the normally speaking children did not change in the bite-block condition, whereas the children with developmental apraxia of speech showed an increase of variability due to the bite-block. In contrast, an increase of within-speaker variability was found in the durational measures of the normally speaking children due to the bite-block, that is, in the consonant and second vowel duration. In children with developmental apraxia of speech only the variability of the consonant duration increased due to the bite-block. When comparing both groups, children with developmental apraxia of speech showed overall larger within-speaker variability than normally speaking children; in all segment durations and in both speaking conditions. This finding could be explained as a lack of durational control in the children with developmental apraxia of speech.

Discussion and conclusion

A possible deviant phonetic *planning* in children with developmental apraxia of speech was discussed in experiment 1 in which the syllable structure was manipulated in an otherwise unchanging context. Whereas systematic durational adjustments to the metrical structure of the syllable were found in the segments of the stressed syllable in normally speaking children, in children with developmental apraxia of speech such systematic effects were missing. This suggests that during speech production in children with developmental apraxia of speech each single segment is processed on its own, without accounting or adjusting for surrounding segments within the syllable. Furthermore, the overall durational patterns suggested that children with developmental apraxia of speech do not process prosodic properties similarly as normally speaking children do. These findings are interpreted as a deficit in phonetic planning, specifically in using prosodic parameters in articulation.

Evidence for a possible deficient use of the syllabary in children with developmental apraxia of speech could not be shown in experiment 1; neither was an effect of syllable frequency observed in normally speaking children.

In a previous study, we suggested that children with developmental apraxia of speech have problems in motor programming (Nijland et al., 2002), which led to longer durations and higher variability. In experiment 2 this was further tested using a bite-block speech condition. Neither normally speaking children nor children with developmental apraxia of speech were able to completely compensate for the bite-block, as shown in both formant values and durational patterns. However, the bite-block effects differed in both groups. In normally speaking children the bite-block hardly affected the extent of anticipatory coarticulation. In contrast, in the speech of children with developmental apraxia of speech large effects of the bite-block were found on vowel quality. This result was interpreted as a clear demonstration of deficient motor programming in developmental apraxia of speech, in a less automated and controlled processing mode. The deviant effect of bite-block on the durations in children with developmental apraxia of speech compared to normally speaking children furthermore supports this interpretation of a motor programming deficit. Thus, the answer to the question we started out with, namely whether children with developmental apraxia of speech show a deficit at either the planning or the programming level, is that *both planning and programming* are involved.

Did our data provide unambiguous answers to the question of what might be the underlying deficit in children with developmental apraxia of speech? As was stated in the introduction, children with developmental apraxia of speech generally present symptoms with various deficits: Besides speech problems (low intelligibility due to inconsistency in consonant substitutions) also soft neurological signs and clumsiness are mentioned (an overview of features of developmental apraxia of speech is given in McCabe et al., 1998). Various researchers discussed the possibility that the speech output of children with developmental apraxia of speech reflects a compensation strategy for a more general disability. And subsequently, it is important to determine for each symptom whether it directly reflects the underlying disorder or is more likely to be the result of a compensation strategy. On the one hand, if a symptom is the result of normal processing then this can be understood as a compensatory symptom. That is, a compensatory symptom is the result of adapted functioning of a normal mechanism under abnormal circumstances or in the presence of a proved disorder at another level. On the other hand, if a symptom could only be explained as the result of deviant mechanism then it must be explained as a symptom of the disorder. This issue of compensatory symptom versus symptom of the impairment is in particular relevant with respect to suprasegmental aspects of speech. It is, for instance, hard to distinguish whether slow speaking rate is a symptom of the disorder or a symptom of compensation. Davis et al. (1998) reported suprasegmental abnormalities in DAS, however, they stated that it is not clear whether these abnormalities are a part of the disorder or a compensation for the impaired ability to produce syllable sequences. Shriberg et al. (1997) showed that children with DAS experience difficulties in using stress. In contrast to Davis et al. (1998), Shriberg et al. (1997) were more explicit and suggested that this difficulty in using stress reflects a problem at a higher level of speech production instead of a compensatory effect.

On the basis of these clinical studies, however, it is impossible to decide whether the suprasegmental abnormalities, such as slow speaking rate and inappropriate use of stress, are resulting from compensatory processing for a deficit at a different level, or from a primary suprasegmental planning deficit. These studies suggested diverse deficits in DAS. Yet another option was proposed by Marion et al. (1993), who discussed the possibility that the deficiencies in speech motor output reflect an ill-formed phonological representation system. Furthermore, Dodd, and McCormack (1995) mentioned that it is difficult to substantiate whether the poor performance of children with DAS on tests of receptive and expressive vocabulary and motor planning for verbal and non-verbal tasks reflect a number of different and distinct underlying deficits, or feedback and feedforward effects from a single deficit. Thus, various studies suggest planning problems in higher linguistic processes in children with DAS (see also Hodge, 1994; McCabe et al., 1998; Velleman & Strand, 1994), which are in accordance with the clinical observations and which indicate comorbidity.

Besides this issue of a deficit at a different level of linguistic processing there might be a more general impairment. Velleman and Strand (1994, p.119–20), for instance, suggested a possible common underlying information processing factor that children with DAS "could be seen as impaired in their ability to generate and utilize frames, which would otherwise provide the mechanisms for analyzing, organizing, and utilizing information from their motor, sensory, and linguistic systems for the production of spoken language". This was interpreted as follows: children with DAS "might 'have' appropriate phonological (or syntactic) elements but are unable to organize them into an appropriate cognitive hierarchy" (p. 120) (for comparison with adulthood apraxia of speech see also Code, this volume, Chapter 7). Combining the results of the two experiments discussed in this chapter, we also suggest a general problem in developmental apraxia of speech (see also Nijland, 2003). That is, the co-occurrence of motoric and higher order psycholinguistic planning deficits, which show similarities with the speech motor planning deficits, suggest a common underlying cause. The results of the experiments could well be explained in the light of a more generalized deficit in sequencing and timing that emerges in speech motor control, phonetic planning and motor programming. There is possibly a common (neurological) substrate that might account for deficits in these areas.

Acknowledgments

Netherlands Organization for Scientific Research (NWO) and Hersenstichting Nederland are gratefully acknowledged for funding this project. This research was conducted while the first author was supported by a grant of the Foundation for Behavioral and Educational Sciences of NWO (575–56–084) and of Hersenstichting Nederland (7F99.06) awarded to the second author. We also thank Roelien Bastiaanse and Frank Wijnen for their constructive comments on earlier drafts of this chapter.

Notes

1 The approach of Varley and Whiteside is an oversimplification and not a direct application of Levelt's model.
2 Note that this might also be true for slips-of-the-tongue. After all, it is true in slips-of-the tongue as well that there are more errors in consonants than in vowels, that there are more errors in clusters than in singleton consonants, and that the word onset is especially error prone as well.

References

Baayen, R. H., Piepenbroek, R., & Gulikers, L. (1995). *The CELEX lexical database [CD-ROM]*. Philadelphia, PA: Linguistic Data Consortium, University of Pennsylvania.

Ballard, K. J., Granier, J. P., & Robin, D. A. (2000). Understanding the nature of apraxia of speech: Theory, analysis, and treatment. *Aphasiology, 14*, 969–95.

Browman, C. P., & Goldstein, L. (1997). The gestural phonology model. In W. Hulstijn, H. F. M. Peters, & P. H. H. M. van Lieshout (Eds.), *Speech production: Motor control, brain research and fluency disorders* (pp. 57–71). Amsterdam: Elsevier Science BV.

Byrd, D. (1995). C-Centers revisited. *Phonetica, 52*, 285–306.

Davis, B. L., Jakielski, K. J., & Marquardt, T. P. (1998). Developmental apraxia of speech: Determiners of differential diagnosis. *Clinical Linguistics and Phonetics, 12*, 25–45.

Dodd, B., & McCormack, P. (1995). A model of speech processing for differential diagnosis of phonological disorders. In B. Dodd (Ed.), *Differential diagnosis and treatment of children with speech disorders* (pp. 65–89). London: Whurr.

Forrest, K., & Morrisette, M. L. (1999). Feature analysis of segmental errors in children with phonological disorders. *Journal of Speech, Language, and Hearing Research, 42*, 187–94.

Fowler, C. A., & Saltzman, E. (1993). Coordination and coarticulation in speech production. *Language and Speech, 36*, 171–95.

Groenen, P., Maassen, B., Crul, Th., & Thoonen, G. (1996). The specific relation between perception and production errors for place of articulation in developmental apraxia of speech. *Journal of Speech and Hearing Research, 39*, 468–82.

Guyette, Th., & Diedrich, W. M. (1981). A critical review of developmental apraxia of speech. In N. J. Lass (Ed.), *Speech and language. Advances in basic research and practice* (pp. 1–49). New York: Academic Press Inc.

Hall, P. K., Jordan, L. S., & Robin, D. A. (1993). *Developmental apraxia of speech.* Austin, TX: Pro-ed.

Hodge, M. M. (1994). Assessment of children with developmental apraxia of speech: A rationale. *Clinics in Communication Disorders, 4*, 91–101.

Hoit-Dalgaard, J., Murry, T., & Kopp, H. (1983). Voice-onset-time production and perception in apraxic subjects. *Brain and Language, 20*, 329–39.

Lehiste, I. (1976). Suprasegmental features of speech. In N. J. Lass (Ed.), *Contemporary issues in experimental phonetics* (pp. 225–39). New York: Academic Press.

Levelt, W. J. M. (1989). *Speaking: From intention to articulation.* Cambridge, MA: MIT Press.

Levelt, W. J. M., Roelofs, A., & Meyer, A. S. (1999). A theory of lexical access in speech production. *Behavioral and Brain Sciences, 22*, 1–75.

Levelt, W. J. M., & Wheeldon, L. (1994). Do speakers have a mental syllabary? *Cognition, 50*, 239–69.

Manuel, S. (1999). Cross-language studies: Relating language-particular coarticulation patterns to other language-particular facts. In W. J. Hardcastle & N. Hewlett (Eds.), *Coarticulation: Theory, data and techniques* (pp. 179–98). Cambridge: Cambridge University Press.

Marion, M. J., Sussman, H. M., & Marquardt, T. P. (1993). The perception and production of rhyme in normal and developmentally apraxic children. *Journal of Communication Disorders, 26*, 129–60.

McCabe, P., Rosenthal, J. B., & McLeod, S. (1998). Features of developmental dyspraxia in the general speech-impaired population. *Clinical Linguistics and Phonetics, 12*, 105–26.

McNeil, M. R., Robin, D. A., & Schmidt, R. A. (1997). Apraxia of speech: Definition, differentiation, and treatment. In M. R. McNeil (Ed.), *Clinical management of sensorimotor speech disorders* (pp. 311–44). New York: Thieme Medical Publishers Inc.

Netsell, R. (1985). Construction and use of a bite-block for the evaluation and treatment of speech disorders. *Journal of Speech and Hearing Disorders, 50*, 103–109.

Nijland, L. (2003). *Developmental apraxia of speech: Deficits in phonetic planning and motor programming.* PhD thesis University of Nijmegen.

Nijland, L., Maassen, B., & Van der Meulen, Sj. (1999). Use of syllables by children with developmental apraxia of speech. *Proceedings of the 14th International Congress of Phonetic Sciences, 3*, 1921–3.

Nijland, L., Maassen, B., & Van der Meulen, Sj. (2003). Evidence for motor programming deficits in children diagnosed with DAS. *Journal of Speech, Language, and Hearing Research, 46*, 437–50.

Nijland, L., Maassen, B., Van der Meulen, Sj., Gabreëls, F., Kraaimaat, F.W., & Schreuder, R. (2002). Coarticulation patterns in children with developmental apraxia of speech. *Clinical Linguistics and Phonetics, 16*, 461–83.

Nijland, L., Maassen, B., Van der Meulen, Sj., Gabreëls, F., Kraaimaat, F. W., & Schreuder, R. (2003). Planning of syllables by children with developmental apraxia of speech. *Clinical Linguistics and Phonetics, 17,* 1–24.

Nittrouer, S., Studdert-Kennedy, M., & Neely, S. T. (1996). How children learn to organize their speech gestures: Further evidence from fricative-vowel syllables. *Journal of Speech and Hearing Research, 39,* 379–89.

Ozanne, A. E. (1995). The search for developmental verbal dyspraxia. In B. Dodd (Ed.), *Differential diagnosis and treatment of children with speech disorders* (pp. 91–109). London: Whurr.

Pollock, K. E., & Hall, P. K. (1991). An analysis of the vowel misarticulations of five children with developmental apraxia of speech. *Clinical Linguistics and Phonetics, 5,* 207–24.

Robin, D. A. (1992). Developmental apraxia of speech: Just another motor problem. *American Journal of Speech-Language Pathology, 1,* 19–22.

Shriberg, L. D., Aram, D. M., & Kwiatkowski, J. (1997). Developmental apraxia of speech III: A subtype marked by inappropriate stress. *Journal of Speech, Language, and Hearing Research, 40,* 313–37.

Shriberg, L. D., & Kwiatkowski, J. (1982). Phonogical disorders II: A conceptual framework for management. *Journal of Speech and Hearing Disorders, 47,* 242–56.

Thoonen, G. (1998). *Developmental apraxia of speech. assessment of speech characteristics.* Dissertation, University of Nijmegen.

Thoonen, G., Maassen, B., Gabreëls, F., & Schreuder, R. (1994). Feature analysis of singleton consonant errors in developmental verbal dyspraxia (DVD). *Journal of Speech and Hearing Research, 37,* 1424–40.

Thoonen, G., Maassen, B., Wit, J., Gabreëls, F., & Schreuder, R. (1996). The integrated use of maximum performance tasks in differential diagnostic evaluations among children with motor speech disorders. *Clinical Linguistics and Phonetics, 10,* 311 36.

Towne, R. L. (1994). Effect of mandibular stabilization on the diadochokinetic performance of children with phonological disorder. *Journal of Phonetics, 22,* 3, 317–32.

Van der Merwe, A. (1997). A theoretical framework for the characterization of pathological speech sensorimotor control. In M. R. McNeil (Ed.), *Clinical management of sensorimotor speech disorders* (pp. 1–25). New York: Thieme Medical Publishers Inc.

Varley, R. A., & Whiteside, S. P. (2001). Forum: What is the underlying impairment in acquired apraxia of speech? *Aphasiology, 15,* 39–84.

Velleman, S. L., & Shriberg, L. D. (1999). Metrical analysis of the speech of children with suspected developmental apraxia of speech. *Journal of Speech, Language, and Hearing Research, 42,* 1444–60.

Velleman, S.L., & Strand, K. (1994). Developmental verbal dyspraxia. In J. E. Bernthal, & N. W. Bankson (Eds.), *Child phonology: Characteristics, assessment, and intervention with special populations* (pp. 110–139). New York: Thieme Medical Publishers Inc.

Walton, J. H., & Pollock, K. E. (1993). Acoustic validation of vowel error patterns in developmental apraxia of speech. *Clinical Linguistics and Phonetics, 7,* 95–111.

Whalen, D. H. (1990). Coarticulation is largely planned. *Journal of Phonetics, 18,* 3–35.

Ziegler, W. (2001). Apraxia of speech is not a lexical disorder. *Aphasiology, 15,* 74–7.

Part III

Theories and models of self-monitoring

9 Critical issues in speech monitoring

Albert Postma and
Claudy C. E. Oomen

Abstract

This chapter reviews some of the central questions pertaining to speech monitoring and the existing theories in the light of recent empirical studies. Temporal analyses indicate that self-repair can occur rather rapidly, demonstrating that speakers can use an internal monitoring channel, in addition to an external (auditory) channel. Both patient data and the comparison of error patterns to repair patterns suggest that there is an essential distinction between these internal and external monitoring channels. Some theoretical implications of these observations are discussed, in particular regarding the normal operation of the perceptual inner loop; the existence of fast, autonomous (production-based) monitoring devices; and the possibility of shifts in the division of labor between external and internal monitoring. That such shifts can occur follows from the changes in monitoring foci reported in the literature.

Introduction

Without doubt, one of our most complex cognitive activities is that of error detection and self-repair. Consider the following classical example from Hockett (1967): "You made so much noise you worke Cor? – wore? – w? – woke Corky up." The speaker of this utterance had to do several things within a limited period of time: Plan and start executing the intended utterance, monitor the progress of the utterance, detect the error (*worke*), interrupt speech (*Cor?* –), edit and initiate a repair attempt (*wore?*), monitor and detect another error in this first repair attempt, and make a further interruption (– *w?*), until finally the speaker succeeds in getting the correctly repaired utterance out (*woke Corky up*).

In the past, speech monitoring and its overt companion error repair have been scarcely studied. So far, theories of self-monitoring and repair have been relatively general and underspecified (although this is rapidly changing, cf. contributions to this volume; Hartsuiker & Kolk, 2001; Oomen & Postma, 2001a, 2002; Postma 2000). In building a more detailed and comprehensive theory, it is necessary to pay attention to a small range of seemingly critical issues, which have hitherto not received sufficient attention. These issues involve (a) what is a viable theory of monitoring; (b) how fast is monitoring; (c) what are the behavioral correlates of monitoring activity; (d) can we manipulate our own monitors; (e) are there individual differences in monitoring capacity?

Theories of speech monitoring

Theories of speech monitoring deal with the enigma of metacognition. Do we have insight in our own cognitive processes? How can we inspect their adequacy? As a consequence, these theories often are quite limited, offering just a general framework or even nothing more than a few elementary principles. Here we will focus on two theoretical approaches that have been best developed. First, there is the perceptual loop theory originally formulated by Levelt (1983, 1989). Basically, the idea is that monitoring takes place in the connections from the speech planning and execution stages to the speech comprehension system, which parses the input from these connections and feeds the results to the conceptualizer. Error detection takes place by the conceptualizer. The monitoring connections in this proposal consist of an inner and an auditory loop,[1] allowing for relatively fast prearticulatory and slower postarticulatory error detection respectively. In short, the perceptual loop monitor is a centrally operated control mechanism, requiring no additional devices for error detection (i.e., both comprehension and conceptualizer exist already for other purposes; see also Hartsuiker, Bastiaanse, Postma, & Wijnen, this volume, Chapter 1).

The second approach to speech monitoring is the production based monitoring theory (Laver, 1973, 1980; Schlenck, Huber, & Willmes, 1987). Actually, several variants have been proposed, none of them too well worked out. Put simply, it is assumed that multiple special purpose monitors exist, distributed over the speech production system. Each one of them is doing only a single job, e.g., checking syntactic structure, and may function relatively autonomously from central attention and capacity. Several arguments have been raised against the concept of production monitoring. One concerns the problem of "information encapsulation". Certain stages of speech production by nature would be closed to inspection by an outside monitor. According to Levelt (1983, 1989) monitors can only look at the end products in the speech production chain: i.e., the speech plan and the overt speech. This criticism is less threatening if one assumes not a central monitor device but rather distributed autonomous specialists, which themselves are encapsulated. A second objection against production monitoring seems more fundamental. Would not our system overflow with monitors if all individual processing steps have their own control device attached? Ideally, a production monitor theory should specify at which levels monitors are postulated. Also bearing on this point, it should be mentioned that most proponents of production monitors actually presume a hybrid model, with loops into the comprehension system underlying perception-based monitoring as well as dedicated production monitors (Postma, 2000).

Temporal characteristics of self-repair

One of the most fruitful lines of research on speech monitoring consists of measuring and manipulating temporal aspects of self-repair behavior. Blackmer and Mitton (1991) observed that self-repair is often characterized by surprisingly fast error-to-cut-off as well as cut-off-to-repair times. The former implies the possibility of prearticulatory monitoring. The second indicates that revision can be planned well before the actual interruption is made.

Rapid self-repair obviously places constraints on a theory of monitoring. We will focus here on the theoretical consequences of a recent study we did on the effect of speech rate manipulations on self-repair behavior (Oomen & Postma, 2001a). In this study, speakers had to describe the route a moving dot was taking through a network of pictures of ordinary objects. Speaking rate was manipulated by speeding up or slowing down the progress of the dot. With higher speaking rates we argued that the perceptual loop theory would predict increased error-to-cut-off and cut-off-to-repair times. The inner loop is supposed to scrutinize the speech plan while it is temporarily held in the articulatory buffer prior to its submission to the articulatory motor system. Effectively, this buffer allows the monitor a look-ahead range, making prearticulatory repair activities possible. When speaking rate is higher, buffering diminishes (Blackmer & Mitton, 1991; Levelt, 1989; Van Hest, 1996). Consequently, the monitor will lag behind the articulation, eventually resulting in longer delays between the moment the error overtly emerges and the interruption and subsequent repair is initiated. Surprisingly, however, we did not find longer monitoring delays, rather the error-to-cut-off times were faster with elevated speech output rates. We concluded that this must mean that besides perceptual loop monitoring there is also a faster, production monitor, which keeps pace with the increases in general speaking rate (Postma, 2000).

In contrast to Postma, in their elegant computer model of speech monitoring Hartsuiker and Kolk (2001) nicely simulated the repair patterns for different speech rates all within the general setting of the perceptual loop theory. To do this, they had to make the following assumptions. First, all stages in the speech production sequence speed up with higher speaking rate, not just articulation. This seems quite plausible (see Dell, 1986). Second, the speed with which the motor system stops on deciding to interrupt should remain constant. Finally, speech comprehension might also become faster in these circumstances. Now this assumption is more disputable. It seems to be an empirical question that can be examined fairly easily (i.e., let listeners detect errors in samples of varying speech rate). Of critical concern is the observation that in our study interruptions were not only issued earlier in time after an error, but also earlier in number of segments (i.e., the interruption point in syllables from the error onset was also earlier) (Oomen & Postma, 2001a). This can only be explained by the Hartsuiker and Kolk model if the speech comprehension system speeds up relatively more than the speech production system (Oomen, 2001). One may wonder how plausible this is.

In short then, knowledge of the temporal constraints of self-repair have led to further specifications of the perceptual loop theory. However, these specifications cannot account for all of the available data. A solution may be to choose for a mixed approach between perception and production monitoring (Oomen & Postma, 2001a). As already noticed, most production monitor theories assume both modes of monitoring – i.e., both perceptual loops and production monitors. While the production monitors might speed up with speaking rate, the part of self-repairs based on perceptual loops should be delayed. As such a variety of net effects can be covered, depending on the ratio between production and perception monitoring and their relative changes by speaking rate. The problem with this solution, however, is that in general theories of production monitoring are utterly underspecified in how exactly the temporal links between production stages and monitoring components proceed.

Patterns of errors or patterns of monitoring?

What are the behavioral correlates of monitoring activity? Whatever the type of monitor responsible for self-repair, it is generally acknowledged that speakers can detect their mistakes before they have emerged in the audible speech. Not only is prearticulatory error detection possible, also the repair can be initiated covertly. This implicates that monitoring activity can have various types of behavioral effects, which, in turn, reflect on the balance between inner and auditory monitoring. As Hartsuiker et al. (this volume, Chapter 1) discuss, this can lead to three results. First, we may have an overt error followed with virtually no delay by the correction (see earlier). Second, disfluencies may occur. The status of disfluencies is controversial, however. Some consider them to reflect repairs of anticipated (sub) segmental speech planning errors (Postma & Kolk, 1993). As the errors themselves remain hidden, the term covert repair is coined. Others, however, typify them as stalling strategies (see Hartsuiker et al., this volume, Chapter 1). In addition, disfluencies such as repetitions have been described to form more or less automatic reactions to temporal disruption in the speech planning mechanisms (Oomen & Postma, 2001b). If a speaker suffers word finding difficulty, she might repeat the previous word, either as a strategic choice to gain time or as an automatic response. Note that all three situations presume the engagement of a monitoring mechanism, even though the initial cause is different. Third, and finally, there may be (covert) repairing without disfluent side-effects or observable overt repairs (Hartsuiker et al., this volume, Chapter 1). Still there are effects, in that the pattern of overt speech errors is changed. By systematically avoiding certain types of errors by means of this "fluent covert repairing", the relative percentage of other types of errors is boosted.

It is this last type of self-repairing that is particularly hard to assess. Nooteboom (this volume, Chapter 10) has provided an excellent attempt to compare error patterns to error repair patterns. A comparison of lexical bias in error patterns with lexical bias in overt self-repairs, reveals that they differ in important respects. Specifically, it seems that overt self-repair is not sensitive to lexical status whereas error patterns (which we take here to reflect the results of "fluent" repairing) generally are. That is, overt correction of erroneous words that form real lexical items is as frequent as correction of errors that do not have lexical status. In contrast, most speech errors form existing words. Nooteboom therefore concludes that it is unlikely that the mechanisms responsible for overt self-repair and error pattern generation are identical. There may be three solutions. First, overt self-repairing and error pattern generation (e.g., lexical bias) both depend on perception monitoring, albeit on different channels, the auditory and inner loop, respectively. If these two channels in some unknown way apply different criteria, their outcomes could diverge. It is not very convincing, however, to assume such a difference in monitoring criteria. Both channels are assumed to feed into the same monitoring system in the conceptualizer. Why would different criteria for the two channels be applied at this relatively late stage? Second, overt repairing might be based on perceptual monitors, whereas the error patterns depend on production monitors (viz resemble the third form of prearticulatory monitoring). Third, error patterns can be the result of intrinsic wiring of the speech production stages – in particular of feedback connections – and have nothing to do with monitoring capacities.

These possible solutions illustrate the difficulty of the problem we are dealing with. Notice that overt repair patterns are not necessarily based on the overt loop, but can derive from prearticulatory and therefore non-perceptual error interceptions as well. Moreover, the distinction between what a feedback connection between successive stages of speech production is doing and how autonomous production monitors operate is not always very clear.

Shifting the monitoring spotlight

What is the monitor exactly looking for, and to what extent can this be changed? If we observe flexibility, what would that teach us about the nature of the monitor process? Some speech slips are clearly more devastating for an utterance than others. A speaker might ignore sloppy articulation, but be very keen to repair phonological or lexical errors. While this could reflect the inherent difficulty to spot certain incidents – i.e., which is a hardwired feature – it could also reflect the adaptivity of the monitoring process. Do speakers shift the focus of their monitor mechanism in specific circumstances? There have been two lines of research regarding this question. One concerns manipulation of monitoring accuracy, either directly or by means of presenting a secondary task concurrently with speaking. In two older studies, Postma and Kolk (Postma & Kolk, 1990; Postma, Kolk & Povel, 1990) changed the aspired quality of speech output in both stutterers and normal speakers by instructions, feedback and training. As expected, the repair rates dropped with lower emphasis on accuracy. An indirect manipulation of accuracy is induced by dual task performance. Oomen and Postma (2002) showed that repair rates decrease when subjects have to perform a dual task concurrently with speaking. Apparently, criteria for error detection might be relaxed or rather heightened depending on the speaking conditions. To some extent both production and perception accounts of monitoring can accommodate these results (Postma, 2000).

Accuracy effects on disfluencies – which some consider covert repairs – appear to be more variable. In particular, dual task loading has sometimes been found to improve fluency in stutterers (Arends, Povel, & Kolk, 1988), sometimes yielded no effect (Thompson, 1985), and sometimes led to increased disfluency in normal speakers (Oomen & Postma, 2001b). Of influence here might be the fact that dual task conditions could not only lower monitoring scrutiny, but at the same time increase the number of events to which a monitor has to react – viz internal speech plan errors – thus yielding zero or variable net disfluency effects (Hartsuiker et al., this volume, Chapter 1). Another relevant factor is the type of dual task employed, specifically the precise change in monitoring focus or effort it brings about.

This brings us to the second line of research on monitoring foci: Can the monitor selectively zoom in on specific classes of errors? Baars and Motley have demonstrated context-dependent semantic and syntactic biases in error monitoring (Baars, Motlet, & MacKay 1975; Motley, 1980; Motley, Camden, & Baars, 1982), suggesting that the type of errors intercepted might vary with the conditions tested. Levelt (1989, 1992) emphasizes that monitoring fluctuates with the distribution of attentional resources. Speakers thus scrutinize different things in different situations.[2] Importantly, speech therapies have tried to change the focus of monitoring in impaired speakers (Marshall et al., 1998). An intriguing study was done by Vasic and Wijnen (this volume, Chapter 13). They argued that hypermonitoring in stutterers for temporal aspects of their speech flow has counterproductive effects, in that it leads to excessive disruption of the temporal patterns of utterances by disfluencies. In line with previous work (Arends et al., 1988) they found a fluency improvement by a generally distracting, nonspeech dual task (see, however, Oomen & Postma, 2001b). Interestingly, a second dual task that elevated monitoring scrutiny but not for a temporal aspect but rather for a particular (lexical) word, also improved fluency. While the "vicious circle" hypothesis by Vasic and Wijnen at present needs further theoretical elaboration, it forms an important target for future research. (See also chapter by Russell, Corley, & Lickley, this volume, Chapter 14.)

Other evidence for the selectiveness of monitoring foci is offered by work on neurological patients. Oomen, Postma and Kolk (this volume, Chapter 12) describe an aphasic patient who normally repairs his semantic errors, but is severely disordered in both detecting and correcting phonological errors. Again this suggests that monitoring can be concentrated on rather specific characteristics of the speech flow. Whether this specificity of the monitoring spotlight is essentially caused by a centrally guided redirecting of the perceptual loops or by selectively turning on or off production monitors is yet unknown. Oomen et al. (this volume, Chapter 12) argued that some support for the latter possibility was offered, because their patient produced many phonological errors that, however, he corrected rather poorly,

Good speakers – bad monitors?

Are there good monitors and poor monitors? Might a problem in speech production not rather be a problem of monitoring? While both language production and comprehension characteristics of speech-language pathologies have been extensively examined, the role of speech monitoring abilities in these pathologies is largely ignored. There are, however, several clinical groups that, as recently has become clearer, might suffer crucial problems of speech monitoring. Research on monitoring skills in these groups can help understand their dysfunctions as well as give further insight in the nature of speech error detection and repair. Table 9.1 provides a provisional list of these groups and their alleged monitoring problems.

We will focus here on the last two groups in Table 9.1. Frith (1987, 1992) and Leudar, Thomas, and Johnston (1992, 1994) have argued that schizophrenics with positive symptoms (e.g. hallucinations) would have defective internal self-monitoring. This would contrast with the recent results we obtained for a group of Broca's aphasics (Oomen, Postma, & Kolk, 2001). We found that patients repaired fewer errors than control subjects in a normal speaking condition, but performed equally well when their auditory feedback was masked by white noise. This intriguing pattern raises at least two possible explanations. First, it clearly suggests that there is a qualitative distinction between prearticulatory and postarticulatory monitoring. Future research

Table 9.1 Clinical groups, alleged monitor dysfunctions, and consequences for speech output

Group	Monitor dysfunction	Consequence
Stutterers	Hyperactive monitoring of temporal speech planning features	Excessive disfluency
Wernicke's aphasics	Defective prearticulatory and postarticulatory monitoring	Poor self-repair. Jargon and fluent aphasia
Schizophrenics	Defective prearticulatory monitoring	Many missed errors when auditory channel is absent
Broca's aphasics	Normal prearticulatory, defective postarticulatory monitoring	Disfluent speech. Fewer late error interceptions

should further examine this distinction by directly comparing the two patient groups on prearticulatory and postarticulatory speech monitoring skills. If the inner and the outer loop feed into a single unitary monitor, as presumed by the perceptual loop theory, this dissociation would have been rather unlikely. Alternatively, it could reflect that the former engages mostly production monitors whereas the latter is solely a function of the perceptual monitor. Broca's aphasics might have a defective perceptual monitoring system while the autonomous production monitors function relatively well. Since self-repairing in a normal speech condition depends on both the inner and outer loop, a defective outer loop would substantially handicap the Broca's patients. In a noise masked condition only the inner loop counts. Hence, the patients would do relatively well. In line with this line of reasoning, Nickels and Howard (1995) reported no correlation between patients' language comprehension skills and their monitoring skills. Such correlation would have been expected if monitoring were solely based on perceptual monitoring. These patient findings thus appear to be most in line with a hybrid model of speech monitoring. Notice, however, that it is peculiar that Broca's patients who have clear deficits in certain stages of speech planning and production, still would have normally operating production monitor devices directly attached to these stages (Oomen et al., 2001).

A second potential explanation for our findings in Broca's patients (Oomen et al., 2001) involves strategic reasons. In line with foregoing section on shifting of monitoring foci, it could be that patients primarily focus their limited resources on internal channels, leading to normal performance when there is only an inner channel, while they cannot profit from an additional external channel under normal speaking conditions.

Conclusions

Let us return to our initial self-repair example. "You made so much noise you worke Cor? – wore? – w? – woke Corky up." How does this speaker know she has made an error? Is she aware of her slip and deliberately issuing the correction? Or is the repair edited more or less automatically, as attested by the trial and error, gradual approximation towards the final target? The question how exactly speech monitoring is operating – perception -based, production based, or both – is not easily answered. We have to take into account not only overt self-repairs, but also disfluencies or covert repairs, and overt error patterns. The critical issues briefly reviewed in this chapter only give us some hints for future research. It is clear from both patient data and the comparison of error patterns to repair patterns that there is an essential distinction between internal and external monitoring. Moreover, temporal analyses suggest that self-repair can sometimes occur rather rapidly. It is unknown yet whether this reflects the existence of fast, autonomous monitoring devices or a shift in the division of labor between the external and internal monitoring. That such shifts can occur, follows from the changes in monitoring foci reported in the literature. Depending on the circumstances we might be more sensitive to lexical, segmental or temporal errors. In addition, speakers can put more effort in internal monitoring – thus emphasizing error prevention – or in external monitoring – concentrating on speech fluency. Speech therapies could particularly target on trying to change the foci of speech monitoring in clinical groups.

Acknowledgements

This study was supported by a grant from the Netherlands Organization for Fundamental Research (NWO, No. 440–20–000).

Notes

1 We ignore the third connection here: The conceptual loop.
2 This flexibility of monitoring focus appears most in line with the perceptual loop theory, although it might be accounted for by certain type of production monitors as well (see Postma, 2000).

References

Arends, A., Povel, D. J., & Kolk, H. H. J. (1988). Stuttering as an attentional phenomenon. *Journal of Fluency Disorders, 13*, 141–51.

Baars, B. J., Motley, M. T., & MacKay, D. G. (1975). Output editing for lexical status in artificially elicited slips of the tongue. *Journal of Verbal Learning and Verbal Behaviour, 14*, 382–91.

Blackmer, E. R., and Mitton, J. L. (1991). Theories of monitoring and the timing of repairs in spontaneous speech. *Cognition, 39*, 173–94.

Dell, G. S. (1986). A spreading-activation theory of retrieval in sentence production. *Psychological Review, 93*, 283–321.

Frith, C. D. (1987). The positive and negative symptoms of schizophrenia reflect impairments in the perception and initiation of action. *Psychological Medicine, 17*, 631–48.

Frith, C. D. (1992). *The cognitive neuropsychology of schizophrenia.* Hove, UK: Lawrence Erlbaum Associates Ltd.

Hartsuiker, R. J., & Kolk, H. H. J. (2001). Error monitoring in speech production: A computational test of the perceptual loop theory. *Cognitive Psychology, 42*, 113–57.

Hockett, C. F. (1967). Where the tongue slips, there slip I. In *To honor Roman Jakobson*, Vol. II (Janua Linguarum, 32) (pp. 910–36). The Hague: Mouton.

Laver, J. D. M. (1973). The detection and correction of slips of tongue. In V. A. Fromkin (Ed.), *Speech errors as linguistic evidence*. The Hague: Mouton.

Laver, J. D. M. (1980). Monitoring systems in the neurolinguistic control of speech production. In V. A. Fromkin (Ed.), *Errors in linguistic performance: Slips of the tongue, ear, pen, and hand*. New York: Academic Press.

Leudar, I., Thomas, P., & Johnston, M. (1992). Self-repair in dialogues of schizophrenics: effects of hallucinations and negative symptoms. *Brain and Language, 43*, 487–511.

Leudar, I., Thomas, P., & Johnston, M. (1994). Self-monitoring in speech production: effects of verbal hallucinations and negative symptoms. *Psychological Medicine, 24,* 749–61.

Levelt, W. J. M. (1983). Monitoring and self-repair in speech. *Cognition, 14,* 41–104.

Levelt, W. J. M. (1989). *Speaking: From intention to articulation.* Cambridge, MA: MIT Press.

Levelt, W. J. M. (1992). The perceptual loop theory not disconfirmed: A reply to MacKay. *Consciousness and Cognition, 1,* 226–30.

Marshall, J., Robson, J., Pring, T., & Chiat, S. (1998). Why does monitoring fail in jargon aphasia? Comprehension, judgment, and therapy evidence. *Brain and Language, 63,* 79–107.

Motley, M. T. (1980). Verification of "Freudian slips" and semantic prearticulatory editing via laboratory-induced spoonerisms. In V.A. Fromkin (Ed.), *Errors in linguistic performance: Slips of the tongue, ear, pen, and hand.* New York: Academic Press.

Motley, M. T., Camden, C. T., & Baars, B. J. (1982). Covert formulation and editing of anomalies in speech production: Evidence from experimentally elicited slips of the tongue. *Journal of Verbal Learning and Verbal Behavior, 21,* 578–94.

Nickels, L., & Howard, D. (1995). Phonological errors in aphasic naming: Comprehension, monitoring and lexicality. *Cortex, 31,* 209–37.

Oomen, C. C. E. (2001). *Self-monitoring in normal and aphasic speech.* Unpublished PhD thesis Utrecht University.

Oomen, C. C. E., & Postma, A. (2001a). Effects of increased speech rate on monitoring and self-repair. *Journal of Psycholinguistic Research, 30,* 163–84.

Oomen, C. C. E., & Postma, A. (2001b). Effects of divided attention on the production of filled pauses and repetitions. *Journal of Speech, Language, and Hearing Research, 44,* 997–1004.

Oomen, C. C. E., & Postma, A. (2002). Limitations in processing resources and speech monitoring. *Language and Cognitive Processes, 17,* 163–84.

Oomen, C. C.E., Postma, A., & Kolk, H. H. J. (2001). Prearticulatory and postarticulatory self-monitoring in Broca's aphasia. *Cortex, 37,* 627–41.

Postma, A. (2000). Detection of errors during speech production. A review of speech monitoring models. *Cognition, 77,* 97–131.

Postma, A. and Kolk, H. H. J. (1990). Speech errors, disfluencies, and self-repairs in stutterers in two accuracy conditions. *Journal of Fluency Disorders, 15,* 291–303.

Postma, A., & Kolk, H. H. J. (1993). The covert repair hypothesis: prearticulatory repair processes in normal and stuttered disfluencies. *Journal of Speech and Hearing Research, 36,* 472–87.

Postma, A., Kolk, H. H. J., & Povel, D.J. (1990). On the relation among speech errors, disfluencies, and self-repairs. *Language and Speech, 33,* 19–29.

Schlenck, K., Huber, W., & Willmes, K. (1987). "Prepairs" and repairs: Different monitoring functions in aphasic language production. *Brain and Language, 30,* 226–44.

Thompson, A. H. (1985). A test of the distraction explanation of disfluency modification in stuttering. *Journal of Fluency Disorders, 10,* 35–50.

Van Hest, G. W. C. M. (1996). *Self-repair in L1 and L2 Production.* Tilburg, The Netherlands: Tilburg University Press.

10 Listening to oneself: Monitoring speech production

Sieb G. Nooteboom

Abstract

According to Levelt (1989) and Levelt, Roelofs, and Meyer (1999) (a) self-monitoring of speech production employs the speech comprehension system, (b) on the phonological level the speech comprehension system has no information about the lemmas and forms chosen in production, and (c) lexical bias in speech errors stems from the same perception-based monitoring that is responsible for detection and overt correction of speech errors. It is predicted from these theoretical considerations that phonological errors accidentally leading to real words should be treated by the monitor as lexical errors, because the monitor has no way of knowing that they are not. It is also predicted that self-corrections of overt speech errors are also sensitive to lexicality of the errors. These predictions are tested against a corpus of speech errors and their corrections in Dutch. It is shown that the monitor treats phonological errors leading to real words in all respects as other phonological, and not as lexical errors and that no criterion is applied of the form "is this a real word?" It is also shown that, whereas there is considerable lexical bias in spontaneous speech errors and this effect is sensitive to phonetic similarity, self-corrections of overt speech errors are not sensitive to lexical status or phonetic similarity. It is argued here that the monitor has access to the intended word forms and that lexical bias and self-corrections of overt speech errors are not caused by the same perception-based self-monitoring system. Possibly fast and hidden self-monitoring of inner speech differs from slower and overt self-monitoring of overt speech.

Introduction: Levelt's model of speech production and self-monitoring

We all make errors when we speak. When I intend to say "good beer" it may come out as "bood beer" or even as "bood gear"; or when I want to say "put the bread on the table" I may inadvertently turn it into "put the table on the table" or into "put the table on the bread". Let us call errors like "bood beer" or "bood gear", where phonemes are misplaced, phonological errors, and ones like "table on the table" or "table on the bread", where meaningful items show up in the wrong positions, lexical errors. Lexical errors supposedly arise during grammatical encoding, phonological ones during phonological encoding (Levelt, 1989). Errors as given in our examples are syntagmatic speech errors, involving two elements in the intended utterance, a source and a target, the source being the intended position of an element, the target being the position where it ends up. So in the intended utterance "bread on the table", underlying the error "table on the table", "table" is the source and "bread" the target. Speakers also make paradigmatic speech errors, involving only a single intruding element, but here I will only be concerned with syntagmatic speech errors (cf. Fromkin, 1973).

The fact that we know that speech errors exist implies that we can detect them. And we not only detect errors in the speech of others, but also in our own speech. In the collection used for the current study, roughly 50 per cent of all speech errors were detected and corrected by the speakers (an earlier analysis of Meringer's, 1908, corpus suggested somewhat higher values; Nooteboom, 1980). Apparently, part of a speaker's mind is paying attention to the speech being produced by another part of the same mind, keeping an ear out for inadvertent errors that may be in need of correction. Let us call this part of the speaking mind the "monitor", and its function "self-monitoring" (Levelt, 1983, 1989). The general question I am focussing on here is: "How is self-monitoring of speech organized, and what information does it operate on?" The question is not new. A firm stand on this issue, based on extensive empirical evidence, has been for example taken by Levelt (1989), and by Levelt et al. (1999). The reason to take their theory as a starting point is that it is the most constrained, most parsimonious, theory of speech production available. In many ways it predicts what it should and does not predict what it should not. Alternative theories will be mentioned in the discussion section.

For the present purposes the following properties of the spreading-activation theory proposed by Levelt and his associates are relevant: (1) Speech production is strictly serial and feedforward only, implying that there is no cascading activation and no immediate feedback from the level of phonological encoding to the level of grammatical encoding; (2) self-monitoring employs the speech comprehension system, also used in listening to the speech of others; (3) the speech being produced reaches the comprehension system via two different routes, the inner route feeding a covert form of not-yet-articulated speech into the speech-comprehension system, and the auditory route feeding overt speech into the ears of the speaker/listener; (4) on the phonological level there is no specific information on intended phonological forms leaking to the speech comprehension system. The monitor must make do with a general criterion of the form "is this a real word?" instead of a criterion such as "is this the word I wanted to say?"; (5) lexical bias in speech errors is caused by the same perception-based self-monitoring system that is responsible for the detection and correction of overt speech errors.

This theory leads to some predictions that can be tested by looking at properties of speech errors in spontaneous speech and their corrections. The following predictions are up for testing:

- The monitor treats phonological errors that lead to real words, such as "gear" for "beer", as lexical errors.
- If spontaneous phonological speech errors show lexical bias, as has been suggested by Dell (1986), then one should also find a lexical bias effect in self-corrections of overt speech errors.

Before testing the first prediction, it should be assessed that so-called real-word phonological errors are indeed caused during phonological and not during grammatical encoding. This question will be dealt with first. Also, it will appear below that there may be a problem in testing the first prediction, caused by the fact that many overtly corrected anticipations, such as "Yew ... New York", may not be anticipations at all, but rather halfway-corrected transpositions. If so, there is no way of telling whether the error triggering the monitor was the real word "Yew" or the non-word "Nork" (cf. Cutler, 1982; Nooteboom, 1980). The question is whether or not this observation potentially invalidates the interpretation of a comparison between correction frequencies of phonological non-word errors, phonological real-word errors and lexical errors. It will be shown that it does. To circumvent this problem, a separate analysis will be made in which non-word and real-word phonological errors are limited to perseverations, such as "good gear" instead of "good beer", because there no part of the error can hide in inner speech. With respect to the prediction concerning lexical bias, it should be noted that reports on the existence of lexical bias in spontaneous speech errors differ. Garrett (1976) did not find evidence for lexical bias, Dell (1986) did, but Del Viso, Igoa, and Garcia-Albea (1991) did not for Spanish, although using a measure for lexical bias that is very similar to Dell's. So before studying lexical bias in self-corrections of overt speech errors, it should be assessed that there really is lexical bias in spontaneous speech errors. As will be seen, there is ample evidence for lexical bias in Dutch spontaneous speech errors. Therefore it makes sense to ask whether or not there is lexical bias in self-corrections in overt speech errors, as predicted from Levelt's theory. The reader will see that there is not. A related question is whether lexical bias is sensitive to phonetic distance between target and error phoneme, as predicted from perception-based monitoring but also from production-based theories, and if so whether the same is true for the probability of self-corrections of overt speech errors. Finally, there is the question whether the structure of the current data rather stems from a collector's bias than from the mechanisms underlying the production and perception of speech.

The following questions will now be dealt with in succession:

- Are alleged real-word phonological errors actually made during phonological or grammatical encoding?
- Does the fact that alleged corrected anticipations might sometimes have been halfway-corrected transpositions hinder the interpretation of comparisons between correction frequencies for non-word and real-word errors?
- Does the monitor treat phonological errors that lead to real words, such as "gear" for "beer", as lexical or as phonological errors?
- Do spontaneous phonological speech errors show lexical bias?
- Do self-corrections of overt speech errors show lexical bias?
- Are lexical bias and probability of self-corrections of overt speech errors equally sensitive to phonetic distance between target and error?
- Do the current data suffer from a collector's bias invalidating otherwise plausible conclusions?

Several possible explanations of the current findings will be discussed in the final section of this chapter.

The corpus

To answer the above questions two different collections of spontaneous speech errors in Dutch were used, the first collection only being used in studying lexical bias, because for these speech errors no overt self-corrections were available.

The oldest collection (AC/SN corpus) is basically the same as the one described by Nooteboom (1969). The errors were collected and noted down in orthography during several years of collecting by two people, the late Anthony Cohen and myself. Unfortunately, corrections were not systematically noted down. Collection of errors continued some time after 1969, and in its present form the collection contains some 1000 speech errors of various types, phonological syntagmatic errors outnumbering other types, such as lexical syntagmatic errors, blends, and intrusion errors. The collection was never put into a digital database and is only available in typed form, each error on a separate card. Selection of particular types of errors for the present purpose was done by hand.

The second collection (Utrecht corpus) stems from efforts of staff members of the Phonetics Department of Utrecht University, who, on the initiative of Anthony Cohen, from 1977 to 1982 orthographically noted down all speech errors heard in their environment, with their corrections, if any (cf. Schelvis, 1985). The collection contains some 2500 errors of various types, of which more than 1100 are phonological syntagmatic errors and some 185 lexical syntagmatic errors. The collection was put into a digital database, currently accessible with Microsoft Access.

Are alleged real-word phonological errors actually made during phonological or grammatical encoding?

Before making any comparisons between non-word phonological errors, real-word phonological errors and lexical errors, we have to make sure that in production alleged real-word phonological errors really arise at the level of phonological encoding and not at the level of grammatical encoding. In Table 10.1 we see confusion matrices for source and target of phonological non-word errors, phonological real-word errors and lexical errors.

These data show that in lexical errors an open-class word is never replaced by a closed-class word and a closed-class word never by an open-class word. In fact, closer analysis shows that syntactic word class is nearly always preserved (cf. Nooteboom, 1969). This is quite different for non-word phonological errors where the distribution of word-class preservation and violation is entirely predictable from relative frequencies and chance. So how do our alleged phonological real-word errors behave? Obviously they behave like non-word phonological errors, not like lexical errors. So we can be reassured that in the bulk of such errors lexical status is purely accidental. Now we are in a better position to ask whether the monitor treats real-word phonological errors as lexical errors, as predicted by Levelt et al., or rather as phonological errors. But first there is this problem with corrected anticipations perhaps being misclassified transpositions.

Corrected anticipations or halfway-corrected transpositions?

It has been observed that relatively many corrected anticipations in collections of speech errors, such as: "Yew. . . . New York", may be misclassified halfway-corrected transpositions (Cutler, 1982; Nooteboom, 1980). If we assume that speech errors can be detected in inner speech before becoming overt, in all these cases the monitor has not one but two opportunities to detect an error, and for all we know the second, hidden, part of the transposition may have been a non-word, as in the current example. This state of affairs potentially upsets any statistical differences we find in a comparison

Table 10.1 Three confusion matrices for source and target being, or belonging to, a closed- versus an open-class word, separately for phonological non-word errors, phonological real-word errors, and lexical errors

	Phonological non-word errors		*Phonological real-word errors*		*Lexical errors*	
Source	Open class	Closed class	Open class	Closed class	Open class	Closed class
Target						
Open class	303	55	169	30	135	0
Closed class	58	21	25	10	0	24

Table 10.2 Numbers of corrected and uncorrected speech errors, separately for perseverations, anticipations, and transpositions

	Perseverations	Anticipations	Transpositions	Total
Corrected	103	*442(?)*	*42(?)*	587
Not corrected	153	238	175	566
Total	256	*680(?)*	*217(?)*	1153

Note: There is a strong interaction between error class and correction frequency (chi^2 = 153; df = 2; p < 0.001). Cursive numbers are suspected not to correspond to what happened in inner speech. Utrecht corpus only.

between lexical and phonological real-word errors. That this is a serious threat may be shown by the following estimates of the relative numbers of anticipations and transpositions in inner speech. Let us assume that the probability of detecting an error in internal speech is not different for antici-pations and perseverations (to the extent that this assumption is incorrect the following calculations will be inaccurate; but if the underlying reasoning is basically sound, they will at least provide a plausible rough estimate). We know the number of uncorrected perseverations, the total number of perse-verations, and the number of uncorrected anticipations (Table 10.2). From the numbers in Table 10.2, using an equation with one unknown, one can easily calculate what the total number of anticipations, and therefore also the number of corrected anticipations, would have been, without the influx of halfway-corrected transpositions. The equation runs as follows:

103 corrected perseverations : 153 not corrected perseverations,
= ? corrected anticipations : 238 not corrected anticipations

The estimate number of corrected anticipations would then be:

$(103 \times 238) : 153 = 160$

The total number of anticipations would be 160 + 238 = 398. The estimate number of misclassified halfway-corrected transpositions is 442 − 160 = 282. Note that this brings the total number of transpositions in internal speech to 282 + 42 + 175 = 499 instead of 217, making transpositions by far the most frequent class of speech errors (Table 10.3). These estimates are further confirmed in the following way: The probability of remaining uncorrected is 0.6 for both perseverations and anticipations. A transposition contains an anticipation plus a perseveration. The probability of remaining uncorrected should therefore be 0.6 × 0.6 = 0.36. The new estimate of the fraction of transpositions remaining uncorrected equals:

$1 - (42 + 282): 499 = 0.35$

Table 10.3 Numbers of corrected and uncorrected speech errors in inner speech, separately for perseverations, anticipations, and transpositions

	Perseverations	*Anticipations*	*Transpositions*	*Total*
Corrected	103	*160*	*324*	587
Not corrected	153	238	175	566
Total	256	*398*	*499*	1153

Note: Cursive numbers are estimated (see text). Utrecht corpus only.

Apparently, still provided that our assumption that the probability of being detected in internal speech is the same for perseverations and anticipations was correct, both parts of the error contribute equally and independently to the probability of remaining uncorrected.

From these calculations, it is at least plausible that a great many corrected anticipations in our corpus originated as halfway-corrected transpositions in inner speech. Of course we have no way of knowing which are and which are not. In all such cases in which the error is phonological we do not know whether the error triggering the monitor was a real word or a non-word. We therefore should treat any comparison between numbers of correction for real-word and non-word anticipations with caution.

Does the monitor treat phonological errors that lead to real words as lexical or phonological?

We know that lexical errors and phonological errors are treated differently by the monitor: Both the distribution of the number of words a speaker goes on speaking before stopping to correct a speech error and the distribution of the number of words a speaker retraces in his correction is different for lexical and phonological errors (Nooteboom, 1980). Our corpus of speech errors noted down with their corrections, makes it possible to compare the distributions of the number of words spoken before the speaker stops for correction, and the number of words included in the correction, between different classes of speech errors. If Levelt et al. are right in assuming that the monitor has no way of knowing whether a particular error was made during grammatical or during phonological encoding, these distributions should be different for non-word and real-word phonological errors, and the same for real-word phonological and lexical errors.

Contrary to this prediction, Figure 10.1. suggests that the distribution of the numbers of words spoken before stopping is very similar for non-word and real-word phonological errors and rather different for real-word phonological errors and lexical errors.

To test these predictions statistically, for the moment neglecting the threat stemming from corrected anticipations being halfway-corrected transpositions, the numbers underlying Figure 10.1 were collapsed into a 2 × 2 matrix

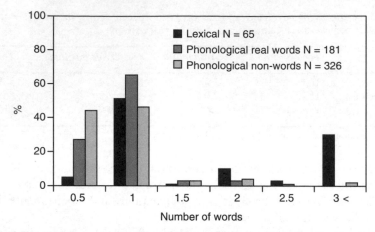

Figure 10.1 Percentage of speech errors as a function of the number of words spoken
before stopping for correcting a speech error, plotted separately for lexical
errors, phonological errors leading to non-words, and phonological errors
accidentally leading to real words.

Table 10.4 Numbers of speech errors as a function of number of words spoken before
stopping to correct a speech error, separately for non-word phonological errors,
real-word phonological errors, and lexical errors

n	*1 or less*	*More than 1*
Phonological non-word	294	32
Phonological real word	163	18
Lexical	36	29

Note: Phonological non-word errors do not differ significantly from phonological real-word
errors ($chi^2 = 0.00217$; df = 1; p > 0.95); real-word phonological errors differ significantly from
lexical errors ($chi^2 = 37$; df = 1; p < 0.0001). Utrecht corpus only.

in order to avoid extremely small expected values, while keeping the relevant
differences. The collapsed matrix is shown in Table 10.4. Phonological real-
word errors differ significantly from lexical but not from phonological non-
word errors. This suggests that the monitor treats the phonological real-word
errors as phonological ones.

Figure 10.2 presents a similar comparison for the number of words
repeated in the correction. The corresponding collapsed matrix of the underlying numbers is given as Table 10.5. Again, these data suggest that the monitor treats phonological real-word errors as phonological and not as lexical
ones.

A great proportion of the data in Tables 10.4 and 10.5 concern corrected
anticipations. As discussed in the previous paragraph, we should treat these
data with some caution. In Tables 10.6 and 10.7 data are presented limited to
phonological non-word and real-word perseverations to be compared with

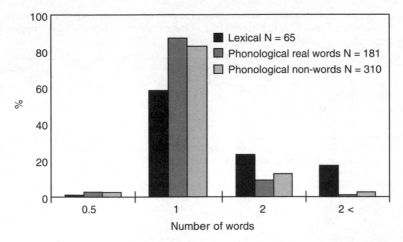

Figure 10.2 Percentage of speech errors as a function of the number of words spoken in the correction, plotted separately for lexical errors, phonological errors leading to non-words, and phonological errors accidentally leading to real words.

Table 10.5 Numbers of speech errors as a function of number of words repeated in the correction, separately for non-word phonological errors, real-word phonological errors and lexical errors

n	*1 or less*	*More than 1*
Phonological non-word	264	46
Phonological real word	161	20
Lexical	39	26

Note: Less than 1 indicates that the speaker not even went back to the beginning of the word containing the error. This occurred only in compounds. Phonological non-word errors do not differ significantly from phonological real-word errors (chi^2 = 1.41; df = 1; p > 0.1); real-word phonological errors differ significantly from lexical errors (chi^2 = 26; df = 1; p < 0.0001). Utrecht corpus only.

Table 10.6 Numbers of speech errors as a function of number of words spoken before stopping for correction, separately for non-word phonological perseverations, real-word phonological perseverations, and lexical errors

n	*Less than 1*	*1*	*More than 1*
Phonological non-word	24	25	0
Phonological real word	15	11	0
Lexical	4	32	29

Note: Less than 1 indicates that the speaker did not complete the word containing the error. Phonological non-word perseverations do not differ significantly from phonological real-word perseverations (chi^2 = 0.52; df = 1; p > 0.3); real-word phonological perseverations differ significantly from lexical errors (chi^2 = 35; df = 2; p < 0.0001). Utrecht corpus only.

Table 10.7 Numbers of speech errors as a function of number of words repeated in the correction, separately for non-word phonological perseverations, real-word phonological perseverations, and lexical errors

n	1 or less	More than 1
Phonological non-word	45	7
Phonological real word	32	6
Lexical	38	27

Note: Less than 1 indicates that the speaker not even went back to the beginning of the word containing the error. Phonological non-word perseverations do not differ significantly from phonological real-word perseverations ($chi^2 = 0.096$; df = 1; p > 0.9); real-word phonological perseverations differ significantly from lexical errors ($chi^2 = 7.3$; df = 1; p < 0.01). Utrecht corpus only.

lexical errors. In a perseveration, no part of the error triggering the monitor can hide in inner speech. Although the data are rather sparse, we find again a significant difference between phonological real-word errors and lexical errors but not between phonological non-word and real-word errors. A concern might be that with real-word errors sometimes syntax is violated, potentially providing an extra cue to the monitor. However, over those phonological real-word anticipations for which it could be assessed whether or not syntax was violated by the error, probability of correction appeared to be equal for errors with violated and with intact syntax (N = 150; $chi^2 = 0.465$; df = 1; p > 0.3). It seems safe to conclude that the monitor treats phonological real-word errors as phonological and not as lexical errors.

Do spontaneous phonological speech errors show lexical bias?

Lexical bias here is taken to mean that, in case of a phonological speech error, the probability that the error leads to a real word is greater, and the probability that the error leads to a non-word is less than chance. Lexical bias has been shown for experimentally elicited speech errors, where chance level could be experimentally controlled (Baars & Motley, 1974; Baars, Motley, & Mackay, 1975). The problem with spontaneous speech errors, of course, is to determine chance. Garrett (1976) attempted to solve this problem by sampling word pairs from published interviews and exchanging their initial sounds. He found that 33 per cent of these "pseudo-errors" created words. This was not conspicuously different from real-word phonological speech errors, so he concluded that there was no lexical bias in spontaneous speech errors. One may note, however, that Garrett did not distinguish between monosyllables and polysyllables. Obviously, exchanging a phoneme in a polysyllabic word hardly ever creates a real word. This may have obscured an effect of lexical bias. Dell and Reich (1981) used a more elaborate technique to estimate chance level, involving "random" pairing of words from the error corpus in two lists of word forms, exchanging of the paired words' initial sounds, and determining how often words are thereby created, normalizing for the frequency of each initial phoneme in each list. They found a significant lexical bias in anticipations, perseverations and transpositions. In the latter, involving two errors ("Yew Nork" for "New York") lexical bias was stronger in the first ("Yew") than in the second ("Nork") error. Del Viso et al. (1991), using a method very similar to Dell's, found no evidence for lexical bias in Spanish spontaneous speech errors. Note, however, that Dell's method is not very straightforward. The greater number of longish words in Spanish as compared with English may have obscured an effect of lexical bias.

In the current study I followed a different approach for assessing lexical bias, restricting myself to single-phoneme substitutions in monosyllables, i.e., errors where a single phoneme in a monosyllable is replaced with another single phoneme, in this way capitalizing on the fact that replacing a phoneme much more often creates a real word in a monosyllable than in a polysyllable. I did not, however, as Garrett (1976) and Dell and Reich (1981) did, restrict myself to initial phonemes, but took all single-phoneme substitutions in monosyllables into account. The two collections of Dutch speech errors together gave 311 such errors, 218 of which were real-word errors and 93 non-word errors. Although these numbers suggest a lexical bias, this may be an illusion, because it is unknown what chance would have given. It is reasonable to assume that a major factor in determining the probability of the lexical status of a phoneme substitution error is provided by the phonotactic alternatives. If, for example, the *p* of *pin*, is replaced by a *b*, the phonotactically possible errors are *bin, chin, din, fin, gin, kin, lin, sin, shin, tin, thin* (with voiceless *th*), *win, yin, *guin, *hin, *min, *nin, *rin, *zin, *zhin, *thin* (with voiced *th*). In this case there are 21 phonotactic alternatives, of which 13 are real words and 8 are nonsense words.

Of course, if all phonotactic alternatives are real words (which sometimes happens), the probability that the error produces a real word is 1; and if all alternatives are nonsense words (which also happens) the probability of a real word error is zero. In the case of *pin* turning into *bin*, the chance level for a real-word error would have been $13/21 = 0.62$. I have assessed the average proportions of real-word phonotactic alternatives for all 311 single-phoneme substitutions in monosyllables (not only initial phonemes), taking only into account the phonotactically possible single phonemes in that position.

The average proportions of real-word and non-word alternatives in this particular set of monosyllables are both 0.5. The expected numbers of real-word and non-word speech errors therefore are both $311/2 = 155.5$, whereas the actual numbers are 218 and 93 (Table 10.8). There is a strong interaction between error categories and expected values based on average proportions of phonotactic real-word and non-word alternatives. Evidently there is a strong lexical bias in spontaneous speech errors.

Table 10.8 Observed numbers of real words and non-words in single-phoneme substitutions in monosyllables only and numbers expected on the basis of the average proportions of real-word and non-word alternatives

	Observed values	*Expected values*
Real words	218	155.5
Non-words	93	155.5

Note: chi^2 = 26; df = 1; p < 0.0001. AC/SN corpus plus Utrecht corpus.

Do self-corrections of overt speech errors show lexical bias?

As we have seen, spontaneous speech errors show a strong lexical bias. If self-monitoring were responsible for lexical bias, by applying a lexicality test, as has been suggested by Levelt et al. (1999), then one would expect the same lexicality test to affect overt self-monitoring. This should lead to non-word errors being more often detected and corrected than real word errors. Indeed, if Levelt et al. were correct in their suggestion that monitoring one's own speech for errors is very much like monitoring someone else's speech for errors, listening for deviant sound form, deviant syntax, and deviant meaning, real-word errors cannot be detected in self-monitoring on the level of phonology. By definition real-word errors would pass any lexicality test, and therefore could only be detected as if they were lexical errors causing deviant syntax or deviant meaning. If, among other criteria, a lexicality test is applied by self-monitoring for phonological errors, we may expect the correction frequency to be higher for non-word errors than for real-word errors. Table 10.9 gives the relevant breakdown for all 315 single-phoneme substitutions in the Utrecht corpus and Table 10.10 gives the relevant breakdown of all 1111 phonological speech errors in this collection.

Obviously, there is no evidence of non-word errors being more frequently corrected than real-word errors. The data in Table 10.10 show that, if we consider all phonological errors instead of single-phoneme substitutions only, the probabilities for correction of real-word and non-word errors are exactly equal. It thus seems very unlikely that a lexicality test is applied in self-monitoring for overt speech errors during spontaneous speech production.

Table 10.9 Numbers of corrected and uncorrected single-phoneme substitutions in monosyllables and polysyllables together, separately for real-word errors and non-word errors

	Real words	*Non-words*
Corrected	99	69
Uncorrected	98	49

Note: chi^2 = 2; df = 1; p > 0.1. Utrecht corpus only.

Table 10.10 Numbers of corrected and uncorrected phonological errors in monosyllables and polysyllables together, separately for real-word errors and non-word errors

	Real words	Non-words
Corrected	218	341
Uncorrected	210	342

Note: chi^2 = 0.117; df = 1; p > 0.7. Utrecht corpus only.

Are lexical bias and probability of self-corrections of overt speech errors equally sensitive to phonetic distance between target and error?

If lexical bias results from editing out of non-words by self-monitoring, one would expect that errors differing from the correct form in only a single distinctive feature would be missed more often than errors differing in more features. The reason is that self-monitoring is supposed to depend on self-perception (Levelt et al., 1999), and it is reasonable to expect that in perception smaller differences are more likely to go unnoticed than larger differences. As lexical bias is supposed to be the effect of suppressing non-words, one expects lexical bias to increase with dissimilarity between the two phonemes involved. To test this prediction I divided the 311 single-phoneme substitution errors in monosyllables into three classes, viz errors involving 1 feature, errors involving 2 features, and errors involving 3 or more features. For consonants I used as features manner of articulation, place of articulation, and voice. For vowels features were degree of openness, degree of frontness, length, roundedness, and monophthong versus diphthong. Table 10.11 gives the numbers of real-word and non-word errors for the three types of single-phoneme substitutions in monosyllables, in the AC/SN corpus and Utrecht corpus together.

These results clearly suggest that lexical bias is sensitive to phonetic (dis)similarity, as predicted both from a perception-based theory of pre-articulatory editing, but also from "phoneme-to-word" feedback (Dell & Reich, 1980; Dell, 1986; Stemberger, 1985). If self-corrections are also sensitive to phonetic (dis)similarity this would favor the hypothesis that both effects stem from the same mechanism. If they are not, this would suggest

Table 10.11 Numbers of real-word errors and non-word errors in monosyllables only, separately for errors involving 1, 2, or 3 or more features

	1 feature	2 features	3 features
Real words	95	96	27
Non-words	59	29	5

Note: chi^2 = 7.29; df = 2; p < 0.01. AC/SN corpus plus Utrecht corpus.

Table 10.12 Numbers of corrected and uncorrected single-phoneme substitutions in monosyllables and polysyllables together, separately for errors involving 1, 2, or 3 features

	1 feature	*2 features*	*3 features*
Corrected	94	85	15
Uncorrected	60	65	19

Note: chi^2 = 3.3; df = 2; p > 0.1; n.s. Utrecht corpus only.

different mechanisms for lexical bias and self-detection of overt errors. Table 10.12 gives the relevant data taken from the Utrecht corpus. Obviously, there is little evidence that self-corrections are sensitive to phonetic (dis)-similarity, although one would predict such an effect from perception-based monitoring. This finding is corroborated by experimental data reported by Postma and Kolk (1992), to be further discussed in the following section. Self-correction of overt speech errors differs in this respect from whatever mechanism is responsible for lexical bias in speech errors.

Do the current data suffer from a collector's bias invalidating otherwise plausible solutions?

Perhaps the current data suffer from a collector's bias, invalidating the otherwise plausible conclusions (cf. Cutler, 1982). Of course, here the two possible sources of such a bias are phonetic similarity and lexical status. It seems unlikely, however, that such biases hold equally for corrected and uncorrected speech errors. The reason is that correction presents a very clear clue to the collector, easily overriding any more subtle difference due to phonetic similarity or lexical status. Thus, if there is a collector's bias due to phonetic similarity or to lexical bias, there should be an interaction between corrected versus uncorrected and lexical status combined with phonetic similarity. The data in Table 10.13 strongly suggest that there is no such interaction. This makes it implausible that the absence of effects of lexical status and phonetic similarity in correction frequencies is due to a collector's bias.

Table 10.13 Numbers of corrected and uncorrected single-phoneme substitutions in monosyllables and polysyllables together, separately for errors involving 1, 2 or more features, and for real-word errors and non-word errors

	1 feature, real word	*1 feature, non-word*	*2/3 features, real word*	*2/3 features, non-word*
Corrected	52	41	47	28
Uncorrected	52	26	53	23

Note: chi^2 = 3.6; df = 3; p > 0.3, n.s. Utrecht corpus only.

That the sensitivity of lexical bias and the insensitivity of self-detection of speech errors to phonetic similarity do not stem from a collector's bias is supported by experimental data provided by Lackner and Tuller (1979), and by Postma and Kolk (1992). Lackner and Tuller had speakers recite strings of nonsense syllables of CV structure, both with and without auditory masking of their own overt speech by noise. Subjects were instructed to press a tele-graph key when they detected an error in their speech. Speakers made many errors with a difference of a single feature between error and target, but hardly any with more than a single feature. Apparently such multifeature errors were suppressed more often. This replicates the sensitivity of lexical bias to phonetic distance, assuming that the repertoire of nonsense syllables to be recited form a temporary lexicon in such an experiment. Because of the lack of multifeature errors, no useful comparisons could be made in terms of detection frequencies. This is different in the experimental data reported by Postma and Kolk. They replicated the Lackner and Tuller experiment, this time with both CV and VC syllables, and with normal speakers and stutterers. They also found many single-feature errors and hardly any multi-feature errors in the CV syllables. Surprisingly, in the VC syllables there were rela-tively many multifeature errors. Whatever the cause of this, detection fre-quencies showed hardly any effect of phonetic distance, precisely as in the current data on self-corrections of spontaneous speech errors. It seems safe to conclude that the current findings cannot be explained away by a collector's bias.

Discussion

In this chapter I have set out to test two predictions derived from the theory of speech production and self-monitoring proposed by Levelt et al. (1999):

- The monitor treats phonological errors that lead to real words, such as "gear" for "beer", as lexical errors.
- If spontaneous phonological speech errors show lexical bias, as has been suggested by Dell (1986), then the same lexical bias should be found in self-corrections of overt speech errors.

Both predictions have been falsified: Real-word phonological errors are clearly treated by the monitor as phonological, not as lexical errors. And although spontaneous speech errors in Dutch show a clear lexical bias, the probability of self-correction of overt speech errors does not show a trace of lexical bias.

The first finding corroborates a finding by Shattuck-Hufnagel and Cutler (1999), who showed that lexical errors tend to be corrected with a pitch accent on the corrected item, whereas both non-word and real-word phonological errors do not. This suggests that the monitor has access to the intended phonological form. Instead of asking, "is this a real word?", it appears to ask, "is this the word I intended to say?" One may note that this may be related to self-monitoring being a relatively slow, conscious, or at least a semi-conscious process (Levelt, 1989). Hartsuiker and Kolk (2001) estimate that the sum of auditory input processing, parsing and comparing is minimally 200 ms, and add another 200 ms for interrupting (cf. Levelt, 1989). Blackmer and Mitton (1991) have provided evidence suggesting that error detection and correction can take place before message interruption, such that speaking and reconstructing the intended message are incremental processes. Both accounts of temporal aspects of self-monitoring do not conflict with the suggestion that overt self-monitoring to some extent may depend on time-consuming conscious processing. Fodor (1983) and Baars (1997) both suggested that consciousness provides access to otherwise hidden subconscious information. In other words, slow and conscious processes are not modular (although they may suffer from limited resources), whereas fast and subconscious processes are often modular. If we take these ideas seriously, self-correction of overt speech errors may have access to intended phonological word forms through (semi-) conscious processing, and therefore has no need for a general criterion of the form "is this a real word?" In this way the current data may be reconciled with the idea that speech production and perception (but not monitoring) are to a large extent modular.

The second main finding of the current study is that lexical bias and self-correction of overt speech errors differ in some important respects, suggesting that they do not stem from the same underlying mechanism. As we have seen, self-correction of overt speech errors is a relatively slow, semiconscious process. Lexical bias must be due to a very fast process that does not interrupt the stream of speech and that never seems to reach consciousness. Self-correction of overt errors does not seem to be sensitive to lexical status, the mechanism responsible for lexical bias obviously is. The latter mechanism is also sensitive to phonetic similarity between target and error, as lexical bias significantly increases with phonetic similarity. In contrast the probability of self-correction of overt speech errors appears to be independent of phonetic similarity. It may be noted that the sensitivity of lexical bias to phonetic similarity in itself is not an argument in favor of either perception-based self-monitoring or a production-based mechanism as the source of the effect, as on the face of it the phonetic-similarity effect is compatible with both explanations. However, the finding that lexical bias is and self-correction of overt speech errors is not sensitive to phonetic similarity suggests that there are two different mechanisms involved.

Because self-correction of overt speech errors obviously is perception based it may be unexpected that there is no effect of phonetic similarity, not only in our data on spontaneous speech but also in the experimental data provided by Postma and Kolk (1992). It seems reasonable to expect that small differences would be more easily not heard than greater differences. Possibly the absence of a similarity effect is related to the assumption that the monitor compares intended with perceived form, instead of checking whether the perceived form is or is not part of the lexicon. One may also note that the absence of a lexicality effect in self-corrections of overt speech errors contradicts a prediction from Mackay's Node Structure Theory (1992). This theory predicts that non-word errors are more easily detected than real-word errors because there is a level where non-word errors are novel combinations, and real-word errors are not.

The properties of the mechanism causing lexical bias in spontaneous speech errors seem to be different from those of self-correction of overt speech errors: Lexical bias is caused by a mechanism that is fast and unconscious, is sensitive to the lexicality of the error and sensitive to phonetic distance between error and intended form. Self-correction of overt errors is time-consuming, and is not sensitive to the lexical status of the error and phonetic distance between error and target. There are several possible explanations for this difference.

One is that lexical bias is caused by a feedback mechanism as suggested by Dell (1986). Dell and Reich (1980) describe the proposed mechanism as follows: "An activated set of phonemes that corresponds to a word is continually reinforced by reverberation with a single word node because most of the activation from the phonemes converges and sums up at that node." Of course, an erroneous set of phonemes would either "reverberate" with the wrong word node, explaining the lexical bias, or with no word at all, explaining the "suppression of non-word outcomes" (Dell & Reich, 1980). A set of phonemes differing minimally from the activated word node would still reverberate" considerably with it, but as the difference increases, "reverberation" would diminish. That lexical bias decreases with phonetic similarity between intended and erroneous form, thus is entirely in tune with the feedback model. Of course, a feedback model is less parsimonious than a strictly serial feedforward-only model. However, it has been shown computationally that lexical bias is consistent with an architecture of speech production in which the interactivity introduced by cascading activation and phoneme-to-word feedback is severely restricted, and thereby seriality to a large extent preserved (Rapp & Goldrick, 2000). An argument against the feedback model, as pointed out by Levelt et al. (1999), is that it does not easily explain that lexical bias is sensitive to contextual and situational information and to social appropriateness (Motley, 1980; Motley, Camden, & Baars, 1982). One may note, however, that an architecture of speech production that is not strictly modular but rather has restricted interactivity, with some "leakage" of information from one module to another, as suggested by Rapp and Goldrick (2000), would more easily allow for such effects.

Alternatively, the current data can be explained by a fast automatic production-based monitor that is completely separate from the perception-based monitor responsible for self-corrections of overt speech errors. Such a production-based monitor has been suggested by Nickels and Howard (1995) and Postma (2000). This would more easily account for the fact that lexical bias is sensitive to contextual and situational information, and social appropriateness (Motley, 1980; Motley et al., 1982), something one would intuitively rather expect from a monitoring system than from a fully automatized speech production system.

A third possibility is that lexical bias is caused by output editing of inner speech, as suggested by Levelt et al. (1999). This would, of course, also account for output editing being sensitive to contextual and situational information and social appropriateness. We then have to assume that output editing of inner speech differs in its properties from output editing of overt speech errors, notably in being fast, unconscious and sensitive to a general criterion of lexicality and to phonetic distance between error and intended form. Perhaps the properties of output editing by the self-monitoring system change as a function of the time the system is allowed to do its job. Fast and hidden editing of unspoken errors remains unconscious, and has to depend on general criteria, slow editing of errors already spoken may become conscious, and may have access to more detailed information about the intended form.

A serendipitous finding of the current study is that the majority of speech errors in inner speech are transpositions or exchanges, contrary to what counting overt speech errors so far suggested. It remains to be seen whether current theories of speech error generation, in as far as they are based on relative frequencies of different types of speech error (cf. Dell, 1986), can easily be retuned in order to accommodate this finding.

The most important conclusions from the current analysis of speech errors and their corrections seem to be the following.

The part of a speaker's mind that watches out for speech errors in order to correct them has access to the intended phonological forms of misspoken words. In this way, contrary to what has been suggested by Levelt et al. (1999), listening for errors in one's own (overt) speech is quite different from listening for speech errors in the speech of other speakers.

Lexical bias in spontaneous speech errors is not caused by the same mechanism that allows for detection and correction of overt speech errors. It may either be caused by an automatic production-based monitor that is quite different from the semi-conscious perception-based monitor that is responsible for self-corrections of overt speech errors (Nickels & Howard, 1995; Postma 2000), or by a phoneme-to-word feedback mechanism, as proposed by Dell (1986) and Dell and Reich (1980), and more recently by Rapp and Goldrick (2000), or by output editing of inner speech as suggested by Levelt (1989) and Levelt et al. (1999). If so, the current results imply that fast and hidden output editing of inner speech, employing a general criterion of lexicality and thereby rejecting nonwords more frequently than real words, is different from output editing of overt speech, comparing the spoken word form with the intended word form. This difference between output editing of inner speech and of overt speech is supported by more recent experimental evidence (Nooteboom, 2003).

Acknowledgements

I am grateful to those who read and commented on earlier versions of this manuscript, and made suggestions for improvements. These are Bernard Baars, Anne Cutler, Gary Dell, Rob Hartsuiker, Pim Levelt, Albert Postma, Ardi Roelofs, Hugo Quené and Frank Wijnen.

References

Baars, B. J. (1997). *In the theatre of consciousness.* New York: Oxford University Press.

Baars, B. J., & Motley, M. T. (1974). Spoonerisms: Experimental elicitation of human speech errors: Methods, implications, and work in progress. *Journal Supplement Abstract Service, Catalog of Selected Documents in Psychology.*

Baars, B. J., Motley, M. T., & McKay D. (1975). Output editing for lexical status from artificially elicited slips of the tongue. *Journal of Verbal Learning and Verbal Behavior, 14*, 382–91.

Blackmer E. R., & Mitton J. L. (1991) Theories of monitoring and the timing of repairs in spontaneous speech. *Cognition, 39*, 173–94.

Cutler, A. (1982). The reliability of speech error data. *Linguistics, 19*, 561–82.

Del Viso, S., Igoa, J. M., & Garcia-Albea, J. E. (1991). On the autonomy of phonological encoding: Evidence from slips of the tongue in Spanish. *Journal of Psycholinguistic Research, 20*, 161–85.

Dell, G. S. (1986). A spreading-activation theory of retrieval in sentence production. *Psychological Review, 93*, 283–321.

Dell, G. S., & Reich, P. A. (1980). Toward a unified model of slips of the tongue, In V. A. Fromkin (Ed.), *Errors in linguistic performance: Slips of the tongue, ear, pen, and hand* (pp. 273–86). New York: Academic Press.

Dell, G. S., & Reich, P. A. (1981). Stages in sentence production: An analysis of speech error data. *Journal of Verbal Learning and Verbal Behavior, 20*, 611–29.

Fodor, J. A. (1983). *The modularity of mind.* Cambridge, MA: Bradford Books, MIT Press.

Fromkin, V. A. (1973). *Speech errors as linguistic evidence.* The Hague: Mouton.

Garrett, M. F. (1976). Syntactic process in sentence production. In R. J. Walker, & E.C.T. Walker (Eds.), *New approaches to language mechanisms* (pp. 231–56). Amsterdam: North-Holland.

Hartsuiker, R. J., & Kolk, H. H. J. (2001). Error monitoring in speech production: A computational test of the perceptual loop theory. *Cognitive Psychology, 42*, 113–57.

Lackner, J. R., & Tuller, B. H. (1979). Role of efference monitoring in the detection of self-produced speech errors. In: W. E. Cooper, & E. C. T. Walker (Eds.), *Sentence processing: Psycholinguistic studies presented to Merrill Garrett* (pp. 281–94). Hillsdale, NJ: Lawrence Erlbaum Associates, Inc.

Levelt, W. J. M. (1983). Monitoring and self-repair in speech. *Cognition, 14*, 41–104.

Levelt, W. J. M. (1989). *Speaking: From intention to articulation.* Cambridge, MA: MIT Press.

Levelt, W. J. M., Roelofs, A., & Meyer, A. S. (1999). A theory of lexical access in speech production. *Behavioral and Brain Sciences, 22*, 1–75.

Meringer, R. (1908). *Aus dem Leben der Sprache.* Berlin: V. Behr's Verlag.

Motley, M. T. (1980). Verification of "Freudian" slips and semantic prearticulatory editing via laboratory-induced spoonerisms. In V. A. Fromkin (Ed.), *Errors in linguistic performance: Slips of the tongue, ear, pen, and hand* (pp. 133–48). New York: Academic Press.

Motley, M. T., Camden, C. T., & Baars, B. J. (1982). Covert formulation and editing of anomalies in speech production: Evidence from experimentally elicited slips of the tongue. *Journal of Verbal Learning and Verbal Behavior, 21*, 578–94.

Nickels, L., & Howard, D. (1995). Phonological errors in aphasic naming: comprehension, monitoring and lexicality. *Cortex, 31*, 209–37.

Nooteboom, S. G. (1969). The tongue slips into patterns. In A. Sciarone, A. J. van Essen, & A. A. van Raad (Eds.), *Nomen, Leyden studies in linguistics and phonetics* (pp. 114–32). The Hague: Mouton. Also in V. A. Fromkin (1973) (Ed.) *Speech errors as linguistic evidence*. (pp. 144–56). The Hague: Mouton.

Nooteboom, S. G. (1980). Speaking and unspeaking: Detection and correction of phonological and lexical errors in spontaneous speech. In V.A. Fromkin (Ed.), *Errors in linguistic performance: Slips of the tongue, ear, pen, and hand* (pp. 87–95). New York: Academic Press.

Nooteboom, S. G. (2003). Self-monitoring is the main cause of lexical bias in phonological speech errors. In R. Eklund (Ed.), *Proceedings of DiSS'03, Disfluency in Spontaneous Speech Workshop*. 5–8 September 2003, Göteborg University, Sweden. *Gothenburg Papers in Theoretical Linguistics, 89*, pp. 25–8.

Postma, A. (2000). Detection of errors during speech production: a review of speech monitoring models. *Cognition, 77*, 97–131.

Postma, A., & Kolk, H. (1992). Error monitoring in people who stutter: Evidence against auditory feedback defect theories. *Journal of Speech and Hearing Research, 35*, 1024–1032.

Rapp, B., & Goldrick, M. (2000). Discreteness and interactivity in spoken word production. *Psychological Review, 107*, 460–99.

Schelvis, M. (1985). The collection, categorisation, storage and retrieval of spontaneous speech error material at the Institute of Phonetics. Utrecht: *PRIPU, 10*, 3–14.

Shattuck-Húfnagel, S., & Cutler, A. (1999) The prosody of speech error corrections revisited [CD-ROM]. *Proceedings of the International Congress of Phonetic sciences in San Francisco, 1–6 August 1999* (pp. 1483–6). San Francisco: Regents of the University of California.

Stemberger, J. P. (1985). An interactive activation model of language production. In A. W. Ellis (Ed.), *Progress in the psychology of language* (Vol. 1, pp. 143–86). Hove, UK: Lawrence Erlbaum Associates Ltd.

11 The division of labor between internal and external speech monitoring

Robert J. Hartsuiker, Herman H. J. Kolk, and Heike Martensen

Abstract

Most theories of verbal self-monitoring assume that we detect speech errors through at least two channels: Overt speech (the external channel) and internal speech (the internal channel). The postulation of two channels raises questions about their relative contribution. We argue that existing proposals for determining this "division of labor" are inadequate: either they fail to take into account that monitoring the internal channel is sometimes slow or they hinge on the unjustified assumption that the two channels are equally accurate. We propose a probabilistic model that expresses a relation between the detection rates of the channels and the frequencies of disfluencies and corrected and uncorrected speech errors. By fitting the model to existing data sets with normal speech and noise-masked speech, acquired from speakers with Broca's aphasia and control speakers, we showed that the internal channel is more effective than the external channel. In fact, the data from Broca's aphasia were compatible with the hypothesis that the external channel is not used at all. Furthermore, the analyses suggest that the external channel is relatively unimportant in the detection of lexical errors, but important in the detection of phonological errors. We propose that the division of labor between channels is under top-down control (selective attention to the internal channel) but also depends on bottom-up influences (access to acoustical or phonetic information).

Introduction

Most theories of monitoring (e.g., Hartsuiker & Kolk, 2001; Levelt, 1983; Levelt, 1989; see Postma, 2000 for review) assume that speakers use at least two information sources: An external and an internal channel. First, speakers can listen to their own overt speech and check whether it contains any discrepancies with intended speech. This implies that the language comprehension system is critically involved in monitoring overt speech. Second, there is convincing evidence that speakers also monitor representations of speech that is not yet articulated through an internal channel. This can be appreciated by considering (1), an English translation of a repair reported by Levelt (1989):

  (1) then you go the v.horizontal line

In this example, the speaker produced a /v/, but interrupts immediately, and repairs with the word "horizontal". Given the context (an experiment in which speakers described routes through networks of colored circles), we can assume that the /v/ was the first sound of "vertical". This error is interrupted so quickly that it is very unlikely that the external channel detected it. The duration of a phoneme such as /v/ is about 70 ms. This leaves little time for auditory recognition of the actual utterance, comparison with target utterance, and halting of the speech apparatus (Hartsuiker & Kolk, 2001). It is much more likely that a representation of "vertical" was corrected internally, before the actual realization of the first sound /v/, but that the interruption took place too late to prevent the error from becoming overt.

There is also experimental evidence for inner monitoring. In one set of studies the participants could not hear their own overt speech, because it was masked by loud white noise[1] (Lackner & Tuller, 1979; Oomen, Postma, & Kolk, 2001, this volume, Chapter 12; Postma & Kolk, 1993; Postma & Noordanus, 1996). These studies consistently showed that speakers are able to detect substantial numbers of speech errors, although they could not use the external channel.

In other studies (e.g., Dell & Repka, 1992; Postma & Noordanus, 1996), speakers were asked to detect errors in *silent* speech. Participants indeed reported errors in inner speech and a similar pattern of error detection was observed as in external speech. This supports the theory of an internal channel, and it suggests that the internal and external channel use similar criteria for error detection.

Motley, Camden, and Baars (1982) inferred the existence of an inner monitor from patterns of speech errors. They used an error elicitation technique that induced many exchange errors, such as *darn bore* instead of *barn door*. They observed that exchanges were much less frequent if they would lead to taboo words (e.g., for *tool kits*), than if they would lead to neutral words. This suggests that exchanges in the taboo condition were intercepted by an internal monitoring channel which prevented them from becoming overt.

Finally, Hartsuiker, and Kolk (2001) implemented a formal model of the time course of incidents associated with monitoring (e.g., the time between the beginning of an error and the moment speech is interrupted). They concluded that in order to account for observed distributions of these intervals, it is necessary to assume that these distributions are the result of a combination of monitoring through the inner channel and outer channel.

The postulation of two monitoring channels raises questions about their relative contribution to error detection and repair (their division of labor). How many (and which) errors are detected by each channel? There are a number of reasons for wanting to separate a given set of error repairs into those that are triggered by the internal and those that are triggered by the external channel. First, such a separation is essential in order to understand how the two channels are coordinated. Do the two channels use the same criteria? Are they using the same checking mechanism? Particularly interesting in this respect is the question whether speakers can exert some strategic control in the division of labor between the channels (Oomen & Postma, 2002). Second, a number of studies suggest that speakers with aphasia have a different division of labor between the two channels than matched control speakers. That is, people with aphasia would predominantly use the internal channel (Oomen, et al., 2001, this volume, Chapter 12; Schlenck, Huber, & Willmes, 1987).

As far as we are aware, there are three proposals for determining the relative contribution of each monitoring channel. First, Schlenck et al. (1987) determined the number of disfluencies (such as filled pauses and part-word repetitions) and overt error repairs in speakers with and without aphasia. Schlenck et al. argued that overt repairs are the result of external monitoring, but that disfluencies are the result of internal monitoring. They called the latter group of incidents "prepairs" (see also Kolk & Postma, 1997; Postma & Kolk, 1993). In line with the terminology used throughout this book, we refer to such incidents as "covert repairs".[2] They observed relatively many covert repairs, but relatively few overt repairs in aphasics. Therefore, they concluded that aphasics have a deficiency in monitoring the external channel but not the internal channel.

Indeed, a stronger reliance on the internal monitoring channel than on the external channel will lead to more covert than overt repairs. But this reasoning cannot be taken to the extreme, where covert repairs are exclusively caused by internal-channel monitoring and overt repairs by external-channel monitoring. It is much more likely that a certain proportion of overt repairs are triggered by the internal channel. This is the case when the internal channel is too slow to intercept the error before onset of articulation, which explains incidents such as *v.horizontal* discussed earlier. Blackmer and Mitton (1991) and Oomen and Postma (2001) showed that in many repairs the time from error to self-interruption was very short (< 200 ms). Although it is arbitrary to assume that all of these errors were detected by the internal channel (see later), it does suggests that the internal channel contributes to a significant proportion of overt self-repairs. In sum, equating covert and overt repairs to exclusive effects of the internal and external channel respectively overestimates the contribution of the external channel.

A similar proposal for determining the relative contribution of each channel was made by Liss (1998). She also reasoned that the internal channel is faster than the external channel, but, as opposed to Schlenck et al., she acknowledged the possibility that errors detected by the internal channel will sometimes surface as overt repairs. Therefore, she considered early self-interruptions (< 500 ms after onset of the error) the result of internal monitoring and late self-interruptions ($\geq$ 500 ms) a result of external monitoring. One can consider this a variant of the Schlenck et al. proposal in which the criterion is shifted from 0 ms (errors never surface, so that each repair is covert) to 500 ms (errors do surface, so that some inner-channel repairs are overt).

However, there is a problem with this proposal. As in any human behavior, one can expect substantial variation in the processes responsible for the timing of interruption. This makes it quite arbitrary to set the criterion at a given value, in particular if the timing distributions of internally and externally triggered interruptions overlap (so that, for example, an interruption after 400 ms results from the external channel, while another interruption after 450 ms results from the internal channel). This would make it impossible to classify interruptions on the basis of their moment of occurrence.

Hartsuiker and Kolk (2001) took a different approach in estimating the division of labor between the two monitoring channels: they proposed a probabilistic model. Instead of trying to classify each individual incident as one that is either triggered by the internal or the external channel, their model estimated the *proportions* of such incidents in a given experiment or experimental condition. These proportions can be estimated from experimental data, because the model specifies a mathematical relationship between observable variables (such as the number of errors that are repaired) and model parameters (such as the error detection rate of the internal channel). Given sufficient assumptions, that model has a unique solution. For example, for the data published by Oomen and Postma (2001), they estimated that 25 per cent (normal speech) to 29 per cent (fast speech) of the overt self-corrections were triggered by the internal channel.

Unfortunately, this model only has a unique solution under the simplifying assumption that *the probability of detecting an error is equal for each channel*. There are, however, reasons to doubt that assumption. According to Wheeldon and Levelt (1995), the input to the internal channel is phonological. For certain phonological contrasts, a minimal phonological difference (e.g., voicing) corresponds to a large phonetic difference. Errors involving such a contrast can be expected to be more easily detectable by the external channel than by the internal channel, and indeed this was confirmed in a noise-masking experiment reported by Lackner and Tuller (1979). This suggests that the external channel is more accurate than the internal channel, at least for certain types of errors. Contrariwise, in normal dialogue one's external speech is often partially masked by environmental sounds and by the voice of one's interlocutor (in overlapping conversational turns). But internal speech is not hindered by masking, which implies that the internal channel is more accurate. Finally, a number of authors assume, contrary to the perceptual loop theory, that the two channels may use different criteria for monitoring (Nooteboom, this volume, Chapter 10; Roelofs, this volume, Chapter 3). That also predicts a difference in accuracy, at least for the errors to which these criteria apply.

In sum, these three proposals (Hartsuiker & Kolk, 2001; Liss, 1998; Schlenck et al., 1987) have shortcomings. The Schlenck et al. and Liss's proposals arbitrarily set the criterion for inner-channel repairs and external-channels at a certain value. Hartsuiker and Kolk assume that both channels are equally effective, an assumption that needs to be tested. In this chapter, we report a new attempt to tease apart the division of labor between the internal and external channels. Furthermore, we compare aphasic and matched control speakers and consider error type (phonological or lexical). We do so by presenting a generalization of Hartsuiker and Kolk's (2001) model. The new model no longer presupposes that the two channels are equally accurate; rather we compare the model's fit to empirical data with or without that assumption and evaluate statistically whether the effectiveness of the two channels differs from equality. The next section expresses this model as a relation between model parameters and proportions of empirically observable incidents. Subsequently, we use the model to estimate the division of labor for speakers with and without aphasia (Oomen et al., 2001) and for lexical and phonological errors (Postma & Noordanus, 1996).

The model

The goal of the model is to estimate the probabilities of four possible processes that can follow the production of an error in the internal speech plan. These processes are: (1) the error is detected by the internal channel and repaired *before* it becomes overt; (2) it is detected by the internal channel, but repaired *after* it becomes overt; (3) it is not detected by the internal channel, but detected by the external channel (and repaired); (4) it is not detected by either channel. The probabilities for these procedures have to be estimated from observable outcomes.

The problem that has to be overcome is that there are only three possible observable outcomes, namely a covert repair; an overt repair; and an error that is not repaired. Procedures (2) and (3) lead to the same outcome, namely an overt repair, and we seek to disentangle the contribution of the inner and the outer channel to this observed outcome.

To understand how the model works, imagine the reversed case: we already know the probabilities for each of these four processes, and we use those probabilities to predict the frequency of each observed category. This case is depicted in Figure 11.1. Notice that Nooteboom (this volume, Chapter 10) follows a similar approach in order to estimate how many phonological exchange errors in the speech plan result in either full exchanges or halfway corrected exchanges (i.e., anticipations) in overt speech.

Figure 11.1 shows our assumption how four processes can lead to the output categories observed in speech-error data. If there is an error in internal speech, the first system that can possibly detect it is the internal channel. There is a certain probability, Di, that the error is detected by this channel, and there is a probability $(1 - Di)$ that the error is missed by this

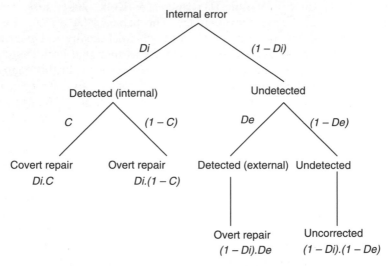

Figure 11.1 (Multinomial) probability tree of a dual-channel self-monitoring system.

channel. If the error is detected by the internal channel, there is a probability C that it is repaired before it is articulated: it becomes a "covert repair". There is a probability $(1 - C)$ that the error becomes overt before speech is interrupted: it becomes an overt repair. Now consider the right hand side of the diagram. The errors that are missed by the internal channel become errors in overt speech. Overt speech is inspected by the external channel and there is a probability De that the error is detected, resulting in an overt error repair. Further, there is a probability $(1 - De)$ that the error is missed, resulting in an uncorrected speech error. If we knew the probabilities for detection by the internal channel (Di), detection by the external channel (De) and correction before an error becomes overt (C), we could calculate the frequencies of our observed outcomes by multiplying the probabilities on the branches leading to each outcome and adding up the probabilities of those branches that lead to the same outcome. These outcome frequencies are listed underneath each of the observed outcomes. For example, the frequency that an error becomes a covert repair is obtained by multiplying Di (the probability that the internal channel detects it) with C (the probability that detection by the internal channel results in covert repair).

Our actual problem however, is exactly the reverse of the situation just described. We know the probability of each of the observed categories and we are searching for a set of values for the parameters that would produce exactly that pattern of observed frequencies. But how can we determine the values of these parameters for a given data set? Given strong assumptions, some (more or less) simple algebra can bring us the solution. Consider the proportion of overt repairs (OR). This will equal the sum of outcome probabilities of internal-channel overt repairs and of external-channel overt repairs (the middle two outcomes in Figure 11.1). Covert repairs are only generated by the internal channel. Therefore, the proportion of covert repairs (CR) equals the first outcome probability in Figure 11.1.

These statements can be expressed algebraically as follows:

$$P(OR) = Di(1 - C) + (1 - Di)De \qquad (1)$$

$$P(CR) = Di.C \qquad (2)$$

By summing these equations, we can express the relation between the two detection parameters (*Di* and *De*) and the empirically observed sum of the overt and covert repair proportions (see also Figure 11.1).

$$P(OR) + P(CR) = Di + (1 - Di)De \qquad (3)$$

This leaves us one equation with two unknowns. Although there are many combinations of values for *Di* and *De* that would not fit this equation, it still has an infinite number of solutions. If we were to assume that both channels are equally accurate (thus *Di* = *De* = *D*), equation (3) can be solved, yielding (4).

$$D = 1 - \sqrt{1 - (P(OR) + P(CR))} \qquad (4)$$

This solution is formally equivalent to the solution provided in Hartsuiker and Kolk (2001, p. 154).

This exercise demonstrates that in order to find unique estimates for *Di* and *De*, we need to reduce its degree of freedom, either by constraining the values that the parameters can take or by forcing the estimated parameters to predict the observed outcomes from different sets of data simultaneously. One constraint on the parameters, as already suggested, is to set *De* and *Di* equal. The model also has a unique solution if either *Di* or *De* is known. In experimental conditions in which the speaker cannot hear herself (e.g., because she is presented with loud noise, which masks speech; see later), we can impose the constraint that *De* = 0, that is the assumption that no errors are detected by the external monitor. With this constraint equation (3) leads again to a unique solution.[3]

So far the models we described were either underspecified (as in equation (3) that has an infinite number of solutions) or saturated as in equation (3) after the introduction of one of the constraints (either *De* = *Di* or *De* = 0). For these saturated models it is always possible to find parameters that perfectly predict the observed frequencies. However, as there is a perfect solution for every possible set of observed frequencies, fitting the model to the data does not test the validity of the model itself.

The situation changes when we try to fit the model to more than one set of outcome frequencies (or more generally, once we have more independently observed categories than parameters to estimate). In that case, we would not expect the parameters to give the exact predictions of the observed frequencies (compare it to tossing a coin 10 times, you would predict 5 heads and 5 tails but you would not be surprised to find 6 heads and 4 tails). Rather the question is: Are there estimates for C, De, and Di that are likely to have produced the observed frequencies in both experiments?

Our approach therefore is to simultaneously estimate the parameter Di in an experimental condition with noise-masking (Constraint: $De = 0$) and without noise masking (De is a free parameter), and then compare the fit of model to both data sets with or without the constraint that in the condition without noise masking both channels are equally effective ($Di = De$). One should consider that constraint as the null hypothesis. If the estimates differ very much, any compromise between the two estimates will not be a very likely source of the observed frequencies in both experiments.

Analysis 1: Aphasic and normal speech

Oomen et al. (2001, this volume, Chapter 12) conducted an experiment in which both speakers with Broca's aphasia and matched control speakers described networks of colored objects in a normal-feedback and a noise-masked condition. The authors recorded and transcribed each description and scored the number of (lexical and phonological) speech errors, the number of these errors that were self-corrected (overt repairs), and the number of repetitions (covert repairs). The frequencies of these incidents are listed in Table 11.1 and Table 11.2 defines the model.

The first four rows of Table 11.2 define the model for the condition with normal auditory feedback. The outcome probabilities correspond to the multiplication of probabilities on the branches of Figure 11.1. In the noise-masked condition only the internal channel is available to the speaker. This means the tree can be pruned: There are no incidents triggered by the external

Table 11.1 Observed frequencies of covert repairs, overt repairs, and uncorrected errors in normal-feedback and noise-masked speech for a group of elderly controls and a group of speakers with Broca's aphasia (Oomen et al., 2001)

	Normal feedback	*Noise masking*
Elderly controls		
Covert repairs	74	60
Overt repairs	157	136
Uncorrected errors	43	86
Total incidents	274	282
People with Broca's aphasia		
Covert repairs	346	333
Overt repairs	274	278
Uncorrected errors	225	270
Total incidents	845	881

channel. The resulting outcome in terms of estimated probabilities are provided in the last three rows of Table 11.2.

Figure 11.2 reports the model estimates for *Di* and *De* for the matched controls (left two bars) and for the speakers with Broca's aphasia (right two bars). The error bars show the 95 per cent confidence intervals.

Figure 11.2 shows that for both groups, the estimated *Di* has a higher value than the estimated *De* and that the confidence intervals do not overlap. The difference is particularly pronounced for the speakers with Broca's aphasia.

How can we evaluate whether a divergence in predicted *Di* reflects just random variation, or whether the internal channel is indeed more accurate than the external channel? We can test this statistically, by considering our model as a *multinomial processing tree* model (e.g., Hu & Batchelder, 1994;

Table 11.2 Multinomial model for monitoring experiments with a normal-feedback and a noise-masking condition

Condition	Outcome	Probability
Normal feedback		
	Covert repair	$Di.C$
	Overt repair	$Di(1 - C)$
	Overt repair	$(1 - Di).De$
	Uncorrected error	$(1 - Di)(1 - De)$
Noise masking		
	Covert repair	$Di.C$
	Overt repair	$Di(1 - C)$
	Uncorrected error	$(1 - Di)$

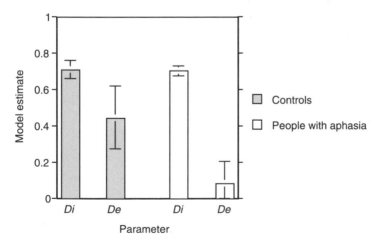

Figure 11.2 Estimated parameter values (*Di* and *De*) and 95% confidence intervals given the unconstrained model, for both elderly controls and people with Broca's aphasia. (Based on data obtained by Oomen et al., 2001.)

Riefer & Batchelder, 1988). This is a class of mathematical model that can be depicted as a tree structure and in which each node represents a processing choice point with a certain choice probability. The endings of the branches represent observable categories (see Figure 11.1). Maximum likelihood estimation of the parameters (the choice probabilities), can be obtained with Hu and Batchelder's Expectation Maximization (EM) algorithm. The likelihood G^2 (or more exactly, the 2*log-likelihood) of the estimated parameters is χ^2 distributed with the degree of freedom as expected value. Given that the degrees of freedom are larger than zero (i.e., there are more observed categories than parameters that have to be estimated), the fit between model and data can be statistically tested. In all analyses reported here, we have used the AppleTree program (Rothkegel, 1999), which implements this parameter estimation and model fitting procedure.

The statistical comparison of the unconstrained model with the constrained model (in which the two channels are equally accurate) shows a significant misfit between model and data in the constrained model (matched controls: G^2 *(2)* = 11.16; p < .01; people with Broca's aphasia: G^2 *(2)* = 140.75; p < .0001), but not in the unconstrained model (matched controls: G^2 *(1)* = 2.50; p = .11; people with Broca's aphasia: G^2 *(1)* = 1.79; p = .18). Thus, for both groups the internal channel is significantly more accurate than the external channel. The discrepancy is particularly large in the speakers with Broca's aphasia, who rely predominantly on the internal channel.

To further explore this difference between the two groups, we fitted the data with a model with the constraint that the external channel did not contribute at all to error detection, neither in normal feedback speech nor (obviously) in noise-masked speech (thus, De = 0).[4] In the case of controls, this adjusted model showed a significant misfit with the data (G^2 *(2)* = 17.47; p < .0005). But in the case of people with Broca's aphasia the adjusted model still fitted with the data (G^2 *(2)* = 3.62; p = .16). Thus, the external channel contributes to error detection in control speakers, but in the case of speakers with Broca's aphasia we cannot the reject the null hypothesis that the external channel detects 0 per cent of the errors.

Finally, we fitted the data with a version of the model in which the accuracy of the internal channel was a free parameter (in other words, the parameter Di could be different in the noise-masking condition as compared to the normal feedback condition). This allowed us to test whether the stronger reliance on the internal channel is an artifact of a shift towards inner-channel monitoring in the presence of noise (e.g., because due to the absence of the external channel, more cognitive resources are available for the internal channel). This model assumed that Di = De in the normal feedback condition and a new parameter was introduced for the accuracy of the inner monitor in the noise-masking condition (Dn). This parameter was allowed to be free. There was a significant misfit with the data (matched controls: G^2 *(1)* = 6.85; p < .01; speakers with Broca's aphasia: G^2 *(1)* = 67.17; p < .000001). Thus, the stronger reliance on the internal channel cannot be explained by a shift towards that channel under noise-masking conditions.

Analysis 2: Lexical and phonological errors

Postma and Noordanus (1996) also tested effects of noise masking on monitoring behavior. Participants were instructed to push a button whenever they detected an error in their own speech. In these experiments, detection of an error by the internal channel will always lead to an overt response (the button is pushed). Therefore, in this task there were no covert repairs. There were only detected errors and undetected errors. Postma and Noordanus reported detection rates for two types of errors: phonological errors (e.g., *dog – dug*) and lexical errors (e.g., *dog – cat*). Table 11.3 lists the observed frequencies of detected and undetected errors for each type of error and Table 11.4 defines the corresponding multinomial model.

The multinomial model for this type of experiment is simpler than the one we used earlier, because covert repairs are not relevant in this context. Therefore, we lose one observed outcome category (covert repairs) and one model parameter (C, the probability that an internally detected error becomes a covert repair). Figure 11.3 depicts the estimated values for Di and De, and

Table 11.3 Observed frequencies of detected and undetected phonological and lexical errors in normal-feedback and noise-masked speech (Postma & Noordanus, 1996)

	Normal feedback	*Noise masking*
Phonological errors		
Detected	224	161
Undetected	80	133
Total incidents	304	294
Lexical errors		
Detected	37	50
Undetected	13	16
Total incidents	50	66

Table 11.4 Multinomial model for error detection experiments with a normal-feedback and a noise-masking condition

Condition	*Outcome*	*Probability*
Normal feedback	Detected error	Di
Normal feedback	Detected error	$(1 - Di).De$
Normal feedback	Undetected error	$(1 - Di)(1 - De)$
Noise masking	Detected error	Di
Noise masking	Undetected error	$(1 - Di)$

(Error detection is indicated by a button press.)

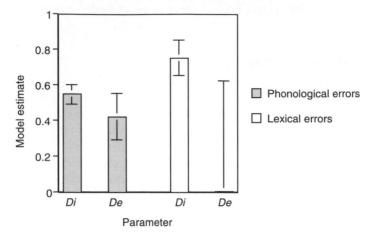

Figure 11.3 Estimated parameter values (*Di* and *De*) and 95% confidence intervals given the unconstrained model, both for phonological and lexical errors. (Based on data reported in Postma and Noordanus, 1996.)

their 95 per cent confidence intervals, for phonological errors and for lexical errors separately.

Figure 11.3 shows large differences between these error types. For phonological errors the estimates of *Di* and *De* have overlapping confidence intervals. But for lexical errors there is a very large difference between the two estimates: The estimated *Di* = .75; the estimated *De* is .0001. Note that although there is a large positive confidence interval for *De*, it does not overlap with the confidence interval for *Di*.

Because we now have removed one model parameter, but also one outcome category for each type of error, we are left with two degrees of freedom in the data and two free parameters in the model. That means we can no longer meaningfully test the model's fit to the data in the unconstrained case (because we are left with 2 – 2 = 0 degrees of freedom, one can always determine a perfect fit; in this case: *Di* = .55, *De* = .42 for phonological errors, and *Di* = .75, *De* = .0001 for lexical errors). However, we can determine the fit between model and data if the constraint of equal accuracy is imposed. For phonological errors, the constrained model's predictions were not significantly different from the data (G^2 *(1)* = 2.52; p = .11). Indeed, the "perfect" estimates for *Di* and *De* had very similar values and overlapping confidence intervals. Thus, for these kinds of error, the hypothesis of equal detection rates cannot be rejected. But with respect to lexical errors, the predictions from the constrained model (*Di* and *De* are both .63) yielded a highly significant misfit with the data (G^2 *(1)* = 23.52; p < .000001). Thus, for these errors the contribution of the internal channel is larger than that of the external channel.

Again, we analyzed the data with a "constrained" model without an external channel. This constrained model showed a significant misfit with the data on phonological errors (G^2 *(1)* = 10.19; p = .001), but not for the data on lexical errors (G^2 *(1)* = .05; p = .83).

To summarize, we estimated the effectiveness of the internal channel and the external channel in four situations: with respect to speech errors, self-corrections, and covert repairs in (1) speakers with Broca's aphasia and (2) matched controls, and with respect to detected and undetected speech errors for (3) phonological errors and (4) lexical errors. The maximum-likelihood estimates from the multinomial model revealed that the best-fitting model has a higher value for *Di* than for *De* in each of the four cases. In three out of the four cases, this difference was highly significant. The only exception occurred with the detection of phonological errors, where the effectiveness of the internal channel did not differ significantly from that of the external channel.

There was a remarkable difference between the speakers with Broca's aphasia and their elderly controls. The estimated probability of detecting errors through the external channel was extremely low for the speakers with aphasia (*De* = .085) and indeed the data are compatible with a model that excludes the external channel altogether. This is in agreement with the conclusions of Oomen et al. (2001) and Schlenck et al. (1987). We will return to that issue in the closing section. Finally, we observed a large discrepancy between the division of labor when detecting phonological errors as compared to lexical errors. The contribution of both channels is (statistically) equal in the detection of phonological errors, but lexical errors are predominantly detected by the internal channel. For these latter errors, the estimate of *De* approached 0 and indeed these data were compatible with a model without an external channel. We will briefly discuss explanations for these findings.

Discussion

We presented a probabilistic model of the division of labor between the internal and the external monitoring channel. The model expresses a relation between the accuracy of each channel and empirically observable variables: the number of covert repairs, and the numbers of repaired and unrepaired overt errors. We applied this model to existing data sets and estimated the division of labor of the two monitoring channels. The data came from experiments which included a noise-masked condition and a normal-feedback condition. Further, we assumed that in the noise-masked condition, the external channel is not available for self-monitoring. On that assumption, the accuracy of the external channel drops to 0. We also assumed that the efficiency of the internal channel was the same in experiments with and without noise masking. With those constraints in place we could estimate the contribution of the two channels and compare the fit of that estimate to the actual data. In three of the four data sets, we observed that the estimated accuracy of the internal channel was higher than that of the external channel (in speakers with aphasia and in normal speakers when all error types are considered; for lexical errors in the normal population). In fact, two out of these three data sets were compatible with the hypothesis that the external channel does not contribute at all to error detection. With respect to the fourth data set (phonological errors), although the estimated accuracy for the internal channel was still higher than that for the external channel, the null hypothesis that the two channels were equally accurate could not be rejected. In sum, the analyses reported here suggest that the internal channel detects a larger proportion of errors than the external channel, that patients with aphasia do not use the external channel, and that the division of labor also varies with error type.

It may be tempting to conclude that the two channels are qualitatively different. For example, the internal channel could be localized in the production system (e.g., Eikmeyer, Schade, Kupietz, & Laubenstein, 1999), there could be *two* internal channels, one that is production based and one that is perception based (Postma, 2000; Vigliocco & Hartsuiker, 2002) or the two channels may be associated with different criteria for error monitoring (Nooteboom, this volume, Chapter 10).

However, that conclusion may be premature. The present model estimates the *actual* effectiveness of each channel, not its *potential* effectiveness. These two types of effectiveness can differ if we consider self-monitoring as an attentional system. If there is one monitoring system, which pays selective attention to only one stream of input at any given time (but switches back and forth between channels), then the effectiveness of any channel is a function of how much selective attention is paid to that channel. Thus, the finding that the internal channel is more effective than the external channel is a result of speakers paying relatively more attention to their internal channel than to their external channel. That would be a sound strategy, as the internal channel allows one to prevent an error from becoming overt, rather than having to repair one when the damage is already done. At the same time, an overreliance on the internal channel may have negative consequences for the fluency of speech, and it disallows speakers to monitor for lower level aspects of speech (loudness, pitch, phonetic realization).

Such an attentional strategy (monitor the internal channel, because prevention is better than repair) can also account for the finding that speakers with Broca's aphasia hardly use the external channel, as suggested by Oomen et al. (2001). These authors first excluded several other explanations (for example, that the aphasic pattern is due to comprehension problems) and then gave an account in terms of selective attention. That account is based on the observation that these patients encounter many morphosyntactic planning problems. In order to prevent that many morphosyntactic errors become overt, they focus on the internal channel, but to an exaggerated extent. Because this focus leads to so much covert repairing, the fluency of speech is compromised: speech becomes slow, effortful and contains many disfluencies. Thus, this explanation accounts for one of the primary symptoms of Broca's aphasia, i.e., disfluent speech (see Kolk, 1995).

Finally, while lexical errors appear to be detected predominantly by the internal channel, phonological errors are detected by both channels with equal accuracy. This cannot be explained by assuming that lexical errors are easier (faster, more accurate) to detect than phonological errors and that they are therefore all intercepted by the internal channel. Oomen and Postma (2002) showed that lexical errors are detected slower, and equally often, as phonological errors in the speech of others and Postma and Noordanus (1996) showed that the detection rate of both types of errors was the same in the normal feedback condition.

An alternative account is that the noise manipulation was not entirely effective in blocking information to the external channel. If the speaker can still hear parts of their utterance, it would benefit the detection of lexical errors (cat → dog) more than phonological errors (cat → cap), as the latter type of error is acoustically more similar to the target. In that case, our model overestimated the contribution of the internal channel for lexical errors. However, given the loud noise levels (90 DB(A)) and given Postma and Noordanus (1996) explicit instruction that speakers should not increase the volume of their speech in the noise-masked condition, this is an unlikely scenario.

We tentatively propose a different account. On this account, the external channel is relatively important for the detection of phonological errors because it is the only channel with access to the phonetic details. Errors in voicing, as in *back → pack* will be more difficult to detect through the internal channel than through the external channel, because the phonological representation is minimally different, whereas the phonetic difference is relatively large. This account, although admittedly speculative, is testable: it predicts that if the phonological errors in Postma and Noordanus' study were assigned to phonetically high and low similarity conditions, the high-similarity errors should be detected less often under masking, but not the low-similarity errors.

Tacit assumptions in the model

There are two assumptions on the aftermath of error detection in our model that merit some discussion. First, if an error is detected by either channel, it will always result in a self-repair. Second, covert repairs correspond to disfluencies (in effect, part-word repetitions). It should be noted that both assumptions only apply to the first two data sets we have evaluated (Oomen et al. (2001) but not to the latter two data sets (Postma & Noordanus, 1996). The latter two data sets only dealt with error detection proper, not with its aftermath.

The first assumption is that errors that are detected, will indeed be repaired. However, it is conceivable that the monitor decides to ignore some of the detected errors. According to Berg (1986), there is a "decision" component in the monitoring system, that evaluates whether the error disrupts communication so much that the utterance needs to be interrupted, and if so, at what point the interruption should be placed. If that is true, our model would overestimate the proportion of missed errors, and hence would underestimate the accuracy of the monitoring system.

However, Berg's proposal implies adding another component to the monitor: A component that considers each error and evaluates its serious-ness. This proposal is based on corpus data suggesting that cut-offs occur at positions that leave the reparandum phonotactically legal. But all those data suggest is that the cut-off is planned; they do not show that there is an evaluation component which decides whether to cut off or not. Furthermore, while it is true that certain errors are more disruptive for communicative success than others, there is a more parsimonious proposal for dealing with that variable impact than postulating an additional component. That proposal solution is a shift in monitoring *focus* (Kolk, 1995; Oomen et al., this volume, Chapter 12; Vasic & Wijnen, this volume, Chapter 13). On a focus account, the monitor would pay particular attention to those errors that most disrupt communication, or which can most successfully be repaired (Oomen et al, this volume, Chapter 12).

The other assumption at the basis of our estimations is that disfluencies are covert repairs and that covert repairs will always reveal themselves as disfluencies. We have presently followed the Oomen et al. approach in exclud-ing filled pauses as disfluencies, but including part-word repetitions. There is substantial support for the hypothesis that filled pauses reflect planning prob-lems (Nickels & Howard, 1995; see also Clark & Fox Tree, 2002; Garrett, 1982). But similar arguments have been made with respect to function-word repetitions (Au-Yeung, Howell, & Pilgrim, 1998; Blackmer & Mitton, 1991; Clark & Wasow, 1998).

Complementary, it is also possible that sometimes a covert repair will not reveal itself as a disfluency. For example, our computational model of the timing of error interruption and repair (Hartsuiker & Kolk, 2001; Hartsuiker, Kolk, & Lickley, this volume, Chapter 15) predicts that error detection and repair can sometimes be completed long before word onset. It is conceivable that in those conditions, a covert repair has no observable consequences. This is consistent with data from Motley et al. (1982), which suggest that taboo words can be covertly edited out without any observable consequences to the fluency of production.[5]

How serious are violations of these assumptions for the current analyses? These assumptions only apply to a subset of the data we considered. To validate the analysis of this subset (the Oomen et al. data) we have run an additional analysis, using a model version without covert repairs. In that analysis, the estimated efficiency of the internal channel (Di) was still larger than the estimated efficiency of the external channel, De (matched control speakers: $Di = .61$; $De = .44$; speakers with aphasia: $Di = .51$; $De = .08$). Thus, the conclusion that the internal channel is more effective does not depend on the covert repair concept. Furthermore, our conclusion that the contribution of the internal channel is larger than that of the external channel, can only be strengthened by finding that some internal error corrections have not been considered in our model.

Of course, the model could be further extended to deal with violations of these assumptions. This would require the incorporation of further parameters (e.g., which proportion of covert repairs become disfluencies) and further assumptions (what if the monitor detects an error through the inner channel and decides not to interrupt; could detection of that error through the external channel lead to the decision to interrupt after all?). But incorporating these parameters and assumptions would yield the model no longer testable. A challenge for further research is rather to test them independently. A promising line of research, for example, is to analyze prosodic aspects of disfluencies. Plauché and Shriberg (2001) for example divided disfluencies into three prosodic categories (based on pausing, duration, and pitch). They suggested that one of these categories, constituting about 30 per cent of function-word repetitions were covert repairs. If this suggestion could be confirmed, it would offer a very promising way of refining the estimates of "covert repairs".

Conclusion

We proposed a probabilistic model that estimated the relative contribution of the internal and external channels with respect to the detection of speech errors. We conclude that the internal channel detects a larger proportion of errors than the external channel does, except in the case of phonological errors where both channels are equally efficient. Speakers with Broca's aphasia do not seem to use the external channel at all. We propose that the division of labor is modulated by selective attention: speakers rather prevent errors than repairing them once the damage is done. Thus, they attend the internal channel relatively more, and the external channel relatively less. Speakers with Broca's aphasia exaggerate this strategy, and as a result their speech is slow and highly disfluent. Finally, a consideration of error types requires that a selective attention account is supplemented. The external channel has access to information to which the internal channel is "deaf" (information about the acoustics and phonetics). We suggest that the external channel is relatively more important in detecting phonological errors because it can exploit the fact that minimal phonological differences are sometimes associated with large differences in phonetics.

Acknowledgements

This research was supported by a grant from the Netherlands Organization for Research (NWO). We thank Peter Howell, Albert Postma, Ulrich Schade, and Frank Wijnen for helpful comments on an earlier version of this chapter. Part of this work was presented at the XII ESCOP conference, Edinburgh, September 2001.

Notes

1   However, notice that there may be other channels for self-monitoring. For example, speakers could be sensitive to proprioceptive feedback (see Postma, 2000, for an overview of possible monitoring channels).
2   But how does one define a "covert repair"? We will follow the convention used by Oomen et al. (2001) to include (part) word repetitions but not filled pauses as covert repairs, and to label these incidents as covert repairs in the tables (but see discussion).
3   We assume that the presence of noise does not affect the internal monitoring channel. This assumption is supported by a study of Postma and Noordanus (1996), which directly compared internal monitoring with and without noise masking. They observed comparable rates of detected disfluencies, phonological errors, and lexical errors across conditions of silent speech, noise-masked speech, and "mouthed" speech, and a higher rate of these incidents in a condition with normal auditory feedback. If noise were to affect the quality of internal monitoring (our parameter *Di*) one would expect participants to report fewer incidents in the noise-masked condition than in the silent speech condition.
4   This suggestion was made by Peter Howell.
5   But these authors did not report disfluency rates.

References

Au-Yeung, J., Howell, P., & Pilgnin, L. (1998). Phonological words and stuttering on function words. *Journal of Speech, Language, and Hearing Research, 41*, 1019–1030.

Berg, T. (1986). The aftermath of error occurrence: Psycholinguistic evidence from cutoffs. *Language and Communication, 6*, 195–213.

Blackmer, E. R., & Mitton, E. R. (1991). Theories of monitoring and the timing of repairs in spontaneous speech. *Cognition, 39*, 173–94.

Clark, H. H., & Fox Tree, J. E. (2002). Using *uh* and *um* in spontaneous speaking. *Cognition, 84*, 73–111.

Clark, H. H., & Wasow, T. (1998). Repeating words in spontaneous speech. *Cognitive Psychology, 37*, 201–42.

Dell, G. S., & Repka, R. J. (1992). Errors in inner speech. In B. J. Baars (Ed.), *Experimental slips and human error: Exploring the architecture of volition*. New York: Plenum Press.

Eikmeyer, H.-J., Schade, U., Kupietz, M., & Laubenstein, U. (1999). A connectionist view of language production. In R. Klabunde, & C. Von Stutterheim (Eds.), *Representations and processes in language production*. Wiesbaden: Deutscher Universitäts-Verlag.

Garrett, M. F. (1982). Production of speech: Observations from normal and pathological language use. In. A. Ellis (Ed.), *Normality and pathology in cognitive function* (pp 19–76). London: Academic Press.

Hartsuiker, R. J., & Kolk, H. H. J. (2001) Error monitoring in speech production: A computational test of the perceptual loop theory. *Cognitive Psychology, 42*, 113–157.

Hu, X., & Batchelder, W. H. (1994). The statistical analysis of general processing tree models with the EM algorithm. *Psychometrika, 59*, 21–47.

Kolk, H. H. J (1995). A time-based approach to agrammatic production. *Brain and Language, 50*, 282–303.

Kolk, H. & Postma, A. (1997). Stuttering as a covert repair phenomenon. In R. Curlee & G. Siegel (Eds.), *Nature and the treatment* of stuttering: *New directions* (2nd ed. pp. 182–203). Needham Heights, MA: Allun & Bacon.

Lackner, J. R. & Tuller, B. H. (1979). Role of efference monitoring in the detection of self-produced speech errors. In: W. E. Cooper & E. C. T. Walker (Eds.), *Sentence processing* (pp. 281–94). Hillsdale, NJ: Lawrence Erlbaum Associates, Inc.

Levelt, W. J. M. (1983). Monitoring and self-repair in speech. *Cognition, 14*, 41–104.

Levelt, W. J. M. (1989). *Speaking: From intention to articulation.* Cambridge, MA: MIT Press.

Liss, J. M. (1998). Error-revision in the spontaneous speech of apraxic speakers. *Brain and Language, 62*, 342–60.

Motley, M. T., Camden, C. T., & Baars, B. J. (1982). Covert formulation and editing of anomalies in speech production.: Evidence from experimentally elicited slips of the tongue. *Journal of Verbal Learning and Verbal Behavior, 21*, 578–94.

Nickels, L. & Howard, D. (1995). Aphasic naming: What matters? *Neuropsychologia, 33*, 1281–1303.

Oomen, C. C. E., & Postma, A. (2001). Effects of time pressure on mechanisms of speech production and self-monitoring. *Journal of Psycholinguistic Research, 30*, 163–84.

Oomen, C. C. E., & Postma, A. (2002). Limitations in processing resources and speech monitoring. *Language and Cognitive Processes, 17*, 163–84.

Oomen, C. C. E., Postma, A., & Kolk, H. H. J. (2001). Prearticulatory and postarticulatory self-monitoring in Broca's aphasia. *Cortex, 37*, 627–41.

Plauché, M. C., & Shriberg, E. E. (1999). Data-driven subclassification of disfluent repetitions based on prosodic features. *Proceedings of the International Congress of Phonetic Sciences.* San Francisco, 1513–16.

Postma, A. (2000). Detection of errors during speech production: a review of speech monitoring models. *Cognition, 77*, 97–131.

Postma, A., & Kolk, H. H. J. (1993). The covert repair hypothesis: Prearticulatory repair processes in normal and stuttered disfluencies. *Journal of Speech and Hearing Research, 36*, 472–87.

Postma, A., & Noordanus, C. (1996). Production and detection of speech errors in silent, mouthed, noise-masked, and normal auditory feedback speech. *Language and Speech, 39*, 375–92.

Riefer, D. M., & Batchelder, W. H. (1988). Multinomial modeling and the measurement of cognitive processes. *Psychological Review, 95*, 318–39.

Rothkegel, R. (1999). AppleTree: A multinomial processing tree modeling program for Macintosh computers. *Behavior Research Methods, Instruments, & Computers, 31*, 696–700.

Schlenck, K.-J., Huber, W., & Willmes, K. (1987). "Prepairs" and repairs: Different monitoring functions in aphasic language production. *Brain and Language, 30*, 226–44.

Vigliocco, G., & Hartsuiker, R. J. (2002). The interplay of meaning, sound, and syntax in sentence production. *Psychological Bulletin, 128*, 442–72.

Wheeldon, L. R., & Levelt, W. J. M. (1995). Monitoring the time course of phonological encoding. *Journal of Memory and Language, 34*, 311–34.

Part IV

Self-monitoring in pathological speech

12 Speech monitoring in aphasia: Error detection and repair behaviour in a patient with Broca's aphasia

Claudy C. E. Oomen, Albert Postma, and Herman H. J. Kolk

Abstract

The present study investigated speech monitoring behaviour of a patient with Broca's aphasia and 11 healthy controls. Speech monitoring was examined in a speaking situation with normal auditory feedback, a speaking situation with white noise, and in a listening situation in which errors had to be detected in the speech of someone else. The results demonstrated that in monitoring his own speech, the patient strongly relied on prearticulatory monitoring, in contrast to the healthy controls. Furthermore, patient G. produced many phonological errors and had trouble repairing these errors, whereas he produced fewer semantic errors and had less trouble repairing these errors. This suggests that there is a relationship between production impairment and monitoring impairment. This could indicate that prearticulatory monitoring in this patient is production based, or that capacity limitations are responsible for the selective monitoring impairment.

Introduction

Spontaneous speech contains numerous errors. Fortunately, many of these errors are detected and repaired by the speaker. The process of online checking the well-formedness of one's own speech is referred to as self-monitoring. Speakers can check their own speech for its linguistic correctness. This includes checking for syntactic, morphological, semantic, and phonological errors. Self-repairs following these types of errors are called "error repairs" (Levelt, 1983). Speakers can also control their speech for contextual and social inadequacies. Self-repairs following such problems are called "appropriateness repairs". In the present study, we will only consider error repairs.

There are different accounts of how error detection takes place. Several researchers have suggested that self-monitoring proceeds through language comprehension (Garrett, 1980; Levelt, 1983, 1989). In Levelt's "perceptual loop theory" of monitoring (1983, 1989), detection of errors in one's own speech is accomplished in the same way as detection of errors in speech produced by others. Speech is parsed by the language comprehension system, after which the output of this parsing process is checked by a central monitor, located in the conceptualizer. Upon error detection, the monitor signals the speech production system to interrupt running speech and to plan a repair. In the perceptual loop theory, error detection proceeds through two different loops. Speakers monitor their speech after it has become overt, which is called auditory loop monitoring or postarticulatory monitoring. In addition, speakers can monitor their internal speech prior to the stage of articulation, which is called inner loop monitoring or prearticulatory monitoring. A prearticulatory detected error can still become overt, because the process of articulation continues while parsing takes place. It is also possible that the error is detected so early, that the self-repair is finished before the error is articulated. In this case, the error is not present in overt speech, but there is a disfluency (e.g., a repetition or a filled pause) resulting from the repairing activity. Therefore, these disfluencies are regarded as "covert repairs" (Levelt, 1983, 1989; Postma & Kolk, 1993). The question whether a disfluency really reflects a covert repair is controversial, however (see Postma, 2000). Nickels and Howard (1995) argue that some types of trouble indicating behaviour coded as "prepairs" (covert repairs) by Schlenck, Huber, and Willmes (1987), such as silent pauses and filled pauses, are indicative of word-finding difficulties rather than of covert repairs.

Whereas it is clear that the language comprehension system is involved in postarticulatory error detection, it is less clear which processes govern prearticulatory error detection. The perceptual loop theory (Levelt, 1983, 1989) postulates that prearticulatory error detection also proceeds through comprehension. An alternative possibility is that prearticulatory error detection is governed by "production-based monitors" that have direct access to the subcomponents of the production process (Laver, 1980; Postma, 2000), for instance, the subcomponents of the formulator (syntactic encoding, lemma selection, phonological encoding).[1] In Schlenck et al. (1987), a hybrid model of monitoring is proposed, in which prearticulatory monitoring is partly comprehension and partly production based.

Speech monitoring impairment in aphasia

Speech monitoring impairments are present in different types of aphasia, for instance in jargon aphasia (Lebrun, 1987; Marshall, Robson, Pring, & Chiat, 1998; Shuren, Smith-Hammond, Maher, Rothi, & Heilman, 1996), in Broca's aphasia, Wernicke's aphasia, and anomic aphasia (Marshall & Tompkins, 1982; Schlenck et al., 1987), and in apraxia of speech (Liss, 1998). In the present study, the speech monitoring performance of a patient with Broca's aphasia was examined. First, we give an overview of the relevant literature.

Several studies on monitoring impairment in aphasia have focused on the relationship between language comprehension skills and monitoring skills. The reason for this is that monitoring deficits can be regarded to result from impaired language comprehension (Lebrun, 1987; Maher, Rothi, & Heilman, 1994). If speech monitoring is completely comprehension based, as proposed in Levelt's perceptual loop theory (1983, 1989), there should be a relationship between language comprehension skills and speech monitoring skills. That is, aphasic speakers with impaired language comprehension skills should also have reduced speech monitoring skills, while speech monitoring skills of aphasic speakers with relatively intact language comprehension should be relatively preserved. Marshall, Neuberger, and Philips (1994) indeed provided evidence for a relationship between language comprehension skills and speech monitoring skills. Patients with high comprehension skills repaired the highest percentage of their errors, and the increase in the percentage of repaired errors was strongest in these patients after speech monitoring therapy.

The results of Schlenck et al. (1987) are more ambiguous, however. In this study, speech monitoring skills of patients with Broca's aphasia, Wernicke's aphasia, and anomic aphasia were examined. Patients with Wernicke's aphasia, who had impaired language comprehension skills, produced few (overt) self-repairs, despite numerous errors. However, this was also the case for the Broca's aphasics, who had relatively intact language comprehension. These findings thus only partly support the idea that monitoring deficits result from impaired comprehension. In addition, all patients produced many covert repairs (resulting from prearticulatory monitoring), in contrast to the healthy controls. Schlenck et al. (1987) suggested that the auditory, post-articulatory monitoring loop is impaired in these patients, whereas prearticulatory monitoring is preserved. The number of covert repairs correlated both with language production skills (i.e., the higher the number of produced errors, the more covert repairs) and with language comprehension skills (i.e., the better language comprehension, the more covert repairs). Schlenck et al. concluded therefore that prearticulatory monitoring is both comprehension and production based. In contrast, Nickels and Howard (1995) found no relationship between language comprehension skills and speech monitoring skills in a study with 15 patients with different types of aphasia. They therefore suggested that prearticulatory monitoring of these patients might be entirely production based. They did not examine the relationship between production skills and speech monitoring skills, however. (See also Roelofs, this volume, Chapter 3.)

Other studies have demonstrated further dissociations between speech monitoring skills and language comprehension skills. The most convincing evidence is provided by case studies describing patients who are aware of their errors and frequently produce self-repairs, despite their impaired comprehension skills. One of the jargon aphasic subjects of Marshall et al. (1998) scored poorly on auditory and written comprehension tests, but frequently produced self-repairs. Marshall, Rappaport, and Garcia-Bunuel (1985) described a patient with severely impaired auditory comprehension, who frequently attempted to repair her phonological errors (but not her semantic errors). In contrast, patients with jargon aphasia fail to detect their errors in spite of good comprehension skills (Maher et al. 1994; Marshall et al., 1998; Shuren et al., 1996). Finally, in a recent group study of Broca's aphasics we reported defective speech monitoring in a normal speaking condition, with relatively intact monitoring in a noise masked speaking condition (Oomen, Postma, & Kolk 2001). Among other things, the latter can suggest the existence of an internal monitor that is not based on comprehension. In a condition which primarily involves this type of monitor, for example, in a noise-masked condition, aphasic patients show fairly adequate self-repairing.

Some of the studies discussed already suggest a link between speech monitoring and language production (Nickels & Howard, 1995; Schlenck et al., 1987). Stark (1988) is most specific about how speech monitoring impairment is related to deficits in language production. A patient was reported with transcortical sensory aphasia who made many semantic errors but rarely repaired these errors. In contrast, she produced considerably fewer phonological errors, while repairing all of these errors. Stark concluded that such selective monitoring impairment in a certain linguistic domain (i.e., lemma selection) results from disorders in the same domain in production. In other words, speech monitoring would be production based.

An alternative explanation for the findings of Stark (1988) is that the patient does *detect* her semantic errors, but that *carrying out* the required repairs is too capacity demanding, because this subprocess of production is impaired. Consequently, patients would refrain from repairing these errors.

It has frequently been proposed that monitoring problems in aphasic patients arise from capacity limitations in performing multiple activities simultaneously, i.e., in speaking and monitoring their own speech at the same time (Lebrun, 1987; Maher et al., 1994; Marshall et al., 1998; Shuren et al., 1996). Consequently, an online speaking situation has frequently been compared to a less capacity-demanding off-line situation, in which patients with jargon aphasia have to detect errors in a recorded sample of their own speech or other-produced speech (Maher et al., 1994; Marshall et al., 1998; Shuren et al., 1996). Interestingly, speakers of jargon aphasia, who are unaware of their speech errors in an online speaking situation, seem to detect a considerably higher percentage of errors in an off-line situation. A reduced capacity to simultaneously perform multiple activities could also account for self-monitoring impairment of patients with Alzheimer's and Parkinson's disease (McNamara, Obler, Au, Durso, & Albert, 1992).

Thus, the literature on speech monitoring impairment in aphasia suggests that the relationship between language comprehension skills and speech monitoring skills is not as evident as predicted from the perceptual loop theory. Several studies indicate that speech monitoring does not exclusively proceed through comprehension, but that prearticulatory monitoring is also (partly) production based. Furthermore, capacity limitations seem to play an important role in aphasic speech monitoring.

Speech monitoring in Broca's aphasia

In the present study we investigated the characteristics of monitoring impairment in a patient with Broca's aphasia. We examined not only the percentage of errors that were repaired ("monitoring accuracy"), but also "self-repair effort" and "self-repair success". Self-repair effort relates to the number of attempts that are made in order to repair an error. A high number of attempts at repair indicates that the production process is very effortful. Self-repair success relates to the percentage of repairs that (eventually) results in a correct utterance. Self-repair effort and success are related to the severity level of aphasia (Farmer, 1977; Farmer, O'Connell, & O'Connell, 1978; Marshall & Tompkins, 1982; Marshall et al., 1994).

We addressed a number of research questions. First, we studied which monitoring channels are used in Broca's aphasia, and to what extent. As already described, Schlenck et al. (1987) proposed that patients with Broca's aphasia primarily concentrate on the prearticulatory monitoring channel. This is in line with the proposal that disfluencies in Broca's aphasia reflect attempts to restart temporally disintegrated sentence representations (Kolk & Van Grunsven, 1985). These temporal disintegrations result from delayed syntactic processing, which affects the encoding of syntactic structures and the selection of grammatical morphology. Kolk (1995) argued that temporal disintegrations are detected and speech is restarted by means of the prearticulatory monitoring channel. Therefore, these disfluencies could be regarded as covert repairs.

In the present study, prearticulatory and postarticulatory monitoring were disentangled by comparing a speaking situation with normal auditory feedback to a speaking situation with white noise. When presented with white noise, speakers can not hear their own speech. Thus, the auditory monitoring channel is cancelled out, and speakers can only monitor prearticulatorily. If individuals with Broca's aphasia primarily concentrate on prearticulatory monitoring, their monitoring performance would not be affected by the presentation of white noise, whereas it would be in normal speakers, who use both monitoring channels. In addition, a speech perception task was conducted, in which errors had to be detected in other-produced speech. In this situation, speech monitoring is necessarily accomplished by means of the auditory loop. If auditory loop monitoring per se is impaired in Broca's aphasia (Schlenck et al., 1987), their monitoring performance (i.e., detection of other-produced errors) should be clearly reduced in a perception situation.

Second, and in contrast to the hypothesis that the auditory loop per se is damaged, we explored if monitoring impairments in Broca's aphasia result from capacity limitations, which make it difficult to perform two activities simultaneously (i.e., speaking and online monitoring), rather than from impaired auditory loop monitoring. Patients with Broca's aphasia might suffer from capacity limitations, as this type of aphasia has been associated with limitations in verbal working memory (Goerlich, Daum, Hertrich, &

Ackermann, 1995). Consequently, error detection in Broca's aphasia might even relatively increase in the off-line speech perception task (when one does not have to do two things at the same time). In turn, capacity limitations could also have particular effects on monitoring performance in the speech production task. If a patient is impaired in certain subprocesses of language production, repairing of these errors could be hampered by capacity demands as well. This would predict a relation between the number of errors resulting from a certain subprocess of production, the percentage of repaired errors of this type, and the self-repair effort and success. That is, the errors that are most frequent should be repaired least, and if a repair attempt is made, it should be more effortful, for example, needing multiple attempts, and often fail in the end, i.e., not reaching a successful continuation.

Third, it is interesting to consider indications of production-based monitoring, as suggested by several of the studies described earlier (Howard, 1995; Schlenck et al., 1987; Stark, 1988). Selective impairments in a certain subprocess of production, which are mirrored by selective monitoring impairments in the same domain, could not only reflect on capacity limitations, but also on production-based monitoring.

Case description

Patient G. is a 71-year-old man, who had suffered a left hemispheric ischaemic stroke approximately three years prior to this study. Patient G. had been diagnosed with Broca's aphasia on the Dutch version of the Aachen Aphasia Test (AAT). He was part of a larger group study with eleven patients with Broca's aphasia, reported in Oomen et al. (2001). Patient G. was selected because he demonstrated selective monitoring impairments in certain subprocesses of production. Eleven healthy controls also participated in this study (mean age 62, age range 42–76).

Table 12.1 shows the scores of patient G. on a subset of AAT tests. The score on "spontaneous speech 2" of the AAT indicates that patient G. was not dysarthric, but that he had a slow speech rate and that his speech was dysprosodic. Furthermore, the score on "spontaneous speech 6" indicates that the patient's speech was agrammatic. The "syntactic off-line" test is a test

Table 12.1 Scores on AAT subtests

	Spontaneous speech 2 (0–5)	Spontaneous speech 6 (0–5)	Syntactic off-line (0–150)	Token test (50–0)
Patient G	2b, 3c	2	104	34

Note: The score on spontaneous speech 2 indicates, on a scale from 0 (very severe disturbance) to 5 (no disturbance), articulation and prosody. 2b: severe dysprosody; 3c: slow speech rate. The score on spontaneous speech 6 indicates the syntactic structure of utterances. A score of 2 indicates that no complex sentences were produced and that function words and inflections are missing.

Table 12.2 Scores on PALPA subtests

	PALPA 2 (0–72)	*PALPA 4 (0–30)*	*PALPA 45 (0–40)*
Patient G	71	30	40
Norm	70.8 (SD 2.0)	29.8 (SD 0.5)	39.8 (SD 0.4)

for syntactic comprehension, a supplement on the standard AAT. When a score exceeds 75, patients are classified as *high comprehenders*. This was the case for patient G.

In order to compare error detection in self- and other-produced speech with more general language perception skills, patient G. performed three subtests of the Dutch edition of the Psycholinguistic Assessment for Language Processing in Aphasia (PALPA), for phonological and semantic auditory word perception: subtest 2 (auditory discrimination: real words), subtest 4 (minimal pairs: picture-word matching, phonologically related distracters), and subtest 45 (word comprehension: spoken picture-word matching, semantically related distracters). The patient's scores on these subtests are given in Table 12.2. The patient's scores were equal to the standardized norm, indicating that his phonological and semantic auditory word perception was intact.

Patient G. and the controls also performed the Corsi Blocks Test, for visuo-spatial short-term memory, and the Digit Span Test (forward) for verbal short-term memory. Patient G.'s score on the Corsi Blocks Test (5) was within two SD from the mean score of the healthy control speakers (5.2, SD 0.9). G.'s score on the Digit Span Test (3), however, was more than 2 SDs from the mean score of the healthy controls (6.2, SD 1.3). This indicates that the verbal working memory of patient G. is reduced, as opposed to his visuo-spatial working memory.

Speech production task: Normal auditory feedback condition and noise-masked condition

In the speech production task, patient G. was required to describe 20 experimental networks, which were presented serially on a computer screen (cf. Oomen et al., 2001). Each network consisted of five coloured pictures of everyday objects. A red dot moved through the network, indicating the route that subjects had to follow in their descriptions. As the results of a pilot study demonstrated that the five-picture networks elicited only few errors in healthy subjects, the healthy controls were required to describe 20 experimental networks consisting of eight coloured pictures of everyday objects.

Subjects were instructed to describe the route of the dot as accurately as possible, at their normal speech rate, and in such a way that it would be understandable for a listener who cannot see the network. They had to indicate the direction of the dot (left/right, up/down), the type of line (curved/straight), and the objects that were passed, including the object colours. Patient G. and the healthy controls received an example description through headphones with a matching network presented on the computer screen (See appendix). The rate of the dot was adjusted to the individual speech rate of each subject. Individual speech rates were determined by presenting first a network for which the route was depicted by the numbers 1 to 5. Subjects had to describe this network at their ordinary rate. Subsequently, the rate of the dot was adjusted to this time. (See also, Oomen & Postma, 2001.)

Two practice networks were administered before the normal auditory feedback condition and before the noise-masked condition, which each contained 10 experimental networks. White noise was generated by a Velleman noise generator, and was presented to the subjects through headphones at a level of 90 dB. At the start of the noise-masked condition, the experimenter gradually increased the noise from 60 to 90 dB. Speech was recorded by a Monarch microphone on a Sony minidisk recorder.

Data analyses

Speech was transcribed and coded by two independent experienced raters. In cases where speech was phonetically or phonologically deviant, speech was transcribed phonetically. Two types of speech error were coded:

1   Semantic errors: when a word is semantically similar to the target:

   Examples: "ijsje *blauw*" (ice-cream *blue*), target: paars (purple)
   "*appel*" (*apple*), target: peer (pear)
   "*links*" (*left*), target: rechts (right)

2   Phonological errors: when the wrong phonemes are selected, or when phonemes are omitted or added:

   Examples: "do*ff*elsteen", target: dobbelsteen (dice)
   "*l*echte lijn", target: rechte lijn (straight line)

Both for semantic and phonological errors the two raters determined:

   The total number of produced errors (repaired and unrepaired).
   The percentage of repaired errors: the total number of repaired errors/ the total number of repaired and unrepaired errors. Multiple attempts at repair and unsuccessful repairs were also coded as "repaired errors":

   Example: "blank . . . bank", target: bank (couch)

   The percentage of multiple attempts at repair (self-repair effort): the number of multiple attempts at repair/the total number of multiple and single attempts at repair.

Successful as well as unsuccessful attempts at repair were included (see lates):

Example: "pappette> kpi . . . parmekt plu", target: paraplu (umbrella)

The percentage of successful self-repairs (self-repair success): the number of (ultimately) successful self-repairs/the total number of successful and unsuccessful self-repairs. Single as well as multiple attempts at repair were included:

Example: "rood nee geel" (red no yellow), target: paars (purple)

In addition, the two raters independently coded the covert repairs. Following Nickels and Howard (1995), the raters adopted a conservative definition of covert repairs and only coded repetitions as covert repairs. Repetitions included sound or part-word repetitions, word repetitions, and multiple word or phrase repetitions. Repetitions that were part of overt self-repairs were excluded. In addition, the proportion of covert repairs was determined for both conditions, by dividing the number of covert repairs by the total number of covert and overt self-repairs.

Speech perception task

For this task, the same 20 experimental networks were used as in the production task. The networks were linked to descriptions that matched the route and the rate of the dot. The descriptions contained errors that were selected from the descriptions of the group study (Oomen et al., 2001). The descriptions were produced by a female native speaker of Dutch, and were presented through headphones. They contained unambiguous phonological (25) and semantic errors (25). The semantic errors included errors of direction, errors on object names, and errors on object colours. Phonological errors included phoneme substitutions, additions and omissions.

Patient G. and the healthy controls were instructed to listen carefully to the descriptions and at the same time watch the dot move through the network. When the description contained an error, for instance if a wrong word was produced (e.g., "red" instead of blue), or if a word contained the "wrong" sounds (e.g., "palasplu" instead of paraplu), they had to say "no" or "wrong" as quickly as possible. When this happened, the experimenter pressed the mouse button in order to stop the dot. Consequently, the subject had to repair the error. In this way, it was clear if the right error had been detected. Both for semantic and for phonological errors, the percentage of repaired errors was determined. The repairs were recorded by a Monarch microphone on a Sony minidisk recorder.

Results speech production task

Typically, patient G. described the objects that were passed by the dot and named the colours of the objects. The direction of the dot and the shape of the line were usually not described. Furthermore, patient G.'s descriptions were agrammatic. Patient G. did not produce complete sentences, and frequently omitted function words and verbs. He produced more phonological and semantic errors than the healthy controls. In particular, the number of phonological errors was substantially and significantly higher ($z = 13.5$, $p <$ .001)[2] (see Table 12.3).

Percentage of repaired errors

Table 12.3 shows that patient G. repaired a lower proportion of his phonological errors than the healthy controls in the condition with normal auditory feedback ($z = 3.0$, $p < .01$), but not in the noise-masked condition ($z = 0.6$, ns). The percentage of repaired semantic errors was also lower for patient G. than for the healthy controls, but these differences were not significant, neither in the normal condition ($z = 1.6$, ns), nor in the noise-masked condition ($z = 0.2$, ns).

Percentage of repaired errors: Normal auditory feedback vs noise

Patient G. repaired a slightly higher percentage of his phonological errors in the noise-masked condition (49 per cent) than in the normal auditory feedback condition (40 per cent). For the semantic errors, the percentage of repaired errors was slightly lower in the noise-masked condition (50 per cent) than in the normal auditory feedback condition (55 per cent). Chi-square

Table 12.3 Errors (means for controls) and self-repairs in the speech production task

	Normal auditory feedback		Noise	
	Patient G	Controls	Patient G	Controls
Number of phonological errors	40	7	45	8
% repaired phonological errors	40	81	49	60
% multiple phonological repairs	63	2	68	1
% successful phonological repairs	38	96	32	97
Number of semantic errors	20	11	16	12
% repaired semantic errors	55	76	50	64
% multiple semantic repairs	55	6	13	3
% successful semantic repairs	64	98	88	100
Number of covert repairs	46	7	35	5
% covert repairs/all repairs	63	30	54	29

tests did not yield significant differences between the two conditions. In contrast to patient G., the healthy controls repaired a lower percentage of their phonological errors in the noise-masked condition than in the normal auditory feedback condition (t(10) = 4.6, p < .001). This was also the case for the percentage of repaired semantic errors (t(10) = 2.7, p < .05).

Covert repairs

Table 12.3 demonstrates that patient G. produced more covert repairs (i.e., repetitions) than the healthy controls, both in the normal auditory feedback condition (z = 3.4, p < .01) and in the noise-masked condition (z = 7.6, p < .001). In addition, the proportion of covert repairs of all (covert and overt) repairs was higher for patient G. than for the normal controls, in the normal auditory feedback condition (z = 2.7, p < .01) as well as in the noise-masked condition (z = 2.1, p < .05).

Self-repair effort and self-repair success

Patient G. exhibited many multiple subsequent attempts at repair. He clearly differed from the healthy controls, who rarely needed multiple attempts at repair after phonological errors (z = 22.2, p < .001) and after semantic errors (z = 4.6, p < .001). In patient G. these events were more frequent after phonological errors than after semantic errors (χ^2 = 4.3, p <. 01). In addition, patient G. produced a lower percentage of successful self-repairs than the healthy controls, both after phonological errors (z = 11.8, p < .001) and after semantic errors (z = 12.2, p < .001). Again, the percentage of successful self-repairs produced by patient G. was lower for phonological errors than for semantic errors (χ^2 = 7.9, p < .01).

Results speech perception task

Table 12.4 shows the results of the speech perception task. In the perception task, the percentage of phonological errors detected and repaired by patient G. did not differ from the percentage of the healthy controls (z = 0.1, ns). In contrast, patient G. repaired a lower percentage of the semantic errors than the healthy controls (z = 4.8, p < .001). Patient G. intercepted a higher percentage of errors in the speech perception task than in the normal auditory feedback condition of the production task. A chi-square test shows a

Table 12.4 Percentage of detected and repaired errors in the speech perception task

	Patient G	*Controls (means)*
% repaired phonological errors	84	86
% repaired semantic errors	60	89

significant difference between the tasks (χ^2 = 8.1, p < .01). For the healthy controls, this was also the case (t(10) = 2.7, p < .05). When comparing the percentages of repaired semantic and phonological errors of patient G., the increase in the percentage of repaired semantic errors in the perception task compared to the production task was very small (5 per cent), and did not reach significance. In contrast, the difference in the percentage intercepted phonological errors between the perception task and the production task was large (44 per cent), and yielded significance (χ^2 = 12.1, p < .001).

Discussion

In the present study, speech monitoring skills of a patient with Broca's aphasia and 11 healthy controls were examined. Compared to the healthy controls, patient G. exhibited impaired speech monitoring skills. In the situation of normal auditory feedback, he corrected a lower percentage of his phonological errors. In addition, patient G. had trouble in issuing the repair proper: he frequently needed multiple attempts to repair and often did not reach a successful solution in doing so, as opposed to the healthy controls.

Use of different monitoring channels

One of the questions addressed in this study concerned the relative contribution of prearticulatory and postarticulatory monitoring in a patient with Broca's aphasia. Patient G. repaired an equal percentage of his semantic and phonological errors in the noise-masked condition and in the condition with normal auditory feedback, in contrast to the healthy controls, who repaired a significantly smaller percentage of these errors with noise masking. This suggests that patient G. primarily concentrates on the prearticulatory, internal monitoring channel, whereas for normal speakers postarticulatory monitoring is crucial as well. The same pattern of results was found in a study with a group of patients with Broca's aphasia (Oomen et al., 2001). The high absolute and relative rate of covert repairs produced by patient G. further confirms the idea that individuals with Broca's aphasia rely relatively more on the prearticulatory monitoring channel than normal speakers. These findings are in harmony with the results of Schlenck et al. (1987) who demonstrated that aphasic patients produced many covert repairs, compared to overt repairs. The large amount of disfluency or covert repairing in Broca's aphasia might reflect attempts to restart temporally disintegrated sentence representations by means of the prearticulatory monitoring channel (Kolk, 1995).

One reason for the presumed primary focus of patient G. on the prearticulatory monitoring channel could be that his postarticulatory, auditory monitoring channel is impaired, as suggested by Schlenck et al. (1987). However, while patient G. repaired a lower percentage of semantic errors than the controls in the perception task, the percentage of repaired phono-logical errors of patient G. in the perception task did not differ from that of the healthy controls. This suggests that the ability to monitor by means of the postarticulatory, auditory monitoring channel per se is not impaired.

Capacity limitations and monitoring impairment

An alternative reason why patient G. would concentrate primarily on prearticulatory monitoring is that his capacity was too limited to concentrate on prearticulatory and postarticulatory monitoring at the same time. This explanation relates to the idea that the self-monitoring impairment in Broca's aphasia is associated with limitations in verbal working memory (Goerlich et al., 1995). It is possible that the restarting of sentence representations by the prearticulatory monitor demands so much capacity that not enough resources are left for postarticulatory monitoring at the same time. Of course, the question remains why the prearticulatory loop is preferred and why not attention is regularly switched between the two channels.

Other findings in the speech production task also indicate that monitoring problems may result from capacity limitations. Monitoring performance of patient G. after phonological errors was more severely impaired than seman-tic error monitoring. Notably, patient G. repaired a lower percentage of phonological errors than the controls, while his semantic error repair rate besides being much higher did not differ from that in controls. In addition, patient G. produced a higher percentage of multiple attempts at repair for phonological errors than for semantic errors, and he was less successful in reaching adequate final repair solutions. These results parallel patient G.'s speech production skills: He produced a larger number of phonological errors than the healthy controls, while the number of semantic errors was small, and did not differ from the controls. Thus, there is a relationship between the severity of patient G.'s production impairment and the severity of his monitoring impairment. Put simply, more monitoring problems seem present for the subprocess of speech production that is more severely impaired. This relationship could derive from capacity limitations. Patient G. could have refrained from repairing (part of) his detected errors because this demands too much capacity.

Capacity limitations can also explain why the proportion of detected phonological errors increased in the speech perception task (compared to the speech production task), whereas the proportion of detected semantic errors did not increase. If patient G. refrained from repairing his phonological errors in the production task because this demands too much capacity, the benefit in the perception task should be relatively large. Not having to speak and monitor at the same time frees more resources for intercepting and re-vising phonological errors in the speech perception task. Repairing semantic errors was less problematic in the speech production task: the percentage of repaired semantic errors and the number of semantic errors produced by patient G. did not even differ from the healthy controls. This implies that repairing semantic errors in speech production is less taxing than repairing phonological errors. Therefore, patient G. might not have gained much for these low demanding incidents in the off-line monitoring situation of the speech perception condition.

Production-based speech monitoring

One problem with the foregoing capacity account, however, is that patient G. repaired as many phonological errors in the noise-masked condition as the normal controls. If he generally refrains from correcting these errors because this would be too demanding, a similar finding should have applied to the noise-masked condition as well. Hence, we need to consider yet another possibility for the present pattern of results, namely production-based speech monitoring. What are the indications for this type of monitoring? Most importantly, it should be noted that patient G. has impaired speech monitoring skills, despite his relatively intact language comprehension skills. A similar dissociation has also been reported in other studies (Maher et al., 1994; Marshall et al., 1998; Shuren et al., 1996). Hence, it is possible that speech monitoring is not exclusively comprehension based, as suggested in Levelt's perceptual loop theory (1983, 1989) but also partly production based. Moreover, the results of the present study clearly demonstrate a selective monitoring impairment regarding a subprocess of production (i.e., phonological encoding), which parallels the selective impairment in phonological encoding in speech production.

Although this pattern might result from capacity limitations, as considered earlier, it could also indicate that speech monitoring of patient G. is (partly) production based. The finding that patient G. primarily concentrates on prearticulatory monitoring is in line with this, as production-based monitoring can only be accomplished prearticulatorily. Furthermore, in the speech production task, patient G. repaired a smaller percentage of phonological errors than the healthy controls, whereas in the speech perception task he repaired a smaller percentage of semantic errors than the healthy controls. This discrepancy might indicate that different monitoring mechanisms are responsible for monitoring self-produced speech (production-based monitoring) than for monitoring other-produced speech (perception-based monitoring). These findings are in line with those of Stark (1988), who also observed a selective monitoring impairment in an aphasic patient, and related this to impairment in the same linguistic subprocess of production.

Why would patient G., whose language comprehension is relatively intact, use a production-based monitor for detecting errors in his own speech? It can be speculated that he does so because production-based monitoring can be accomplished relatively automatically, as opposed to comprehension-based monitoring, which demands more central resources (cf. Oomen & Postma, 2002). In line with this, Nickels and Howard (1995) propose that some aphasic patients abandon comprehension-based monitoring (and adopt production-based monitoring) because errors that are detected cannot be successfully repaired. In this view, the distinction between comprehension-based and production-based monitoring is integrated with capacity limitations (see also Postma, 2000).

Conclusions

In the present study we investigated monitoring behaviour of a patient with Broca's aphasia and 11 healthy controls. We considered which monitoring loops the patient concentrated on, whether monitoring deficits result from capacity limitations, and whether there are any indications for production-based monitors. The results demonstrate that in the speech production task, the patient primarily concentrated on the prearticulatory monitoring loop, as opposed to the healthy controls. What is particularly interesting in this patient is the selective impairment in producing and repairing phonological errors. The finding that patient G. produced many phonological errors and had trouble repairing these errors, whereas he produced fewer semantic errors and had less trouble repairing these errors, suggests a relationship between production impairment and monitoring impairment. This relationship may indicate that prearticulatory monitoring in this patient is production based, and that central capacity limitations are responsible for such selective monitoring impairment. In a normal speaking situation patient G. cannot effectively use his comprehension-based monitor to repair phonological errors, because this takes too much central capacity. There still is the possibility to repair these errors by a relatively intact automatic, production based (internal) monitor mechanism. Under noise masking the monitoring advantage of healthy controls is levelled off because the comprehension-based monitor can no longer be used. Thus, in general, in a noise masked condition speakers tend to engage hardly the comprehension-based monitor, at least for certain types of errors (e.g., phonological errors).

Acknowledgements

Albert Postma was supported by a grant from the Netherlands Organization for Fundamental Research (NWO, No. 440–20–000).

Notes

1 Recently, Levelt, Roelofs, and Meyer (1999), see also Roelofs (this volume), adjusted the original perceptual loop theory. Although monitoring is still considered to proceed through perception, Levelt et al. (1999) suggest that the comprehension system (i.e., the inner loop) can also have access to the phonological code. This poses problems, however, for the concept of a centrally governed monitoring device that cannot access the subcomponents of production (the phonological code), but only its outcome (cf. Kolk & Postma, 1996; Postma, 2000).

2 Z-scores (z = score individual patient – mean score healthy controls/SD healthy controls) were calculated to compare patient G. with the healthy controls. To compare differences within the patient, Chi-square tests were conducted (cf. Shuren et al., 1996). For instance, the number of repaired and unrepaired errors in the normal auditory feedback were compared to the number of repaired and unrepaired errors in the noise-masked condition.

Appendix: Example description (translated from Dutch)

"You start off at the purple skate. Then you go to the left with a straight line to the green audio tape. Then you take a diagonal line down to the left to the yellow duck. From there you go up with a curved line on the left to the red strawberries. Then you go to the right with a straight line to the green tape. And from there you go up with a bow on the right to the blue children's bed."

References

Farmer, A. (1977). Self-correctional strategies in the conversational speech of aphasic and non-aphasic brain damaged adults. *Cortex*, *13*, 327–334.

Farmer, A., O'Connell, P. F., & O'Connell, E. J. (1978). Sound error self-repairs in the conversational speech of non-fluent and fluent aphasics. *Folia Phoniatria*, *30*, 293–302.

Garrett, M. F. (1980). Levels of processing in sentence production. In B. Butterworth (Ed.), *Language production*, Vol. 1. London: Academic Press.

Goerlich, C., Daum, I., Hertrich, I., & Ackermann, H. (1995). Verbal short-term memory and motor speech processes in Broca's aphasia. *Behavioural Neurology*, *8*, 81–91.

Kolk, H. H. J. (1995). A time-based approach to agrammatic production. *Brain and Language*, *50*, 282–303.

Kolk, H., & Postma, A. (1996). Stuttering as a covert repair phenomenon. In R. F. Curlee and G. M. Siegel (Eds.), *Nature and treatment of stuttering*. Boston: Allyn & Bacon.

Kolk, H. H. J., & Van Grunsven, M. F. (1985). Agrammatism as a variable phenomenon. *Cognitive Neuropsychology*, *2*, 347–84.

Laver, J. D. M. (1980). Monitoring systems in the neurolinguistic control of speech production. In V. A. Fromkin (Ed.), *Errors in linguistic performance: Slips of the tongue, ear, pen, and hand*. New York: Academic Press.

Lebrun, Y. (1987). Anosognosia in aphasia. *Cortex*, *23*, 251–63.

Levelt, W. J. M. (1983). Monitoring and self-repair in speech. *Cognition*, *14*, 41–104.

Levelt, W. J. M. (1989). *Speaking: From intention to articulation*. Cambridge: MA: MIT Press.

Levelt, W. J. M., Roelofs, A., & Meyer, A. S. (1999). A theory of lexical access in speech production. *Behavioural and Brain Sciences*, *22*, 1–75.

Liss, J. M. (1998). Error revision in the spontaneous speech of apraxic speakers. *Brain and Language*, *62*, 342–60.

Maher, L. M., Rothi, L. J. G., & Heilman, K. M. (1994). Lack of error awareness in an aphasic patient with relatively preserved auditory comprehension. *Brain and Language*, *24*, 297–313.

Marshall, J., Robson, J., Pring, T., & Chiat, S. (1998). Why does monitoring fail in jargon aphasia? Comprehension, judgment, and therapy evidence. *Brain and Language*, *63*, 79–109.

Marshall, R. C., Neuburger, S. I., & Philips, D. S. (1994). Verbal self-correction and improvement in treated aphasic clients. *Aphasiology*, *8*, 535–47.

Marshall, R. C., Rappaport, B. Z., & Garcia-Bunuel, L. (1985). Self-monitoring behavior in a case of severe auditory agnosia with aphasia. *Brain and Language*, *15*, 292–306.

Marshall, R. C., & Tompkins, C. (1982). Verbal self-repair behaviors of fluent and non-fluent aphasic subjects. *Brain and Language*, *15*, 292–306.

McNamara, P., Obler, L. K., Au, Durso, R., & Albert, M. L. (1992). Speech monitoring skills in Alzheimer's disease, Parkinson's disease, and normal ageing. *Brain and Language*, *42*, 38–51.

Nickels, L., & Howard, D. (1995). Phonological errors in aphasic naming: Comprehension, monitoring and lexicality. *Cortex*, *31*, 209–37.

Oomen, C. C. E., & Postma, A. (2001). Effects of time pressure on mechanisms of speech production and self-monitoring. *Journal of Psycholinguistic Research*, *30*, 163–84.

Oomen, C. C. E., & Postma, A. (2002). Resource limitations and speech monitoring. *Language and Cognitive Processes*, *17*, 163–84.

Oomen, C. C. E., Postma, A., & Kolk, H. H. J. (2001). Prearticulatory and postarticulatory self-monitoring in Broca's aphasia. *Cortex*, *37*, 627–41.

Postma, A. (2000). Detection of errors during speech production. A review of speech monitoring models. *Cognition*, *77*, 97–131.

Postma, A., & Kolk, H. H. J. (1993). The covert repair hypothesis: Prearticulatory repair processes in normal and stuttered disfluencies. *Journal of Speech and Hearing Research*, *36*, 472–87.

Schlenck, K., Huber, W., & Willmes, K. (1987). "Prepairs" and repairs: Different monitoring functions in aphasic language production. *Brain and Language*, *30*, 226–44.

Shuren, J. E., Smith-Hammond, C., Maher, L. M., Rothi, L. J. G., & Heilman, K. M. (1996). Attention and agnosia: The case of a jargon aphasic with unawareness of language deficit. *Neurology*, *45*, 376–78.

Stark, J. A. (1988). Aspects of automatic versus controlled processing, monitoring, metalinguistic tasks, and related phenomena in aphasia. In J. A. Stark, & W. U. Dressler (Eds.), *Linguistic analyses of aphasic language*. New York: Springer Verlag.

13 Stuttering as a monitoring deficit

Nada Vasiç and Frank Wijnen

Abstract

Stuttering is a well-studied phenomenon ascribed by various scholars to problems that arise during speech planning and/or the execution of a speech plan. This study focuses on self-monitoring, a crucial accessory to normal speech production, as sketched by Levelt (1983, 1989). We propose that stuttering stems from a malfunctioning monitoring process. An experimental study is presented in which the monitoring process was put under scrutiny in dual task conditions. The results indicate that (1) performing a secondary, non-linguistic task during speaking suppresses disfluency, particularly blocking, in persons who stutter; (2) forcing the monitor's focus toward the lexical content of the output of the production mechanism also reduces disfluency. These findings are explained by assuming that individuals who stutter habitually allocate too much processing resources to monitoring, and that, in doing so, the focus of their monitoring is maladaptively rigid. Our conjecture is that monitoring in stuttering individuals is focused on the temporal flow of speech, in an attempt to prevent any type of discontinuity surfacing in overt speech.

Introduction

Ask anyone to describe the speech of a person who stutters and she will mention blocks, repetitions, particularly of word parts, and prolongations. These are the primary symptoms of stuttering. In addition to these, there is a variety of clinical phenomena that we will call the secondary characteristics of stuttering. Each of these has to do with variation in the degree of disfluency, both within utterances and in the speaker's verbal output at large as a result of external conditions. Within utterances, disfluencies tend to concentrate at, first, the beginning of clauses (Koopmans, Slis & Rietveld, 1992) and, second, accented content words. As to output at large, it has long been known that the overall amount of disfluency within a person can vary substantially (see, e.g., Bloodstein, 1972). Even the most severe stutterers report that they occasionally experience almost stutter-free periods. In some clinical handbooks (e.g., Baker & Cantwell, 1995), fluctuations in disfluency under the influence of social context, speech situation or speech partner, content of the message, emotional condition, etc. is mentioned as a distinctive feature of stuttering. Finally, an interesting feature of stuttering is its temporary amelioration as a result of changes in the manner of speaking, such as whispering, singing or choral reading, or as a result of manipulations of auditory feedback (in experimental or clinical settings).

In this chapter, we sketch a psychological hypothesis that can account for both the primary symptoms and many of the secondary characteristics of stuttering. The basis of this hypothesis is a well-established model of the human language-production mechanism, Levelt's *blueprint of the speaker* (Levelt, 1989). This blueprint, which outlines the processing modules that in a serial incremental fashion transform a pre-verbal message into a series of articulatory movements, has served as a cornerstone of much research. Over the years the model has been refined and extended, specifically in the domain of word selection and phonological encoding (see e.g., Levelt, Roelofs, & Meyer, 1999, Roelofs, 2002). We will not present the model in any detail, but concentrate on the one component that is crucial to our story, the *monitor*. The monitor is a device that checks the correctness of both content and form of the output of the production mechanism. Levelt portrays it as a part of the conceptualizer. Unlike the formulator sub-components, which create linguistic representations, and are considered to be highly automatic, the conceptualizer is (partly) under conscious control. Levelt does not detail the inner architecture of the monitor. It would seem to comprise minimally two components, one of which attends to the output of the speech-programming process, and a second one that compares this output with some standard. If the output does not satisfy a particular criterion, the monitor initiates a self-correction. A self-correction typically consists of three phases: (a) interrupting speech; (b) repairing the error (i.e., construction of a new speech plan); and finally, (c) restarting of the articulation at the point where the interruption occurred, or at a point prior to the interruption (see Hartsuiker & Kolk, 2001).

Levelt proposes that the monitor uses two input channels. It keeps track of the realized speech, through the so-called "outer loop", and it has direct access to the output of the formulator before this is transformed into audible speech, through the "inner loop". Note that the monitor is assumed to use the normal language-perception system. In contrast, other authors have argued that various types of monitoring should be viewed as the function of feedback systems within the production mechanism (see Postma, 2000; Postma & Oomen, this volume, Chapter 9). One of the advantages of the perceptual loop hypothesis of monitoring is that it is economical; it does not postulate any processing architecture beyond what we know must be present. Consequently, it allows us to formulate strong predictions. In particular, we must assume that it is constrained by the principles related to discrimination, sensitivity and attention that we see at work in all perceptual systems. These will be dealt with later in greater detail.

Stuttering as covert repairing

An influential hypothesis that has associated stuttering with monitoring is the *Covert Repair Hypothesis* (Kolk, 1991; Postma & Kolk, 1993; Postma, Kolk, & Povel, 1990). It states that speech disfluency (both in stuttered and in "normal" speech) reflects the interrupting and restarting that result from pre-articulatory detecting and repairing of an error in the utterance plan. Restarting at a point before the interruption produces a repetition. Another possibility is that the speaker halts articulation until a new (repaired) speech plan is available. In such cases, an observer will hear a pause, a block or a tensed prolongation. Note that on this hypothesis, the error locus is not in the speech fragment that is repaired, but in some part of the speech plan that is still waiting to be uttered.

What errors lead to the covert repairs we perceive as disfluencies, and why are there so many of them in the speech of persons who stutter? Several researchers claim that stuttering is related to a problem in phonological encoding (e.g., Bosshardt, 1999; Postma, Kolk, & Povel, 1990). One of the findings that has fostered this hypothesis is a high co-morbidity of stuttering and phonological problems in early childhood (St. Louis, 1991; Wolk, Edwards, & Conture, 1993; Yaruss & Conture, 1996). Postma and Kolk (1993; Kolk, 1991) have proposed that the actual dysfunction underlying stuttering resides in selecting phonemes for utterance plans. This process has been modelled as activation spreading in a connectionist network (see e.g., Dell, 1988). Building a phonological output representation is realized through the association of phonemes with slots in a metrically defined frame. Normally, if a slot in the frame needs to be filled, the phoneme that has the highest activation level at the critical time point is selected. In a person who stutters, however, activation spreading is slow. This means that when a specific slot needs to be filled, it is likely that competition among candidate phonemes has not settled. Consequently, a misselection may occur. Many such misselections are pre-articulatorily detected and repaired, which yields interruptions and restarts in overt speech. Thus, the primary symptoms of stuttering reflect the response of the monitor to the encoding problem.

The Covert Repair Hypothesis (CRH) yields a number of interesting predictions. One is that if, due to whatever conditions, disfluency is suppressed, overt speech errors should increase in frequency. The reverse prediction also holds: The more overt stuttering, the less phonological errors should be observable. Of course, these two predictions hinge on the assumption that the average frequency of errors in phonological encoding (i.e., covert and overt) is constant (which may not be true). A second prediction is that stuttering individuals and normal speakers should differ on indices that reflect the phonological encoding process.

Postma and Kolk (1990) addressed the trade-off prediction. They asked persons who stutter and control subjects to read tongue-twister sentences in two conditions: High accuracy (avoid all errors) and normal accuracy. The high accuracy condition yielded markedly fewer speech errors in both subject groups than the normal condition, but the frequency of self-corrections and disfluencies was not affected. Thus, the accuracy instruction raised the *ratio* of disfluencies to speech errors. The high accuracy instruction also induced a relative increase of self-corrections following overt speech errors. According to Postma and Kolk, the parallelism between these two patterns indicates that disfluencies in fact are self-corrections[1] – i.e., covert repairs. That stuttering individuals produce many more disfluencies in proportion to the number of overt errors than normal speakers must mean, therefore, that their encoding system generates more speech errors – which are pre-articulatorily repaired. An alternative interpretation, perhaps not as elegant, but still consistent with the data, is that the disfluencies have nothing to do with the apparent trade-off between slips of the tongue and self-corrections. This implies that the higher number of disfluencies observed in stuttering individuals is not a result of a higher number of phonological errors, but of something else, which needs to be identified.

In follow-up studies, Postma and Kolk (1992a, 1992b) found that noise masking reduced the number of disfluencies and self-corrections in normal speakers. There was no concomitant increase of speech errors, however. When asked to speak very accurately, subjects were able to do so, but this did not raise the rate of disfluencies and self-corrections. Postma and Kolk argue that two complementary processes underlie the effect of the accuracy instruction. First, the error rate goes down, presumably because the subjects allot more resources to encoding. Second, there is an overall increase in covert corrections – but as error rate goes down, this is hardly visible. Note that, again, the alternative interpretation is that disfluencies are not related to errors in the speech plan. This can explain why their number, in contrast to the number of speech errors, is not influenced by the accuracy instruction. Moreover, this account is not embarrassed by the observation that disfluency decreases under noise masking while speech error rate does not go up concomitantly, as the covert repair hypothesis predicts.

Is there any direct evidence for phonological encoding problems in stuttering speakers? Wijnen and Boers (1994) used the *implicit priming* technique (Meyer, 1991) in an attempt to answer this question. Their results suggested that phonological encoding in stutterers does not proceed in the same way as in non-stuttering individuals. When the initial consonants of words to be spoken in response to visual cues were identical (as in *baker* – *buddy* – *bible*), reaction times in stuttering individuals were statistically indistinguishable from those in a condition in which all initial consonants were different. In the control subjects, by contrast, response times were shorter when the initial consonants were identical. When the initial consonant *and* the subsequent vowel were identical (*bible* – *bias* – *bylaw*), a significant and approximately equal priming effect was obtained in both groups of speakers. In a subsequent experiment, however, Burger and Wijnen (1999) were unable to replicate these results. An overview of the individual data of the Wijnen and Boers study indicated that the average pattern reported is representative for only 4 out of 9 stuttering subjects. The other 5 stuttering participants performed just like the non-stuttering subjects. A cautious conclusion to be drawn from this work is that in *some* stuttering speakers, phonological encoding may be deviant.

In their study on stuttering and phonological disorders in children Yaruss and Conture (1996) found that the predictions of the CRH regarding the co-occurrence of speech disfluencies and speech errors were supported for non-systematic (slips of the tongue) speech errors, but not for systematic (phonological rule based) speech errors. Their results also indicated that, unlike the CRH would predict, utterances produced with faster articulatory speaking rates or shorter response latencies were not more likely to contain speech errors or speech disfluencies. Therefore, their findings suggest that speech disfluencies may not result from self-repairs of systematic speech errors produced during conversational speech.

In summary, the experimental evidence pertinent to the CRH appears to be inconclusive. Neither a trade-off between disfluencies and overt speech errors nor phonological encoding problems in stutterers have been indisputably demonstrated. We are quite aware that a case cannot be built on absence of evidence, but it seems that a malfunction of phonological encoding in people who stutter quite conspicuously fails to find support in various studies (Hubbard & Prins, 1994; Prins, Main, & Wampler, 1997). Some other observations need to be considered as well. It is well known that speakers are capable of detecting speech errors in sub-vocal speech (e.g., Dell, 1980). If stuttering is to be traced back to frequently occurring errors in the speech plan, one should expect that people who stutter should be able to report these errors. However, they generally cannot. Stuttering persons often stress that they are focused on the problems that might arise in their overt speech, which seems to suggest that they put a lot of energy in monitoring their own production. Furthermore, we already mentioned that stuttering can disappear, under the right circumstances. This, too, would seem difficult to reconcile with the notion of a hard-wired processing defect.

Inadequate monitoring

We are inclined to abandon the assumption that phonological encoding is perturbed in stuttering persons. At the same time, we would like to keep the core assumption of the CRH, notably the assumption that disfluencies are covert self-corrections. The question then is, if it is not segmental errors that are corrected, what is it? Before we venture to answer this question, we have to specify some basic characteristics of monitoring.

In Levelt's (1989) conception, monitoring is modulated by attention.

The observation that many speech errors are not corrected (Levelt, 1983; Nooteboom, 1980) would seem to be a clear indication of this. Furthermore, Levelt (1983) observed that the likelihood of repairing an error increases as it occurs closer to the end of a phrase. Levelt's explanation is that as the realization of an utterance proceeds, less attention needs to be invested in planning, and hence more resources are free for output monitoring. Some indirect evidence that monitoring can be under strategic control comes from an elicited speech error experiment by Baars, Motley, and MacKay (1975). They found that fewer non-word errors were produced when the stimulus materials contained existing words than when they consisted of nonsense items. This can be interpreted as a task-induced increased vigilance for non-word output (but see Hartsuiker, Corley, & Martensen, 2002; Humphreys & Swendsen, 2002).

Thus there are indications that the amount of attention invested in self-monitoring can vary. Additionally, everyday experience suggests that attention can be directed to a specific attribute of the speech output. When there is a lot of ambient noise, speakers are forced to monitor clarity or loudness, which in more favourable acoustic circumstances is unnecessary. When delivering a formal speech, it is likely that the speaker will closely monitor the semantic cohesion of the discourse, whereas in, e.g., a conversation with a friend, this may be less prominent. In formal social situations, e.g., conversations with a superior or an unfamiliar person, it is important to avoid inappropriate phrases, whereas in an informal conversation this may well be unimportant. For the amount of resources allocated to monitoring, we will use the term *effort*. The selective aspect of monitoring, by way of contrast, will be referred to as *focus*. In line with general assumptions, we assume that attentive resources are limited. This means that when more attention is focused on inspection of a particular characteristic of the produced speech, e.g., cohesion, there will be fewer resources available for monitoring of other factors, e.g., articulatory clarity.

A third parameter of monitoring will be referred to as the *threshold*. This parameter relates to the criteria the output needs to satisfy in order to be acceptable. Two types of criteria can be distinguished, absolute and relative. Absolute criteria can be associated with, for instance, grammatical well-formedness. Relative criteria may apply to, e.g., message coherence or articulatory clarity. With regard to relative criteria, speakers can determine a threshold value relative to the task they must perform and the strategic decisions they make in that situation. If the produced speech does not exceed the threshold, a self-correction needs to be performed.

It has been suggested that stuttering results from the detection and correction of non-existing speech errors (Sherrard 1975). However, as Janssen (1994) has pointed out, no explicit account has ever been offered as to how the perceptual system would "hallucinate" speech errors.[2] Conceivably, under Sherrard's hypothesis, and presupposing a perception-based monitor, persons who stutter would experience many "slips of the ear"

(Bond, 1999), not only when self-monitoring, but also when listening to others. However, as far as we know, there is no evidence in support of this prediction. Postma and Kolk (1992b) report that stuttering and non-stuttering persons detect slips of the tongue equally fast and accurately, which at least suggests that error detection is unimpaired in people who stutter. Rather than being the result of a processing defect, dysfunctional monitoring could be the result of an inadequate setting of (one of) the parameters, effort, focus or threshold.

Evidence that stuttering is correlated with excessive attention for one's own speech is provided by some dual task experiments. An example is a study conducted by Arends, Povel, and Kolk (1988). They used three speech tasks with an increasing difficulty level: Counting out loud (from 20 to 99), counting backwards in threes (97, 94, 91, etc.), and spontaneous speaking. In the dual task conditions, a demanding perceptual-motor task (*pursuit rotor tracking*) had to be performed at the same time as speaking. Arends et al. found, first, that disfluency rate was influenced by the difficulty of the speech task. Second, performing the secondary task suppressed disfluency in severe stutterers. Other studies within the dual task paradigm (Bosshardt, 1999; Kamhi & McOsker, 1982) yielded results that are less clear-cut, but generally compatible with the excessive self-monitoring hypothesis. In contrast, Oomen and Postma (2002) report that when normally fluent speakers were performing a tactile recognition task while speaking, they produced more filled pauses and (word) repetitions in a dual task condition, than in a single (speaking) condition.

Excessive monitoring can only account for the core symptoms of stuttering if it is maintained that disfluencies represent self-corrections. The next step then is to determine what the monitor perceives as errors. What does the monitor *focus* on, and where does the boundary of the output's acceptability (*threshold*) lie? Our proposal is, paradoxically, that individuals who stutter do so because they are trying to avoid it. We surmise that stuttering individuals have a tendency to *focus* on cues related to temporal or rhythmic disruption, both in planning and in overt speech. In doing so, they apply overly strict acceptability criteria. It appears, therefore, that stutterers indeed try to correct non-existent errors, not because of faulty perceptual processing, but because of a faulty evaluation process. Normal speech abounds with discontinuities and temporal variation. Discontinuities in speech planning and delivery may arise as a result of transient difficulties in word finding or formulating. Variations in the temporal domain include prolongations of sounds that stem from the dynamics of articulation, or from linguistically or discursively conditioned prominence (word stress and sentence accent). The realization of certain classes of speech sounds (e.g., plosives) necessarily involves brief interruptions of the articulatory flow. Individuals who stutter are inclined to perceive each of these phenomena as the onset of a disfluency. They interrupt themselves in order to prevent the supposed incidents from surfacing. Since such interruptions are perceived as disfluencies as well (and in this case rightfully so), they give rise to new interruptions, and the undesired result can be a series of repetitions or blocks. In such situations, the monitor enters a loop, a vicious circle resulting in a complete halt of speech delivery.

Vicious Circle Hypothesis

Our hypothesis, then, is that the three attention parameters of the monitor: Effort, focus and threshold are inappropriately set in persons who stutter: (1) more effort is invested in monitoring than is required for adequate speech production; (2) the monitor focuses habitually on temporal fluctuation and discontinuity; (3) the threshold for acceptable output is set so high that even normal and unavoidable discontinuities and temporal fluctuations are perceived as disfluencies (false positives). A number of straightforward predictions can be derived:

> *ad 1. Effort.* If the resources available to the monitor are reduced, disfluency will decrease.
> *ad 2. Focus.* If a person who stutters is forced to monitor something other than temporal discontinuity, given that resources are limited, the chance of detecting discontinuities or temporal fluctuations will decrease. Consequently, disfluency will decrease.
> *ad 3. Threshold.* Since we assume that monitoring is based on perceptual processing, we predict that also in listening to speech from someone else, stutterers will entertain a more conservative standard with respect to fluency than non-stutterers.

Prediction 3 is addressed by Russell, Corley, & Lickley (this volume, Chapter 14). In what follows we describe a dual task study, aimed at testing predictions 1 and 2.

The experiment

Participants

In our study 22 stuttering (mild to severe) and 10 non-stuttering persons took part. All were native Dutch speakers. Of the 22 stuttering individuals, 14 were males and 6 females, which is close to the 2:1 ratio that we find in this population in general. Persons who stutter had been diagnosed as such by a speech therapist, and they considered their disfluency to be a problem. The control group consisted of individuals who had never seen a speech therapist and who did not stutter and had no other speech-related problem.

Tasks

The experiment comprised four conditions, a speaking-only (baseline) condition and three conditions in which speaking was accompanied with one of the secondary tasks now described. To elicit semi-spontaneous speech, subjects were asked to read a newspaper article prior to each trial in order to retell its content. In case they stopped talking, the experimenter would call out a cue word/topic, such as "holidays", "family", "hobbies" etc. and the subjects had to elaborate on the topic.

The first distraction task was the computer game *PONG*, a virtual table tennis game, which engages visual-motor skills. Two parameters in *PONG* can be adjusted to influence the difficulty of the game: Initial speed of the ball, and acceleration. Each time the ball is hit it accelerates by a set value, and when the player misses, the next ball will move at the speed set as initial. The initial values of the speed and acceleration parameters were tailored to each subject's skill. In the "Pong simple" (PS) condition, these parameters were kept constant throughout the trial. In the "Pong difficult" (PD) condition, speed was raised in order to make the distraction task more demanding. In both conditions, the computer monitored the subject's performance on the task.

The second distraction task was designed to redirect the monitor's focus. This task required subjects to monitor for the occurrence of a particular word in their output. The word was *die* (*that* – indexical and relative pronoun), which occurs frequently. Subjects were instructed to press a button each time they detected *die*. A computer recorded their responses.

Each trial lasted 10 minutes. The order of presentation of trials was completely counterbalanced across participants. Subjects were tested individually and were all paid for their participation. They were told that the experiment was designed to investigate their ability to perform another task while speaking. Each subject was taped on a digital audio recorder. After reading the instructions with a short description of the experimental tasks subjects were screened for *PONG*. This was used to determine the level for *PONG* in the PD condition.

Transcription and coding

Speech produced by subjects in each of the conditions was transcribed and coded for disfluencies with a cut-off point after 7 minutes. Disfluencies were transcribed and classified as blocks, self-corrections, prolongations, repetitions, senseless sound insertions, word breaks, unfilled pauses or filled pauses. Any audible tense fixation on any part of a word was coded as a block. A self-correction was identified by an interruption, followed by a retracing and/or an alteration of the original utterance, as in [[*I went to see a*] *went to see the doctor . . .*]. Some stuttering individuals tended to prolong segments in an unnatural way; such incidents were coded as prolongations.

Repetitions were coded as several different types, namely, repetitions of the initial segment of a word, of a syllable in a word, of a whole word, or a word string. Additionally, combinations of several of these were described as complex repetitions. Some stutterers inserted sounds between particular words/ segments, which are clearly not related to the words that are uttered after them, e.g., *He told me to* [*s:*] *go home*. These instances were coded as "senseless sound insertions". Word breaks were defined as interruptions of words without completion or retracing. Finally, two different types of pause were coded. Filled pauses were pauses accompanied with a sound usually transcribed as *uh*, *um* or *hm*, and unfilled pauses were all unnaturally long soundless breaks that occurred between speech segments. Several occurrences of one type of disfluency on the same position were counted as one disfluency. However, disfluencies of a different type that occurred on the same segment were coded and counted separately.

Transcribing and coding was done in the CLAN program originally designed for the CHILDES database (MacWhinney, 1995). CLAN enables fast and efficient data analysis. We counted the number of words and the number of disfluencies per condition. Disfluency was, therefore, determined in terms of the number of disfluencies per condition in relation to the number of words uttered in each condition. Additionally, phonetic, morphological and syntactic speech errors were also coded, but these will not be discussed in this report because they occurred too scarcely.[3] Filled pauses were not included in the analysis, as they appear to be strongly associated with macro-planning and conceptualizing, rather than formulating (Goldman-Eisler, 1968; Swerts, Wichmann, & Beun 1996). The total number of observations (words for all conditions for all subjects) for the whole sample that we analyzed was 55,177.

Data analysis

As in the population at large, stuttering severity varied considerably in our sample of subjects. We had no preconception as to how stuttering severity would interact with the experimental manipulations, and we therefore did not have any a priori way to model subject variability. However, rather than treating subject variability as random noise, as a traditional statistical analysis (e.g., analysis of variance) would have forced us to do, we decided to perform an analysis that takes subject variability into account, viz multilevel analysis (Goldstein, 1995). This approach is optimally tailored to a full exploration of data such as ours, since it allows a more complex structure of the error variances, such that both differences between subjects and within subjects (between different conditions) can be removed from the residual error variance. A more detailed outline of the statistical model we used to analyze the data is given in the appendix.

In order to determine whether the experimental conditions affected disfluency, the amount of disfluency was calculated in proportion to the number of words produced in each condition. To this end, each individual word a particular subject produced was coded as fluent or as not fluent. Using the MLN computer program (Prosser, Rasbash, & Goldstein, 1995), a two-level regression model was fitted on the data with variance between subjects as level 1 and variance within subjects as level 2. The model produced population estimates of mean disfluency per condition expressed in logits (which can be easily translated into estimated proportions), and estimates of the variances associated with the means. Differences between conditions were evaluated by testing the differences between the regression weights in the fitted model that correspond to each of the conditions. Under H0, the test statistic t has a large sample χ^2 distribution with degrees of freedom equaling the number of conditions compared, minus one.

Results

In Table 13.1, the estimated mean proportions of disfluencies are given for each condition. These estimates are derived from the logit values calculated by the model. Clearly, the baseline condition (speaking only) yields a higher mean proportion of disfluencies than the other three conditions. This difference is small; nevertheless, it is significant ($\chi^2_1 = 11.98$, $p < .01$). The difference between the three dual task conditions in the proportions of disfluencies is not significant ($\chi^2_1 = 3.84$, $p > .05$). Since we would like to generalize across the population of stuttering individuals we checked whether the observed measurements correspond to the values predicted by the model. If this is the case, we would be able to claim that our results follow the pattern predicted for the population. The correlation between the observed and the predicted measurements is high enough (0.66) for the estimates generated by the model to be accepted as a true reflection of the population observed.

The second step in our analysis was to look more closely at the different types of disfluency produced by subjects. It could be that some disfluencies, particularly the ones that are very typical of the speech of stutterers exhibit the effect predicted by our model more so than other types of disfluencies, e.g., the ones that are less typical of stuttering. As already noted, a range of different types of disfluencies was coded, counted and for each

Table 13.1 Estimated population values of proportions of disfluencies per condition, and the associated logits (stuttering individuals)

Parameter	Proportion	Logit (standard error)
Speech only	.191	−1.451 (0.124)
Pong simple	.173	−1.559 (0.124)
Pong difficult	.172	−1.576 (0.124)
Monitoring *die*	.170	−1.575 (0.124)

different type we calculated and compared the means. The results are given in Table 13.2.

Eleven different types of disfluency were coded and counted, and as can be seen in Table 13.2, some of these occurred very infrequently. Additionally, the differences across conditions in the number of particular types of disfluency were often not significant. Therefore, we decided to focus on the most frequent ones, namely, blocks and word repetitions. Blocking most clearly distinguishes stuttering from normal disfluency. Word repetitions, contrariwise, are common in stuttering individuals as well as in non-stuttering persons when they are forced to speak and perform a secondary task at the same time.

Blocks were the most frequent type of all disfluencies (close to 10% across conditions), with the exception of the *die* monitoring condition. There was a significant difference in the mean number of blocks between all dual conditions and the baseline condition ($\chi^2_1 = 4.27$, $p < .01$). The proportion of blocks in the baseline condition is significantly higher than in each of the experimental conditions. Additionally, in the *die* monitoring condition subjects produced a significantly lower number of blocks in comparison to the other two dual task conditions.

Word repetitions were also numerous with a significant difference between Pong difficult condition and the baseline condition ($\chi^2_1 = 8.68$, $p < .01$); subjects produced more word repetitions in the baseline condition. It is interesting to note that there were significantly more disfluencies in monitoring *die* versus all other conditions. Similar results were found for *word string* repetitions. There was an increase in the number of word string repetitions in the monitoring *die* condition in comparison to all other conditions.

Table 13.2 Proportions of disfluently uttered words in persons who stutter, broken down over disfluency types (in multiples of 10^{-2})

	Speech only (proportion)	Pong simple (proportion)	Pong difficult (proportion)	Monitoring die (proportion)
Blocks	9.934	9.160	9.335	5.455
Corrections	.998	.671	.723	1.048
Prolongations	.161	.298	.077	.274
Rep: Initial segment	.350	.284	.295	.601
Rep: Initial syllable	1.045	1.115	1.213	1.567
Rep: Complex	.077	.120	.081	.042
Rep: Word	3.296	2.944	2.734	3.868
Rep: Word string	1.609	1.431	1.580	2.471
Senseless sound insertions	.663	.489	.316	.625
Unfilled pauses	.258	.277	.265	.419
Word breaks	.712	.523	.677	.670
Total	19.103	17.312	17.296	17.040

Table 13.3 Estimated population values of proportions of disfluencies per condition, and associated logits (control subjects)

Parameter	Proportion	Logit (standard error)	Word repetitions only (prop.)
Speech only	.039	−3.201 (0.141)	.020
Pong simple	.031	−3.427 (0.144)	.016
Pong difficult	.029	−3.507 (0.141)	.011
Monitoring *die*	.047	−2.993 (0.140)	.026

Table 13.3 reports the same analysis for the control group.

The baseline condition is significantly more disfluent than the two distraction conditions. The difference between baseline condition and Pong difficult condition was significant ($\chi^2_1 = 11.26$, $p < .01$). Similarly, the baseline condition and the Pong simple condition differed from each other significantly ($\chi^2_1 = 6.41$, $p < .01$). No difference was found between the two distraction conditions (Pong difficult vs Pong simple) in which the resources were taken away from monitoring of speech production. Finally, the experimental condition in which the monitor's focus was shifted was the most disfluent. This particular condition was significantly different from all other conditions ($\chi^2_1 = 6.37$, $p < .01$).

We examined the different types of disfluency and compared their means across conditions. Only four types occurred in the speech of the non-stuttering control group, namely, *self-corrections* and three different types of *repetitions* – word initial segments, words, and strings of words. Of all four types of disfluency, only one type exhibited a difference across conditions, viz *word repetitions*. In the monitoring *die* condition non-stuttering subjects produced the most word repetitions. There was a significant difference between the baseline and monitoring *die* condition ($\chi^2_1 = 5.81$, $p < .01$). There was no difference between the baseline and Pong simple condition. The latter differed significantly from the Pong difficult and monitoring *die* ($\chi^2_1 = 6.00$, $p < .01$) conditions. In the Pong difficult condition subjects produced the lowest number of word repetitions, with a significant difference between this condition and all other conditions ($\chi^1_1 = 18.12$, $p < .01$).

Discussion

We set out to test two predictions derived from the Vicious Circle Hypothesis. The first is that performing an additional task during speaking (but unrelated to it) reduces the amount of disfluency in people who stutter. This is based on the assumption that stuttering people spend an excessive amount of attentional resources on monitoring, and that a secondary task will take some of these resources away, preventing the monitor from being overly vigilant. The second prediction was based on our proposal that a stuttering person's monitor habitually focuses on discontinuities and indices of temporal variability.

If we would succeed in pushing away the monitor from its habitual focus, speech should become less disfluent.

The first prediction was tested in a dual task experiment in which the secondary task was designed to be demanding enough to engage much of the participant's attentional resources. The results support the prediction: When distracted by a visual-motor task, stutterers produce less disfluency. The effect is small, but significant. The results of previous dual task studies are somewhat inconsistent (see Arends et al., 1988), and this may be related to the degree to which the secondary task can continuously engage the subjects' attention. In our experiment, the degree of difficulty of the visual-motor secondary task was varied in order to verify this claim. The results indicate that even a task that is not very demanding – the simple version of Pong – can be effective. The effectiveness of the secondary task appears to hinge on its capacity to continuously engage attentive processing (see e.g., Arends et al., 1988; Thompson, 1985). We think that we may have underestimated the demands made by the Pong game, particularly for relatively inexperienced players. At the very least, the game requires continuous visual attention in order for it to be played successfully.

The second prediction – pertaining to the stuttering person's habitual monitoring focus – was confirmed as well. It is important to emphasize that the manipulation we used to redirect focus is principally different from the one in the Pong conditions. The visual-motor distracter task is entirely unrelated to the process of speaking, and only intended to take away resources from the general pool. By contrast, the instruction to monitor for a particular word does not reallocate attention resources to a different process. It changes the way in which the processing resources used by the monitor are deployed.

The non-stuttering subjects exhibited a different pattern than the stuttering subjects. Both Pong conditions led to a slight decrease of disfluency, and the more demanding condition yielded fewer disfluencies than the simple condition. Directing the monitor's focus to lexical content of the output led to a significant *increase* in disfluency, contrasting with the effect in the stuttering subjects.

It should be noted that the decrease of disfluency in the dual task conditions might be related to reduction in speech rate. However, although we did not systematically measure speech rate, our impression was that it did not differ much across conditions. Nevertheless, it is certainly a point worth considering in follow-up studies. We consider it unlikely, however, that speech rate could have played a major role in the present results, particularly in the light of the differential effects of the dual task conditions on different types of disfluency, to be further detailed later.

Different types of disfluencies responded differently to the two types of secondary tasks in the stuttering group. We focused on the two most prominent types, blocking and word repetitions. In the persons who stutter the frequency of blocks decreased in all three dual task conditions as compared to the baseline. By contrast, the amount of repetitions dropped in the Pong conditions, but appeared to rise in the *die* monitoring condition. Similarly, the control group exhibited a rise in the number of (word) repetitions in the *die* monitoring condition, and a decrease in the difficult Pong condition. This result contrasts in part with the result reported by Oomen and Postma (2002), who found and increase of filled pauses and repetitions in normal speakers when they performed a perceptuo-motor secondary task. However, it is possible that the tactile recognition task Oomen and Postma employed is less continuously attention demanding than our visual-motor task. Consequently, their subjects may have adapted a different way of dealing with the task demands than ours.

The crucial difference between the stuttering and non-stuttering speakers is in blocking. It is the most frequent type of disfluency in stuttering subjects whereas controls do not produce any blocks. It is precisely this type of non-fluency that proved to be most sensitive to the experimental conditions. This gives rise to the idea that blocking most directly reflects the habitual, maladaptive monitoring behavior that persons who stutter have acquired. Clinical analyses of the development of stuttering in children (e.g., McDearmon, 1968; Yairi and Lewis, 1984), generally argue that emergence of blocking indicates that the "physiological" disfluency of the immature child has turned into a problem. Johnson (1956, 1959) wrote that the emergence of blocking is correlated with the child's emerging awareness of his disfluency.

Reiterating previously articulated material (repeating), contrariwise, is a normal, natural response of the language production system to trouble in planning or delivery as can be seen from the data obtained from the non-stuttering speakers (see Howell & Sackin, 2000, for a related proposal). We assume that part of the repetitions in stuttering are these "normal" reactions of the language production system. Another part may be due to the maladaptive monitoring process we hypothesize. Naturally occurring disfluency is sensitive to the "amount of work" in the production system: It rises as the speech task gets more difficult (Arends et al., 1988).

Thus, the differences in behaviour between stuttering and control subjects are consistent with our hypothesis. The perceptual-motor secondary task we used takes away processing resources across the board. In comparison to the baseline condition (speaking only), this secondary task does not put additional "pressure" on the language-production system itself. By performing this task, stutterers are prevented from following their habit of excessive monitoring. This has a beneficial effect on their speech, most conspicuously with regard to the most pathological of all disfluencies, blocks. The non-stuttering subjects become less disfluent when performing a secondary perceptual-motor task as well. However, in contrast to the persons who stutter, the effect in the non-stuttering subjects was found in the repetitions.

The focus-directing task appears to have two simultaneous effects: (1) What it is supposed to do, namely drawing the stuttering person's monitor away from what it normally focuses on, and (2) by doing so, increasing the load on the production system. Consider what it means to be instructed to explicitly report every occurrence of a particular word in your speech output. It means consciously controlled monitoring. It is very likely that this will interfere with normal speech planning and delivery, and that, therefore, the number of normal disfluencies will rise, and more so than the distracting effect will suppress them, as can be seen from the results of the control group. From this perspective, it is very meaningful that in persons who stutter the decrease is in the non-normal type of disfluency, whereas the rise is in the class of disfluencies that (at least in part) can be considered normal. This observation may provide support for our interpretation that in fact two processes co-occur, one that affects the normal ("healthy") part of the language production system (more repetitions) and one that affects the "pathological" part, what we have named maladaptive monitoring (less blocking).

Summarizing, our results support two predictions derived from the Vicious Circle Hypothesis. In this volume, Russell, Corley, and Lickley (Chapter 14) supply further corroborative evidence, pertaining to the conjectured badly tuned *focus* and *threshold* parameters of the monitor in persons who stutter. One question that remains, is whether the VCH can account for what we called the "secondary characteristics" of stuttering. We conclude our chapter by briefly discussing this issue.

It has repeatedly been noted that the distribution of stuttering incidents over utterances is highly similar to that of disfluencies considered normal. Normal disfluency tends to peak at the beginning of utterances (see Maclay & Osgood, 1959; Schilperoord, 1996; Wijnen, 1990). Most likely, such disfluencies reflect normal planning operations. The Vicious Circle Hypothesis predicts that stuttering individuals try to prevent oncoming discontinuities by (paradoxically) interrupting the speech flow. This can explain why stuttering is most dense at utterance beginnings. In a similar vein, the fact that stuttering frequently occurs on accented words (Burger & Wijnen, 1998; Prins, Hubbard, & Krause, 1991) can be explained by assuming that a stuttering person's monitor evaluates the normal segmental prolongations associated with accentuation (Eefting & Nooteboom, 1993) as imminent disfluency.

In persons who stutter, external timing of speech production, as in singing and chanting, usually suppresses disfluency (Brady 1969; Brayton & Conture, 1978; Fransella 1967; Fransella & Beech, 1965; Howell & El-Yaniv, 1987). These experiments strongly suggest that the effect cannot be due to mere distraction, or the reduction of speech tempo. Rather, it appears to be *rhythm* that is responsible for the effect. Following an externally defined rhythm most likely requires a particular kind of monitoring (continuously checking whether the output is rhythmically aligned with the input). In the terminology of the Vicious Circle Hypothesis, externally timed speech production forces a reorientation of the monitor's focus. Singing imposes the additional task of checking the produced pitch. It has also been noted that whispering improves fluency in stutterers. Most likely, whispering engages the monitor in keeping the loudness/voice quality at a desired level, and thus prevents it from focusing on discontinuities.

Third, a well-known phenomenon is the (temporary) amelioration of stuttering by delayed auditory feedback (DAF; Goldiamond, 1965) and frequency altered feedback (FAF), where the speech signal is played back with an altered fundamental frequency (Ingham, Moglia, Frank, Ingham, & Cordes, 1997). The effect of DAF may be related to the fact that the cues to which the stuttering person's monitor is oriented are shifted in time and therefore rendered useless. In the case of FAF, however, these cues stay intact. Conceivably, frequency altered speech fed back to the speaker attracts attention, as a result of the mismatch with the speaker's expectancy (or internal representation). This conjecture appears to be confirmed by results obtained in a neuro-imaging study by McGuire, Silbersweig, and Frith (1996). As FAF "diverts" the attention, so to speak, the VCH predicts that its effect will be temporary. Due to habituation, the signal will lose its attraction after a while, and the speaker will relapse into the normal pattern. This prediction is supported by the results obtained by Ingham et al., (1997).

We believe that the Vicious Circle Hypothesis can provide a unified explanation of a range of seemingly divergent observations on stuttering in terms of maladaptive monitoring. Obviously, this must lead to the inevitable question of how monitoring maladaptation arises. The answer to this question should be looked for in the realm of developmental psychology. Stuttering most commonly originates in childhood, evolving from normal developmental disfluency. Early developmental stuttering comprises an increase of hesitations and self-corrections, possibly related to an imbalance between language development and the maturation of the speech production system (Wijnen, 1994). In most cases, children overcome this phase in language development. However, in children in whom this imbalance is somewhat stronger, an awareness of their own disfluency may develop. It is also possible, as Johnson (1959) argued, that someone either consciously or unconsciously draws the child's attention to his frequent hesitations and interruptions.[4] Nevertheless, regardless of how it comes about, a heightened awareness of "failing" could be a possible cause of an eventually maladaptive setting of the monitoring parameters. There have hardly been any studies that have looked into the awareness of stuttering in stuttering children. Needless to say that more research is required in order to provide convincing evidence that children can be oversensitive to their own stuttering behaviour. It has also been pointed out that children who stutter often exhibit delayed or abnormal phonological development (Wolk et al., 1993). It is possible that children with a phonological delay frequently attempt to correct themselves, both overtly and covertly. The effect of this is an increase in speech disfluency, which in itself could possibly draw the monitor's attention. All these suggestions are highly speculative, of course, but at the same time they indicate how the Vicious Circle Hypothesis may unify divergent views on the ontogenesis of stuttering.

Acknowledgements

The research reported in this chapter was supported by the Netherlands Organization for Scientific Research (NWO), through grant number 525–21–002. We are grateful to Huub van den Bergh for his extensive help with statistical matters, and to Albert Postma, Rob Hartsuiker, Ulrich Schade, and Zenzi Griffin whose insightful comments have helped us tremendously in shaping this contribution.

Appendix

In order to estimate the mean number of disfluencies (or proportions) per condition several peculiarities of the data at hand have to be reckoned with. First, the number of disfluencies varies between speakers due to either his or her disposition or to the number of observations made in this individual. In traditional statistical analyses, all observations are considered as independent. However, as mentioned earlier, whether or not a disfluency is observed depends on characteristics of the speaker. More specifically, observations of different speakers are not exchangeable. Translated into statistical terms this means that a two-step sampling procedure is in operation. First, individuals are selected and in the second step observations are made (in four different conditions) on these individuals. In order to test whether the differences between conditions are significant, estimates of the variances between observations (within speakers) as well as the variance among speakers are necessary. Failing to take into account either of the two variance components results in underestimation of the variance and hence in an overoptimistic estimate of the standard errors (and H0 is rejected too easily).

Additionally, the number of observations per speaker is relevant. We are in need of a precise estimate of the proportion of disfluencies per speaker. The (expected) difference between two samples of spontaneous speech of a subject is a function of the number of observations made on that subject. More specifically, if the samples are small, relatively large differences are to be expected, but if the samples are large, small differences will reach significance. In order to combine both demands, a multilevel model with observations (i) nested within speakers (j) is specified. In this model, it is assumed that the variance within speakers is binomially distributed as only disfluencies versus nondisfluencies are observed, and the differences between speakers are normally distributed. A standard method to circumvent estimates outside the parameter range (0,1) is to use a logit link.[5] Such a logit link has, in fact, two advantages. First, parameter values are always within the permitted range. Second, especially near the end of the "proportion scale" it is extremely difficult to show (significant) differences between conditions. That is, as proportions are either near zero or near unity it becomes hard to show differences between conditions, due to a restriction of the range of proportions. A logit transformation stretches the range of proportions thereby circumventing this peculiarity of the data. Hence, for all four conditions, the logit of the mean proportion is estimated. And the differences between conditions are tested by means of a chi-square distributed testing statistic (Goldstein, 1995).

Notes

1 Oomen and Postma (2002) report that the ratio of disfluencies to speech errors increased when speakers had to perform a tactile recognition task simultaneously with speaking, in comparison to only speaking. According to the authors, this result argues against the idea that disfluencies are exclusively reactions to segmental errors.

2 If the speech recognition system is to be modelled as comprising a network of phoneme nodes, analogous to what has been proposed for production, it is conceivable that a node different from the one corresponding to a certain input segment reaches an activation threshold earlier than the correct one, for instance, as a result of noise in the system. This would constitute the proximal cause of misidentification.

3 The Covert Repair Hypothesis predicts that when disfluency is suppressed the number of speech errors should rise. The number of speech errors in our data was too low to run a statistical analysis.

4 It should be mentioned, however, that Johnson's Diagnosogenic Theory has recently received sharp criticism questioning the ethics and the findings of one of the influential studies supporting it (see Ambrose & Yairi, 2002).

5 Remember: Logit (proportion$_j$) = Log (proportion$_j$ / [1 − proportion$_j$]) which equals Log [Frequency$_j$ / Nj − Frequency$_j$]), with N$_j$ being the number of observations (words) on the jth individual.

References

Ambrose, N. G., & Yairi, E. (2002). The Tudor study: Data and ethics. *American Journal of Speech-Language Pathology, 11*, 190–203.

Arends, N., Povel, D. J., & Kolk, H. (1988). Stuttering as an attentional phenomenon. *Journal of Fluency Disorders, 13*, 141–51.

Baars, B., Motley, & MacKay, D. G. (1975). Output editing for lexical status in artificially elicited slips of the tongue. *Journal of Verbal Learning and Verbal Behavior, 14*, 382–91.

Baker, L., & Cantwell, D. P. (1995). Stuttering. In H. I. Kaplan & B. J. Sadock (Eds.), *Comprehensive textbook of psychiatry*, (Vol. 2, 6th ed.). Baltimore, MA: Williams & Wilkins.

Bloodstein, O. (1972). The anticipatory struggle hypothesis: implications of research on the variability of stuttering. *Journal of Speech and Hearing Research, 15*, 487–94.

Bond, Z. S. (1999). *Slips of the ear*. San Diego, CA: Academic Press.

Bosshardt, H. G. (1999). Effects of concurrent mental calculation on stuttering, inhalation and speech timing. *Journal of Fluency Disorders, 24*, 43–72.

Brady, J. P. (1969). Studies on the metronome effect on stuttering. *Behavior Research and Therapy, 7*, 197–204.

Brayton, E. R., & Conture, E. G. (1978). Effects of noise and rhythmic stimulation on the speech of stutterers. *Journal of Speech and Hearing Research, 21*, 276–84.

Burger, R., & Wijnen, F. (1998). *The effects of accent, linear word position and consonant-vowel transition on stuttering.* Poster presented at the ESCoP Conference, Jerusalem.

Burger, R., & Wijnen, F. (1999). Phonological encoding and word stress in stuttering and nonstuttering subjects. *Journal of Fluency Disorders, 24,* 91–106.

Dell, G. S. (1980). *Phonological and lexical encoding: an analysis of natural occurring and experimentally elicited speech errors.* Doctoral dissertation University of Toronto.

Dell, G. S. (1988). The retrieval of phonological forms in production: Test of predictions from a connectionist model. *Journal of Memory and Language, 27,* 124–42.

Eefting, W., & Nooteboom, S. G. (1993). Accentuation, information value and word duration: Effects on speech production, naturalness and sentence processing. In V. J. van Heuven, & L. C. W. Pols (Eds.), *Analysis and synthesis of speech: Strategic research towards high-quality text-to-speech generation.* Berlin: Mouton.

Fransella, F. (1967). Rhythm as a distractor in the modification of stuttering. *Behaviour Research and Therapy, 5,* 253–5.

Fransella, F., & Beech, H. R. (1965). An experimental analysis of the effect of rhythm on the speech of stutterers. *Behaviour Research and Therapy, 3,* 195–201.

Goldiamond, I. (1965). Stuttering and fluency as manipulable operant response classes. In L. Krasner, & L. Ullman (Eds.), *Research in behavior modification.* New York: Holt, Rinehart & Winston.

Goldman-Eisler, F. (1968). *Psycholinguistics: Experiments in spontaneous speech.* New York: Academic Press.

Goldstein, H. (1995). *Multilevel statistical models.* London: Arnold.

Hartsuiker, R., Corley, M., & Martensen, H. (2002). *Lexical bias in spoonerisms. A related beply to Baars et al. (1975).* Paper at the ESCoP Conference, Edinburgh.

Hartsuiker, R., & Kolk, H. (2001). Error monitoring in speech production: A computational test of the perceptual loop theory. *Cognitive Psychology, 42,* 113–57.

Howell, P., & El-Yaniv, N. (1987). The effects of presenting a click in syllable-initial position on the speech of stutterers: Comparison with a metronome click. *Journal of Fluency Disorders, 12,* 249–56.

Howell, P., & Sackin, S. (2000). Speech rate modification and its effects on fluency reversal in fluent speakers and people who stutter. *Journal of Development and Physical Disabilities, 12,* 291–315.

Humphreys, K. R., & Swendsen, A. (2002). *Asymmetric lexical bias in speech errors.* Poster presented at CUNY 2002, New York.

Hubbard, C. P., & Prins, D. (1994). Word familiarity, syllabic stress pattern, and stuttering. *Journal of Speech and Hearing Research, 37,* 564–71.

Ingham, R. J., Moglia, R. A., Frank, P., Ingham, J. C., & Cordes, A. K. (1997). Experimental investigation of the effects of frequency altered auditory feedback on the speech of adults who stutter. *Journal of Speech, Language and Hearing Research, 40,* 361–72.

Janssen, P. (1994). De etiologie van stotteren: Theorieën, modellen, hypothesen en speculaties. *Stem-, Spraak- en Taalpathologie, 3,* 3–41.

Johnson, W. (1956). *Stuttering.* In Johnson, W., Brown, S. J., Curtis, J. J., Edney, C. W., & Keaster, J. (Eds.), *Speech handicapped school children.* New York: Harper.

Johnson, W. (1959). *The onset of stuttering: Research findings and implications.* Minneapolis, MN: University of Minnesota Press.

Kamhi, A., & McOsker, T. (1982). Attention and stuttering: Do stutterers think too much about speech? *Journal of Fluency Disorders, 7*, 309–21.

Kolk, H. (1991). Is stuttering a symptom of adaptation or of impairment? In Peters, H. F. M., Hulstijn, W., & Starkweather, C. W. (Eds.), *Speech motor control and stuttering*. Amsterdam: Elsevier/Excerpta Medica.

Koopmans, M., Slis, I. H., & Rietveld, T. C. M. (1992). Stotteren als uiting van spraakplanning: Een vergelijking tussen voorgelezen en spontane spraak. *Stem-, Spraak- en Taalpathologie, 1*, 87–101.

Levelt, W. J. M. (1983). Monitoring and self-repair in speech. *Cognition, 14*, 41–104.

Levelt, W. J. M. (1989). *Speaking: From intention to articulation*. Cambridge, MA: MIT Press/Bradford Books.

Levelt, W. J. M., Roelofs, A., & Meyer, A. S. (1999). A theory of lexical access in speech production. *Behavioral and Brain Sciences, 21*, 1–38.

Maclay, H., & Osgood, C. E. (1959). Hesitation phenomena in spontaneous English speech. *Word, 15* 19–44.

McDearmon, J. R.(1968). Primary stuttering at the onset of stuttering: A reexamination of data. *Journal of Speech and Hearing Research, 11*, 631–7.

McGuire, P. K., Silbersweig, D. A., & Frith, C. D. (1996). Functional neuroanatomy of verbal self-monitoring. *Brain, 119*, 101–111.

McWhinney, B. (1995). *The Childes project*. Hillsdale, NJ: Lawrence Erlbaum Associates, Inc.

Meyer, A. S. (1991). The time course of phonological encoding in language production: phonological encoding inside a syllable. *Journal of Memory and Language, 30*, 69–89.

Nooteboom, S. G. (1980). Speaking and unspeaking: Detection and correction of phonological and lexical errors in spontaneous speech. In V. A. Fromkin (Ed.), *Errors in linguistic performance: Slips of the tongue, ear, pen, and hand*. New York: Academic Press.

Oomen, C., & Postma, A. (2002). Resource limitations and speech monitoring. *Language and Cognitive Processes, 17*, 163–84.

Postma, A. (2000). Detection of errors during speech production: A review of speech monitoring models, *Cognition, 77*, 97–131.

Postma, A., & Kolk, H. (1990). Speech errors, disfluencies, and self-repairs of stutterers in two accuracy conditions. *Journal of Fluency Disorders, 15*, 291–303.

Postma, A., & Kolk, H. (1992a). The effects of noise masking and required accuracy on speech errors, disfluencies and self-repairs. *Journal of Speech and Hearing Research, 35*, 537–44.

Postma, A., & Kolk, H. (1992b). Error monitoring in people who stutter. Evidence against auditory feedback defect theories. *Journal of Speech and Hearing Research, 35*, 1024–1032.

Postma, A., & Kolk, H. (1993). The covert repair hypothesis: Prearticulatory repair processes in normal and stuttered disfluencies. *Journal of Speech and Hearing Research, 36*, 472–87.

Postma, A., Kolk, H., & Povel, D. J. (1990). On the relation among speech errors, disfluencies, and self-repairs. *Language and Speech, 33*, 19–29.

Prins, D., Hubbard, C. P., & Krause, M. (1991). Syllabic stress and the occurrence of stuttering. *Journal of Speech and Hearing Research, 34*, 1011–1016.

Prins, D., Main, V., & Wampler, S. (1997). Lexicalization in adults who stutter. *Journal of Speech, Hearing and Language Research, 40*, 373–84.

Prosser, R., Rasbash, J., & Goldstein, H. (1995) *MLN software for multilevel analysis*. London: University of London, Institute of Education.

Roelofs, A. (2002). Storage and computation in spoken word production. In Nooteboom, S., Weerman, F., & Wijnen, F. (Eds.), *Storage and computation in the language faculty*. Dordrecht: Kluwer.

Schilperoord, J. (1996). *It's about time: Temporal aspects of cognitive processes in text production*. Doctoral dissertation Utrecht University.

Sherrard, C. A. (1975). Stuttering as false alarm responding. *British Journal of Disorders of Communication, 10*, 83–91.

St. Louis, K. (1991). The stuttering/articulation disorders connection. In Peters, H. F. M., Hulstijn, W., & Starkweather, C. W. (Eds.), *Speech motor control and stuttering*. Amsterdam: Elsevier/Excerpta Medica.

Swerts, M., Wichmann, A., & Beun, R.-J. (1996). *Filled pauses as markers of discourse structure*. Paper presented at the Fourth International Conferences on Spoken Language Processing. Philadelphia, PA, 3–6 October.

Thompson, A. H. (1985). A test of the distraction explanation of disfluency modification in stuttering. *Journal of Fluency Disorders, 10*, 35–50.

Wijnen, F. (1990). The development of sentence planning. *Journal of Child Language, 17*, 651–75.

Wijnen, F. (1994). Taalproduktie en ontwikkeling. *Toegepaste Taalwetenschap in Artikelen, 48*, 39–46.

Wijnen, F., & Boers, I. (1994). Phonological priming effects in stutterers. *Journal of Fluency Disorders, 19*, 1–20.

Wolk, L., Edwards, M. L., & Conture, E. (1993). Co-existence of stuttering and disordered phonology in young children. *Journal of Speech and Hearing Research, 36*, 906–917.

Yairi, F., & Lewis, B. (1984). Disfluencies at the onset of stuttering. *Journal of Speech and Hearing Research, 27*, 154–9.

Yaruss, J. S., & Conture, E. G. (1996). Stuttering and phonological disorders in children: Examination of the covert repair hypothesis. *Journal of Speech and Hearing Research, 39*, 349–64.

14 Magnitude estimation of disfluency by stutterers and nonstutterers

Melanie Russell, Martin Corley, and Robin J. Lickley

Abstract

Everyone produces disfluencies when they speak spontaneously. However, whereas most disfluencies pass unnoticed, the repetitions, blocks and prolongations produced by stutterers can have a severely disruptive effect on communication. The causes of stuttering have proven hard to pin down – researchers differ widely in their views on the cognitive mechanisms that underlie it. The present chapter presents initial research that supports a view (Vasic & Wijnen, this volume, chapter 13) that places the emphasis firmly on the self-monitoring system, suggesting that stuttering may be a consequence of oversensitivity to the types of minor speech error that we all make. Our study also allows us to ask whether the speech of people who stutter is perceived as qualitatively different from that of nonstutterers, when it is fluent and when it contains similar types of minor disfluencies. Our results suggest that for closely matched, naturally occurring segments of speech, listeners rate the speech of stutterers as more disfluent than that of nonstutterers.

Introduction

Research into stuttering often seems to fall at the first hurdle: That of defining what constitutes a stutter, in contrast to the disfluent speech that everyone produces. As of yet there is no consensus on a formal definition: Researchers such as Perkins (1995) emphasize the speaker's feelings of loss of control; others, such as Postma and Kolk (1993), prefer definitions in terms of the frequencies of particular *types* of disfluency. However, a consensus is slowly emerging that some of the symptoms associated with stuttering can be accounted for within a model of speech developed to account for normal hesitations, speech errors, and self-corrections (e.g., Levelt, 1983).

Self-monitoring in stuttering

Self-monitoring can be described as "the process of inspecting one's own speech and taking appropriate action when errors are made" (Hartsuiker & Kolk, 2001). Levelt's (1983, 1989) theory assumes that both overt speech and an internal speech plan are monitored. Postma (2000) summarizes a number of common speech errors and identifies evidence for two types of self-monitoring: Overt speech repairs (where speakers correct themselves mid-utterance) support the monitoring of external speech, whereas covert repairs (where there is no overt error, but a repair can be inferred from a hesitation in the speech output) supply evidence for the internal monitor. In fact, evidence suggests that the repair is often ready before the error is articulated (e.g., Blackmer & Mitton, 1991), and that errors can be made in the absence of articulatory activities or spoken output (for example, when imagining that one is articulating a tongue-twister: Dell & Repka, 1992). Thus the self-monitoring system would appear to have components which are distinct from the monitoring of motor systems (such as articulation) and from the auditory channel. Importantly, the speech that we produce has *already* been affected by self-monitoring; there is no external record of the original, possibly imperfect, speech plan.

Recent theorists have taken this view on board. For example, Postma and Kolk (1993) hypothesize that stuttering results from covert detection and correction of errors in the articulatory plan through the internal self-monitor. Covert self-correction would prevent the speech error from becoming overt, but would, as a side-effect, compromise the fluency of speech. Evidence for this Covert Repair Hypothesis is inconclusive (for details, see Hartsuiker, Kolk, & Lickley, this volume, Chapter 15; Vasiç & Wijnen, this volume, Chapter 13), but still supported by current studies (e.g., Melnicke, Conture, & Ohde, this volume, Chapter 6, who suggest that not only phonological encoding, but syntactic and semantic processes may be impaired in the formulation of speech by children who stutter).

Blackmer and Mitton (1991) also ascribe a role to monitoring. According to these authors, rapid subsyllabic repetitions, a key symptom of stuttering, occur when the monitor detects a lack of input, and consequently "restarts" previous articulatory movements.

More recently, Wijnen (2000; Vasiç & Wijnen, this volume, Chapter 13) has placed the emphasis entirely on the self-monitoring system, by proposing that stuttering is the direct result of an overvigilant monitor. Paradoxically, the repairs made often introduce disfluencies rather than prevent them: "Stutterers stutter because they try to avoid it" (Wijnen, 2000). Such a view can be easily extended to account for aspects of stuttering such as context dependency and linguistic distribution.

These proposals have in common the assumption that stuttering is related to self-monitoring; they also share, to a greater or lesser degree, the entailment that there is a continuity between stuttered and normal disfluencies (in contrast to, e.g., Perkins, 1995). Arguably, the most parsimonious view is that of Vasiç and Wijnen (this volume, Chapter 13); since there are no differences in planning processes (Postma & Kolk, 1993) or timings (Blackmer & Mitton, 1991) between stutterers and nonstutterers, all differences between the two groups must be attributed to the self-monitor. Given an appropriate experimental paradigm, we should be able to find direct evidence for the self-monitor's sensitivity in those who stutter. By a similar process of inference, we would expect there to be continuity between the speech of stutterers and nonstutterers: It is not errors in planned speech, but how many repairs are initiated, which differentiates the two groups.

Sensitivity of the self-monitor

According to Vasiç and Wijnen, there are three specific ways in which the speech monitor may be "oversensitive" to (potential) speech errors. First, too much cognitive effort may be invested in monitoring. Second, the focus (as distinct from effort) of the monitoring system may be rigid and unadaptive. Third, the threshold of the monitor may be too low: A "hypersensitivity" to minor speech distortions that nonstutterers would tolerate (or in other words regard as within the bounds of "normal" speech) increases the likelihood of stuttering. The first two assertions are addressed in Vasiç and Wijnen's chapter; in this chapter we focus on the third.

There are three basic proposals for the nature of the self-monitoring system. The first (Levelt, 1983, 1989) supposes that the mechanisms (at the conceptual, phonetic, and auditory levels) that understand language produced by others are shared with the self-monitoring system. The second (Laver, 1973, 1980) assumes multiple monitoring devices attuned specifically to production, including the potential to monitor the articulatory motor processes themselves. A third view (MacKay, 1987, 1992a, 1992b) suggests that error awareness arises from the prolonged activation of otherwise uncommitted nodes in the system for speech production. In an extensive review, Postma (2000) concludes that current evidence largely favours the view of Levelt (1983, 1989) in which the systems responsible for language perception and for self-monitoring are shared. If we accept this view, then people who stutter should show increased sensitivity to disfluencies in others', as well as their own, speech. In the simplest case, this sensitivity would be manifest whatever the provenance of the disfluent speech – i.e., whether it is uttered by a stutterer or a nonstutterer.

The current study addresses this issue by eliciting, from a group of stutterers and a comparison group of nonstutterers, ratings of the "severity of disfluency" of recorded speech fragments. The fragments are excerpted from recordings made of dialogues between pairs of stutterers, and between matched pairs of nonstutterers. This allows us simultaneously to address the second, continuity, assumption of many single-model accounts. Few studies have directly assessed the sensitivity of people who stutter to disfluency in the speech of others. Postma and Kolk (1992) come close, by comparing the abilities of people who stutter and fluent subjects to detect errors (rather than disfluencies) in sequences of CV and VC syllables produced by another speaker. Their finding was that people who stutter were less successful than controls in detecting errors under these conditions. In addition, they found that the two groups did not differ in their ability to detect their own errors in the production of CV and VC sequences. The results are taken as evidence that self-monitoring via auditory feedback is not impaired in people who stutter. In our study, we ask listeners to rate severity of disfluency, rather than error, in samples of spontaneous speech, rather than non-word strings.

Continuity between stuttered and normal disfluencies

To some researchers (e.g., Bloodstein, 1970), the difference between the clinical disorder of stuttering, and "normal" speech disfluency is simply a matter of degree. Stuttering is recognized by the frequency and severity of syllable-sound repetition. "There is no test for determining the precise point at which speech repetitions stop being 'normal' and become 'stuttering'. We cannot specify where the wall of an igloo ends and the roof begins. It is not a scientific question" (Bloodstein, 1970). In order to strengthen his argument, Bloodstein (1970) describes what he calls the "Consistency Effect": The distribution of disfluencies in the speech sequence is supposedly similar for stutterers and nonstutterers. Cross (n.d.) agrees that a categorical differentiation between stutterers and nonstutterers is both unnecessary and invalid, because the nature and degree of the problem vary from one individual to the next. He concludes that the issue is not whether the person is a stutterer or not, but whether the form or frequency of speech disruptions interferes with their ability to convey a message.

However, Perkins (1990) insists that a qualitative categorical distinction *does* exist between stutterers' and nonstutterers' speech. He suggests that there are two definitions of stuttering. The observer's viewpoint corresponds to the continuity hypothesis, whereas the stutterer's viewpoint corresponds to a categorical judgement. According to this perspective, speakers *know* when they stutter, but listeners can only *guess*. So, disfluency in nonstutterers is concerned with the motor control aspects of speech, whereas disfluency in stutterers seems to involve additional psychological aspects such as loss of control and feelings of helplessness.

In order to disentangle these views, the current study obtains ratings of fluent and disfluent speech fragments recorded from dialogues between stutterers and between nonstutterers. We should be able to ascertain whether there is a general distinction to be made between stutterers' and nonstutterers' speech, and (based on Levelt's, 1983, view of self-monitoring outlined earlier) whether stutterers perceive a discontinuity where others perceive a continuum.

The present study

The present pilot study investigates the phenomenon of stuttering *perceptually*, in contrast to previous work (e.g., Vasiç & Wijnen, this volume, Chapter 13) which has posited self-monitoring accounts of stutterers' speech *production*. In the experiment reported in this chapter, we asked judges who stuttered to rate the fluency or otherwise of short extracts from recordings made in naturalistic circumstances of dialogues between pairs of stuttering participants or pairs of nonstuttering controls. For each type of dialogue, half of the extracts were of fluent speech, and half were of mildly disfluent speech, where the onset of a word was repeated a single time. We would not expect either set of judges to rate extracts obtained from dialogues between stutterers as more disfluent *overall* than those obtained from nonstutterers' dialogues; we expect there to be little or no *qualitative* difference between the speech of the two groups. However, to test Vasic and Wijnen's hypothesis directly, the ratings given by our judges were compared with those from a second group of judges without stutters. If Vasic and Wijnen are correct, the judges who stutter should be more sensitive to disfluency. This sensitivity could manifest itself in one of two ways: If the judges who stutter detect and are sensitive to minor infelicities in the fluent speech extracts, we might expect them to rate these (as well as the disfluent samples) as worse. By the same token, an increased sensitivity to disfluency may make people who stutter likely to *differentiate more* between fluent and disfluent speech.

There are two justifications for the approach taken here: First, we avoid prejudging whether disfluent speech should be considered as "normal" or "stuttered", an absolute distinction which many researchers dispute; and, second, if we accept Levelt's view that the processes responsible for self-monitoring are also responsible for the processing of others' speech, we are in a position *directly* to compare the sensitivities of stutterers and nonstutterers to disfluencies in speech. The approach relies on using a rating system sensitive enough to capture small differences in listeners' perceptions of the fluency of recorded speech. We have chosen to use magnitude estimation, an approach used increasingly in linguistic studies where fine judgements are required, which we now outline.

Magnitude estimation

"Until stuttering can be identified qualitatively, we have no way of knowing what it is we have studied. Empirical evidence is needed to determine the best appropriate measures" (Perkins, 1995). The technique of magnitude estimation promises to be an extremely useful way of accessing fine judgements about the severity of disfluency in speech. This method was developed by psychophysicists to make the best use of participants' ability to make fine judgements about physical stimuli, and has since been used in a number of linguistic acceptability tasks (Bard, Robertson, & Sorace, 1996; Keller, 2000). Participants are instructed to assign any number to a given stimulus (the modulus), and rate the following stimuli proportionately. This can be compared to traditional "Likert scale" measures, where participants are asked to assign a number on a discrete scale (often 1–7). The disadvantage of such interval scaling is that there is no way of knowing in advance if people's sensitivities to the data provided are limited to a seven-way distinction any more than to a four-way one (Bard et al., 1996). In contrast, in magnitude estimation, raters' responses are unconstrained; categorical judgements can be revealed rather than imposed. This method has been demonstrated to result in robust but fine distinctions. In previous research on stuttering, it has been argued that magnitude estimation has greater construct validity than other methods (Schiavetti, Sacco, Metz, & Sitler., 1983). Experience with internet studies using magnitude estimation (e.g., Keller & Alexopolou, 2001) demonstrates that it can be used consistently by untrained readers and listeners.

Method

Speech corpora

All stimuli used in the experiment were unedited samples of spontaneous speech taken from task-oriented dialogues. The HCRC Map Task Corpus (Anderson et al., 1991) was used as a model. In the map task, both speakers have a similar map and one speaker (instruction giver) has a route marked on their map, which they have to describe to the other (follower). Discrepancies between the two maps provide occasions for discussion and negotiation. The HCRC Map Task Corpus has proven to be a rich source of disfluent speech in nonstutterers, both as instruction giver and as follower (Branigan, Lickley, & McKelvie, 1999; Lickley, 2001).

To provide natural samples of speech by stutterers, two dialogues involving two pairs of speakers who stutter were recorded. The stuttering speakers were recruited with the help of a local speech and language therapist and a self-help group in Edinburgh. Recordings took place in a quiet studio, with speakers sitting at tables facing each other about five metres apart, their maps raised on easels at an angle so that neither participant's map was visible to the other. Speakers were fitted with clip-on microphones and recorded onto separate channels on digital audio tape and SVHS videotapes.

Nonstuttering control stimuli came from two sources. The first source was the speech of two speakers from the HCRC corpus itself, which involved speakers with Scottish accents and was recorded in very similar conditions to the new corpus. These two speakers provided matches for the stimuli produced by the two Scottish stuttering speakers. Since the other two stuttering speakers were not Scottish speakers, nonstuttering speakers with very similar accents were recruited to record another dialogue, so as to counter any biasing effects of regional accent in the experiment.

The HCRC Map Task Corpus has full transcriptions and disfluency annotation time aligned with the digitalized speech signal. The new dialogues were transcribed and annotated for disfluency using signal processing software on Unix workstations. Disfluency annotation was performed with reference to the HCRC disfluency coding manual (Lickley, 1998), which was adapted to include disfluencies associated with stuttering (multiple repetitions, prolongations and blocks). The same software was used to excise the experimental stimuli from the dialogues into separate files.

Stimulus selection

For the purposes of the current study, we attempted to match the stimuli produced by stutterers with similar stimuli produced by nonstutterers. This strategy meant that the type of disfluency we could use in stimuli was restricted to a small subset of the types of disfluency that are produced by people who stutter: Single repetitions of part words, rather than multiple repetitions. While they are a common characteristic of the speech of people who stutter, multiple repetitions are somewhat rare in the speech of non-stutterers. In the HCRC Map Task Corpus (described in Anderson et al., 1991), we find nearly 2000 disfluent repetitions, only 161 of which consist of more than one repetition and only 19 of more than two. Of these, only one is a part-word repetition, consisting of progressively shorter repetitions of the onset of a three syllable word (undernea- under- und- un- no underneath).

Perceptual studies on nonstuttered speech using nonstuttering listeners suggest that minor disfluencies such as single part-word repetitions are harder to detect and more often missed altogether by listeners than other types of disfluencies (Bard & Lickley, 1998): Nonstutterers, at least, appear to find such disfluencies unobtrusive.

Restricting the stimuli in our study to this type of disfluency has a bearing on our interpretation of the results. If stutterers are more sensitive even to such minor disruptions than are nonstutterers, this will serve to emphasize their oversensitivity and support the notion that their acceptability threshold for errors is significantly higher. In addition, if we find that listeners judge these minor disfluencies differently for stutterers and nonstutterers, we will have evidence that contradicts the continuity hypothesis, suggesting that there is a qualitative difference even between the "normal" disfluencies for the two sets of speakers.

Materials

A total of 64 stimuli were selected from the corpora described so as to include sets of 32 disfluent and 32 fluent stimuli. Half of these came from the four stuttering speakers and the other half from four nonstutterers. All the disfluent stimuli contained single repetitions of word onsets. Each stimulus produced by a stutterer was matched as closely as possible with a stimulus from a nonstutterer with the same regional accent. Disfluent stimuli were matched for phonetic content of the repeated segment wherever possible (e.g., *that s-section* was matched with *going s-straight up*). Fluent stimuli were matched for their lexical and syntactic content, as far as possible (e.g., *then you go up* was matched with *then you go straight up*). However, finding precisely matched controls from a small corpus of spontaneous speech is virtually impossible. Where such a precise match was not possible, the most liberal criterion used was that speech segments should be of equivalent length. No patterns likely to bias experimental outcomes could be detected in the less precisely matched stimuli.

One stimulus, a disfluent item produced by a nonstutterer, was selected as modulus, and headed each of three blocks of 21 other stimuli. Apart from this stimulus, the items were presented in different random orders for each subject.

Subjects

Subjects in the listening experiment consisted of 16 nonstutterers (9 female, 7 male) and 6 stutterers (1 female, 5 male), with an age range of 20–45. None reported having hearing deficits. None had previous experience of the task of giving fluency judgments.

Procedure

The experiment was carried out using Psyscope (Cohen, MacWhinney, Flatt, & Provost, 1993) on an Apple Macintosh computer. Stimuli were played over headphones to subjects seated in sound-proofed listening booths.

Instructions were presented on the computer screen in several short sections. Subjects were told that their task was to give a numerical response that matched their perception of the severity of speech disfluency for each segment of speech that they heard. They were asked to rate *more disfluent* segments with *higher* numbers and *less disfluent* segments with *lower* numbers and to relate their judgments to their score for the modulus segment. They were encouraged not to base their ratings on anything other than fluency (e.g., speaker accent, grammaticality) and to respond as quickly as possible. Subjects responded by typing their responses on a computer keyboard. The presentation of stimuli was self-paced: A new stimulus was played when the subject hit the "return" key on the keyboard.

The experiment was preceded by a practice session to familiarize the subjects with the magnitude estimation task. The practice session consisted of judgments of tone duration, rather than line length, which is the measure usually used in magnitude estimation, in order to maintain the auditory aspect of the experiment.

Following the practice session, subjects performed the experiment without interruption, typically completing the task in about 15 minutes. Responses, consisting of typed numbers corresponding to the three repetitions of the modulus, together with 63 other comparative ratings, were recorded in data files generated by Psyscope.

Results

Each participant's ratings were divided by the value they had given to the modulus stimulus, to make the scores comparable. Since the ratings were ratios (how much more or less fluent than the modulus) they were then log-transformed. A transformed rating of zero thus indicated that the participant had judged a stimulus to be equivalently fluent to the modulus; scores greater than zero indicated increased disfluency, and scores less than zero indicated that the stimulus had been rated as relatively fluent.

The analysis of the transformed scores was, however, made more difficult by a design flaw in the study. Participants rated each modulus three times, but no attention was drawn by the experimenters to the fact that the two repetitions should be given the initial modulus rating. This lack of "anchoring" resulted in an appreciable drift in participants' scoring throughout the experiment; of 22 participants in total, only five gave the modulus item the same score on all three occasions. In other words, the results from 17 participants introduced additional, non-systematic, error variance into the study (and because the modulus ratings did not appear to change in predictable ways, there is no obvious way to compensate for this). The analysis by participants reflects these problems, and will not be reported here. However, because the experimental stimuli were randomized, each stimulus had an equal chance of occurring early in the experiment (before the onset of drift). This means that the error variance due to drift should be approximately equally partitioned across items, and a by-items analysis can be used to give a clearer picture of the outcome of the experiment.[1]

The analysis reported here included the (matched) stimuli as a random factor, and explored the effects of rater (with or without stutter), speaker (with or without stutter), and type of utterance (fluent or disfluent) as within-item factors. All means reported are of log-transformed adjusted ratings.

Only two of the variables had independent effects: Unsurprisingly, disfluent utterances were judged to be more disfluent than fluent utterances (0.10 vs -0.57; $F(1,15) = 153.17$, $p <. 001$); and speakers with stutters were rated slightly less fluent overall (0.13 vs -0.34; $F(1,15) = 7.29$, $p = 0.003$). There was no independent effect of rater (that is, raters appeared to use similar ranges of scores, whether or not they had stutters themselves). Interestingly, there was no interaction between speaker and utterance type, suggesting that disfluent or fluent utterances from speakers with stutters were perceived equivalently to similar utterances from nonstuttering speakers; the interaction between speaker and rater, and the three-way interaction, also failed to reach significance.

However, the interaction between rater and utterance type did reach significance ($F(1,15) = 23.41$, $p < 0.001$). As can be seen from Figure 14.1, this reflects the fact that raters with stutters differentiated more between disfluent and fluent utterances than did raters without stutters, suggesting

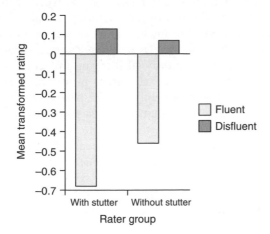

Figure 14.1 Mean transformed ratings of fluent and disfluent utterances by raters with and without stutters.

that people with stutters discriminate more sensitively between fluent and disfluent speech. We return to this point in the discussion.

Discussion

It is widely agreed that despite the inclusiveness of the label, people who are described as, or describe themselves as, stutterers often display very different symptoms and coping strategies. In this context, results from a small-scale study such as that reported here need to be treated with caution: It is too early to make any claims about a single cause of stuttering. However, taken together with the studies reported by Vasic and Wijnen, the findings from the present study converge to implicate the self-monitor in stuttering. In a direct test of sensitivity to disfluency, stutterers were found to differentiate more between disfluent and fluent speech than nonstutterers, regardless of whether that speech had been originally uttered by someone considered to have a stutter or someone who was a nonstutterer. This evidence is consistent with one interpretation of Vasic and Wijnen's hypothesis. It would be premature however to conclude that people who stutter do not rate *fluent* speech as worse; given the small numbers of participants, comparisons of *absolute* ratings between groups must be treated with caution. However, the evidence clearly indicates a difference in *relative* ratings, consistent with either version of the hypothesis; further, we can assume that since participants were explicitly instructed to rate the recordings for fluency, the focus and cognitive effort devoted to the task were maximized, and have little role to play in the outcome.

In contrast, it is important to note that the continuity hypothesis was not directly supported: Excerpts from dialogues between stuttering participants were rated as worse than those from nonstutterers, regardless of whether they were fluent or not, and regardless of who was doing the rating. In fact, there is evidence that both the disfluent and the fluent speech of stutterers may involve abnormal motor activity, both in laryngeal dynamics (e.g., Adams, Freeman, & Conture, 1985) and in the supralaryngeal organs (Wood, 1995). Using electropalatography, Wood found that stutterers produced greater degrees of lingual-palatal contact while producing alveolar plosives in fluent speech than did nonstutterers. It seems likely that such indications of muscular tension in the speech production apparatus (for example "hard contacts" in Van Riper's, 1982, terms) may be perceptible to listeners. If they were present in our experimental materials, subjects may have reflected this in their fluency judgements. In itself, this supposition does not contradict a self-monitor-based explanation of stuttering: Sensitivity to the likelihood of stuttering, and a hypersensitivity to potential repairs, may be reflected in motor activity.

The study reported here is also limited in that it only addresses onset repetitions: One of several symptoms associated with stuttering. One reason for investigating repetitions first is because the silent interval can be measured objectively, and can therefore be used as a reliable measure of stuttering for clinicians (stutterers tend to have a shorter silent interval). Although Wijnen (2000) argues that the Vicious Circle Hypothesis also applies to other symptoms such as prolongations and blocks, further research is needed before we are able to rule out counterexplanations of these manifestations. Another limitation is the number of subjects in this study: We are addressing this in a larger study currently nearing completion.

In contrast to the more "objective" view presented here, Perkins (1995) claims that it is the speaker's feelings of loss of control over their speech that truly defines stuttering, rather than particular types or frequencies of disfluency. He argues that taking averages of averages and trying to obtain a quantitative description of an essentially qualitative issue loses most of the sensitivity and original quality of the data. The issue of subjectivity is of crucial importance in this area of research – to what extent can the diverse speech behaviour of stutterers be quantified in controlled experiments? We would contend that using a sufficiently sensitive task such as magnitude estimation avoids some of the pitfalls that Perkins envisages, and allows us to make important insights into the nature of stuttering. This approach has little to say about the pathology of stuttering (as yet, there is no account of what *causes* hypersensitivity in the self-monitor), but much to say about its manifestation, and by implication, about some possible therapeutic approaches. In particular, the findings reported here and in Vasiç and Wijnen's earlier chapter suggest that stuttering may be ameliorated by encouraging clients to tolerate, rather than attempt to avoid, the speech errors that all speakers are prone to make.

Author note: The order of the second and third authors is arbitrary. Correspondence concerning this chapter should be addressed to either Martin Corley or Robin Lickley.

Note

1 Note that we can consider the stimuli used in this experiment to be a subset of the infinite population of comparable disfluencies. Thus a by-items analysis does not fall subject to the criticism of Raaijmakers, Schrijnemakers and Gremmen (1999).

References

Adams, F. R., Freeman, F. J., & Conture, E. G., (1985). Laryngeal dynamics of stutterers. In R. F. Curlee, & W. H. Perkins, (Eds.), *Nature and treatment of stuttering: New directions*. San Diego, CA: College-Hill Press.

Anderson, A. H., Bader, M., Bard, E. G., Boyle, E., Doherty, G., Garrod, S., Isard, S., Kowtko, J., McAllister, J., Miller, J., Sotillo, C., Thompson, H., & Weinert, R. (1991). The HCRC Map Task Corpus. *Language and Speech, 34*, 351–66.

Bard, E. G., & Lickley, R. J. (1998). Graceful failure in the recognition of running speech. *Proceedings of the 20th Annual Meeting of the Cognitive Science Society*. University of Wisconsin-Madison, USA, 108–13.

Bard, E. G., Robertson, D., & Sorace, A. (1996). Magnitude estimation of linguistic acceptability. *Language, 72*, 32–68.

Blackmer, E. R., & Mitton, J. L. (1991). Theories of monitoring and the timing of repairs in spontaneous speech. *Cognition, 39*, 173–94.

Bloodstein, O. (1970). Stuttering and normal nonfluency: A continuity hypothesis. *British Journal of Disorders of Communication*, 30–9.

Branigan, H., Lickley, R. J., & McKelvie, D. (1999). Non-linguistic influences on rates of disfluency in spontaneous speech. *Proceedings of the ICPhS, International Congress on Phonetic Sciences* (pp 387–90). San Francisco.

Cohen, J. D., MacWhinney, B., Flatt, M., & Provost, J. (1993). Psyscope: A new graphic interactive environment for designing psychology experiments. *Behavioral Research Methods, Instruments, and Computers, 25*, 257–71.

Cross, D. E. (n.d.) *A systems approach to stuttering*. Retrieved 30 October 2002, from http://www.ithaca.edu/cross/SPECIALIZATIONS/STUTTERING/Stuthome.html

Dell, G. S., & Repka, R. J. (1992). Errors in inner speech. In B. J. Baars (Ed.), *Experimental slips and human error: Exploring the architecture of volition*. New York: Plenum Press.

Hartsuiker, R. J., & Kolk, H. H. J. (2001). Error monitoring in speech production: A computational test of the perceptual loop theory. *Cognitive Psychology, 42*, 113–57.

Keller, F. (2000). *Gradience in grammar: Experimental and computational aspects of degrees of grammaticality*. Unpublished doctoral dissertation, University of Edinburgh.

Keller, F., & Alexopoulou, T. (2001). Phonology competes with syntax: Experimental evidence for the interaction of word order and accent placement in the realization of information structure. *Cognition, 79*, 301–72.

Laver, J. D. M. (1973). The detection and correction of slips of tongue. In V. A. Fromkin (Ed.), *Speech errors as linguistic evidence*. The Hague: Mouton.

Laver, J. D. M. (1980). Monitoring systems in the neurolinguistic control of speech production. In V. A. Fromkin (Ed.), *Errors in linguistic performance: Slips of the tongue, ear, pen, and hand*. New York: Academic Press.

Levelt, W. J. M. (1983). Monitoring and self-repair in speech. *Cognition*, *14*, 41–104.

Levelt, W. J. M. (1989). *Speaking: From intention to articulation*. Cambridge, MA: MIT Press.

Lickley, R. J. (1998). *HCRC disfluency coding manual*. HCRC Technical Report. HCRC/TR-100, Human Communication Research Centre, University of Edinburgh.

Lickley, R. J. (2001). Dialogue moves and disfluency rates. In *Proceedings of DiSS '01: Disfluency in spontaneous speech*, ISCA Tutorial and Research Workshop, University of Edinburgh, 93–96.

MacKay, D. G. (1987). *The organization of perception and action: A theory for language and other cognitive skills*. New York: Springer Verlag.

MacKay, D. G. (1992a). Awareness and error detection: New theories and research paradigms. *Consciousness and Cognition*, *1*, 199–225.

MacKay, D. G. (1992b). Errors, ambiguity, and awareness in language perception and production. In B. J. Baars (Ed.), *Experimental slips and human error: Exploring the architecture of volition*. New York: Plenum Press.

Perkins, W. H. (1990). What is stuttering? *Journal of Speech and Hearing Disorders*, *55*, 370–82.

Perkins, W. H. (1995). *Stuttering and science*. San Diego, CA: Singular Publishing Group.

Postma, A. (2000). Detection of errors during speech production: A review of speech monitoring models. *Cognition*, *77*, 97–131.

Postma, A., & Kolk, H. H. J. (1992). Error monitoring in people who stutter: Evidence against auditory feedback defect theories. *Journal of Speech and Hearing Research*, *35*, 1024–1032.

Postma, A., & Kolk, H. (1993). The covert repair hypothesis: Prearticulatory repair processes in normal and stuttered disfluencies. *Journal of Speech and Hearing Research*, *36*, 472–87.

Raaijmakers, J. G. W., Schrijnemakers, J. M. C., & Gremmen, F. (1999). How to deal with "The language-as-fixed-effect fallacy": Common misconceptions and alternative solutions. *Journal of Memory and Language*, *41*, 416–26.

Schiavetti, N., Sacco, P. R., Metz, D. E., & Sitler, R. W. (1983). Direct magnitude estimation and interval scaling of stuttering severity. *Journal of Speech and Hearing Research*, *26*, 568–73.

Van Riper, C. (1982). *The nature of stuttering*. Englewood Cliffs, NJ: Prentice-Hall.

Wijnen, F. (2000). Stotteren als resultaat van inadequate spraakmonitoring [Stuttering as the result of inadequate speech monitoring]. *Stem-, Spraak- en Taalpathologie*, *9*.

Wood, S. (1995). An electropalatographic analysis of stutterers' speech. *European Journal of Disorders of Communication*, *30*, 226–36.

15 Stuttering on function words and content words: A computational test of the covert repair hypothesis

Robert J. Hartsuiker, Herman H. J. Kolk, and Robin J. Lickley

Abstract

The covert repair hypothesis (CRH) of stuttering (Postma & Kolk, 1993) considers disfluencies to be the result of covert self-monitoring and self-repair of speech errors. In this chapter, we consider how well this hypothesis accounts for an interaction between lexical type and position in a phonological unit on stuttering frequency (Au-Yeung, Howell, & Pilgrim, 1998). We show that the CRH predicts this interaction when it is supplemented with a formal model of the time-course of self-monitoring, which relates observed symptoms to the moments in time when errors in speech plans are intercepted and repaired.

Introduction

There is increasing attention for the hypothesis that the disfluencies typically occurring in stuttering (e.g., blocks, prolongations, hesitations, (part-) word repetitions, and self-corrections) are related to self-monitoring processes, the processes with which speakers inspect the quality of their own speech. In a nutshell, this hypothesis entails that people who stutter detect many planning problems in their internal speech. Disfluencies are the result of reactions to these problems, for example attempts to self-correct an internal error.

There are a number of variations of this hypothesis, differing in two respects. First, what kinds of problem would the monitor detect?[1] According to Kolk and Postma (1997) the monitor detects errors in an internal representation (i.e., a phonological code), but according to Clark and Wasow (1998) the monitor detects upcoming delays in planning. Howell, Au-Yeung, and Sackin (1999) postulate a low-level detection device, which is sensitive to asynchronies between planning and execution. Second, given that the monitor detects a problem, why would a disfluency ensue? On Kolk and Postma's account, it results from self-correction of phonological speech errors. Clark and Wasow (1998) view it as a strategy to signal the occurrence of delays in planning. Howell et al. (1999) extended this hypothesis: Some disfluencies result from a stalling tactic, whereas others occur when the stalling tactic is not used and an incomplete speech plan is executed.

In this chapter, we will evaluate one monitoring theory of stuttering in some detail: Postma and Kolk's (1993; Kolk & Postma, 1997) "covert repair hypothesis" (CRH). We will put this theory to the test by formalizing it and assessing whether it is consistent with empirically observed data. This theory considers disfluencies to be a reaction to internal speech errors, both in people who stutter and in people who do not. Kolk and Postma (1997) proposed that phonological encoding in stuttering is excessively error prone, as a result of disturbed timing of this process. If phonological units are selected too fast, there will be relatively many speech errors. Indeed, formal models of phonological encoding (Dell, 1986; see also Dell & Kim, this volume, Chapter 2) predict that phonological substitution errors are more frequent with decreased time for selection. These predictions were confirmed in experiments that manipulated speech rate (Dell, 1986; see also Oomen & Postma, 2001b). Thus, the CRH assumes that problems in the timing of phonological encoding result in many errors in a representation of internal speech. The self-monitoring system will often detect these errors before they are articulated. On error detection, the monitor interrupts speech and repairs errors. These "covert repairs" disrupt the fluent delivery of speech, resulting in incidents we perceive as disfluencies.

Postma and Kolk (1993) also proposed an account for the *types* of disfluency one observes, in particular for disfluencies at the level of the syllable. They assumed that disfluencies are a function of how much of the syllable is realized before the moment of interruption. This proposal is illustrated in Table 15.1, adapted from Postma and Kolk (1993).

Suppose a speaker intends to produce the syllable "SIP", but there is an error of phoneme selection, yielding a phonological code for "SIT". Table 15.1 relates the extent to which the error SIT is realized before interruption to the types of disfluency. If the interruption takes place before the syllable

Table 15.1 Covert repairing in intra-syllabic interruptions: The relation between how far a syllable is planned or executed and the type of resulting disfluency (adapted from Postma & Kolk, 1993)

Erroneous plan: SIT executed plan	*Intended syllable: SIP observed (intrasyllabic) disfluency*
(No audible sound)	##..SIP (block)
S	SSSSIP (prolongation)
S	S..S..SIP (repetition)
SI	SI..SIP (repetition)
SI	SIIIIP (drawl)
SI	SI#P (broken word)
SIT	SIT. . .SIT (repetition)
SIT	SIT. . .SIP (error + overt repair)

onset it results in a block. If interruption occurs right after the first phoneme there will be a prolongation or consonantal repetition (S.S.SIP or SSSSIP). Interruption after the vowel leads to a part-syllable repetition (SI-SIP) or a broken word (SI #P). If the interruption occurs later, there will be a syllable repetition (SIT SIT) or an overt repair (SIT SIP).

What is the evidence for the CRH? Before turning to the model, we will briefly review two lines of research. The first of these considers manipulations aimed at directly affecting the self-monitor. According to Levelt (1989) self-monitoring requires attention. Thus, manipulations affecting the availability of attentional resources will affect the performance of the monitor. Arends, Povel, and Kolk (1988) exploited this putative property of the monitoring system. Participants who stutter produced speech in conditions with or without a simultaneous (visuo-motor) secondary task. If the secondary task takes away attention for monitoring, one would expect fewer disfluencies in that condition. This counterintuitive prediction was confirmed, at least for the speakers who stuttered most severely. Secondary task effects on stuttering rates were also observed by Vasiç and Wijnen (this volume, Chapter 13).

Contrariwise, Bosshardt (2001) found no effects of a "semantic or phonological judgement" secondary task on stuttering rate. Similarly, Oomen and Postma (2002), testing people who do not stutter, observed that the proportion of disfluencies per correct word was not affected by the presence of a "random number tapping" secondary task. Consistent with the CRH, however, the number of phonological errors increased in the presence of a double task. Finally, Oomen and Postma (2001a) observed *more* disfluencies in the presence of a secondary task, again testing speakers who do not stutter. This is in contrast with the predictions from the CRH. Thus, the empirical support from this line of research is inconclusive.

The second line of research considers the relationship between phonological encoding and disfluency (see also Melnick, Ohde, & Conture, this volume, Chapter 6). The CRH predicts that disfluencies occur most frequently on phonologically complex words (e.g., words containing a string of consonants, or late-acquired consonants), assuming that these words are more likely to lead to internal speech errors. Howell and Au-Yeung (1995) found no effect of these variables when controlling for the phonological factors suggested by Brown (1945) (such as word class, word length, and whether the word began with a consonant or vowel). Subsequent work, however, revealed that phonological complexity did influence stuttering rate, depending on the locus in the word of the complex consonants (Howell, Au-Yeung, & Sackin, 2000).

Other studies considered the co-occurrence of phonological problems and disfluencies. If phonological encoding problems really underlie disfluency, one might expect such a co-occurrence. Yaruss and Conture (1996) tested children who stutter and divided them into groups with normal phonological abilities and disordered phonological abilities. They concluded that speech errors and disfluencies co-occur for incidental speech errors ("slips of the tongue"), but not for systematic speech errors ("phonological processes"). Wolk, Blomgren, and Smith (2000), however, focussing on the level of the syllable rather than the utterance, observed that disfluencies occurred equally often in syllables with and without phonological errors. The only exception constituted syllables with word-initial consonant clusters. In these syllables, there were more disfluencies if the syllable contained a phonological error.

Wijnen and Boers (1994) used a psycholinguistic paradigm to test for phonological planning deficits in people who stutter and people who do not. In this task (Meyer, 1990; Roelofs & Meyer, 1998), participants first learn to associate word pairs. In the test phase, the first word of a pair serves as a cue for the production of the second word (the "target word"), and these words are produced in sets of five words. Meyer and colleagues showed that if all target words in a set begin with the same consonant, or consonant and vowel, there is a reduction in word production latencies.

Wijnen and Boers (1994) observed that control speakers had shorter naming latencies if the target words appeared in a set where each word began with the same consonant. There was a larger effect when both consonant and vowel were shared. For stuttering participants, however, an effect occurred only when both the consonant and vowel were shared. This suggests a phonological planning deficit, possibly related to the retrieval of the vowel. However, Burger and Wijnen (1999) did show a priming effect for people who stutter when only the consonant was shared. They also concluded that the data pattern observed by Wijnen and Boers was representative for only a subset of participants.

To summarize, both the evidence for the role of the self-monitor in stuttering, and for the hypothesis that phonological problems underlie disfluency is inconclusive. Why is it so difficult to find support for the CRH? We think there are problems with each of the approaches commonly taken. The CRH is based on the interaction of two "hidden" processes: Speech planning and self-monitoring. Since the net result of successful monitoring is to remove an internal error, we cannot establish whether an internal error really underlies a given disfluency. Therefore, the studies using secondary task paradigms aimed at isolating the monitoring component. All things being equal, a decrease in the quality of monitoring should lower the rates of disfluencies. But are all things equal? The logic collapses if attentional manipulations affect speech planning processes as well as the quality of monitoring. Notice that there is empirical evidence (e.g., Fayol, Largy, & Lemaire, 1994; Hartsuiker & Barkhuysen, 2001; Jou & Harris, 1992; Oomen & Postma, 2002) that speech errors occur more frequently under secondary task conditions. But if the secondary task both *increases* the number of internal speech errors and *decreases* the proportion of those errors that are covertly repaired, then the covert repair hypothesis does not make any clear predictions about the proportion of disfluencies: There could be more, fewer, or equal numbers of speech errors in the secondary task condition, depending on which component is affected the most.

There is an analogous problem with the approach that tests for co-occurrence of phonological problems and stuttering, as pointed out by Wolk et al. (2000). If the monitor detects phonological errors before they are produced, then the net effect of covert repair is to remove these phonological errors. Because of this trade-off, co-occurrence of disfluency and phonological errors is not necessarily predicted.

There is a different problem with the studies by Burger and Wijnen (1999) and Wijnen and Boers (1994) who tested for phonological encoding deficits in people who stutter. This approach avoids the trade-off problem, as it only considered fluent speech (thus, speech that was accepted by the monitor). However, it is unclear whether their priming task taps into the component that is hypothesized to be deficient. In the model of word form encoding proposed by Levelt, Roelofs, and Meyer (1999), the benefits of priming take place during a process in which selected phonological segments are attached to a metrical frame for the word. But this is not the process that Kolk and Postma (1997) assumed to be deficient. According to them, the phonological encoding problem in stuttering lies in the *selection* of phonemes, a process preceding the attachment to the lexical frame. Thus, implicit priming may not be the most appropriate tool to test the covert repair hypothesis.

In this chapter, we will propose a different approach for evaluating the CRH. Our approach comprises the testing of predictions from a formal model of self-monitoring (Hartsuiker & Kolk, 2001). This model aimed to precisely account for the time-course of self-monitoring. In the CRH, the occurrence of a disfluency depends on the time-course of error detection and self-repair relative to the onset of speech. Therefore, our model allows us to make predictions about the likelihood that an error in the speech plan leads to a disfluency or not, and if so, what kind of disfluency it is most likely to be.

We will apply this model to data on disfluency rates for different types of word and for different positions in the utterance. We used data reported by Au-Yeung et al. (1998) and by Howell et al. (1999). We will show that the CRH can account for their data pattern, given two plausible assumptions. The first assumption concerns the time course of speech planning for words of different types. We assume that the production of *function* words is less time consuming than the production of *content* words (see later). Au-Yeung et al. (1998) share this assumption with us. The second assumption concerns the situation in which an error is detected long before articulation. We assume that in such cases, the error can be edited out of the speech signal without leaving any auditory trace. This assumption is supported by empirical findings (Motley, Camden, & Baars, 1982; Timmermans, Schriefers, & Dijkstra, submitted).

An interaction between lexical type and position in phonological word on disfluency

Let us first consider the 1998 findings of Au-Yeung et al. These authors analyzed the frequency of stuttering on words of different lexical classes and at different positions in the utterance. As disfluencies, they counted word repetitions, part-word repetitions, and prolongations of segments and syllables. Speech was collected from people who stutter in several age groups, ranging from very young children to adults.

Two types of lexical class were considered: *Function* words, which are important for the syntax, but bear little or no intrinsic meaning (e.g., pronouns and determiners) and *content* words, which do bear intrinsic meaning (e.g., nouns, verbs, and adjectives). This distinction is important in linguistics for several reasons; for example, function words have different phonological and syntactic properties from content words. The lexical class distinction also plays an important role in theories of sentence production (e.g., Garrett, 1982) and aphasiology (e.g., Bradley, Garrett, & Zurif, 1980). It is interesting to note that there are age differences with respect to stuttering on function and content words: Whereas adults are more likely to stutter on content words (Brown, 1945), young children who stutter are more likely to be disfluent on function words (Bloodstein & Grossman, 1981). Howell et al. (1999) showed a developmental trend towards content-word stuttering in a single experiment.

Important for our present purposes, Au-Yeung et al. (1998) also showed that the position of function and content words in a larger prosodic unit affects the probability of disfluencies. They divided utterances into "phonological words", which consist of a content word and zero or more preceding and consecutive function words (Selkirk, 1984). Parsing of utterances into phonological words is based on semantic coherence. For example, in "the plane flew away to Brussels", the particle "away" would be clustered with the verb "flew", but the preposition "to" would be clustered with the proper name "Brussels". There were more disfluencies on function words in *initial* positions of the phonological word than on function words in *later* positions. In particular, there were many disfluencies on function words preceding content words, but hardly any disfluencies on function words following content words (see also Howell et al., 1999). There was no effect of position on the number of disfluencies affecting content words.

Au-Yeung et al. (1998) interpreted their findings as follows. A function-word disfluency is a stalling tactic to compensate for the unavailability of the plan for the upcoming content words. But disfluencies on content words are due to word-intrinsic factors, such as phonological complexity. They occur when the stalling tactic is not used, and the speaker attempts to execute an incomplete plan (see Howell & Sackin, 2000, for a more elaborate version of this proposal).

Like the CRH, this account postulates that disfluencies are an interaction between problems in speech planning and reactions to these problems. But unlike the CRH, it assumes two different reactions, leading to two different surface forms of disfluency: A stalling tactic is either invoked or ignored. A more parsimonious account would postulate only a single reaction. We will present an alternative explanation that assumes that disfluencies are a result of only one reaction: Covert self-repair.

Modeling the lexical type by position interaction

Au-Yeung et al. (1998) reported (1) an effect of the position within the phonological word on function word disfluencies, but not on content word disfluencies; (2) an enhanced position effect on function word disfluencies when a content word intervenes between two function words. The aim of our simulations is to test whether the position effects reported by Au-Yeung et al. follow from the Hartsuiker and Kolk (2001) model. The comparison of interest is that between different positions in the phonological word for each lexical type; it is *not* a purpose of the simulation to account for differences in overall number of disfluencies between different lexical types. In this section, we will use Hartsuiker and Kolk's (2001) model of self-monitoring to predict the moment of self-interruption relative to the onset of speech. These moments of interruption are mapped onto types of symptoms, using a set of rules similar to those in Table 15.1.

Model architecture

The architecture of the model is illustrated in Figure 15.1.

The model is a formalization and elaboration of Levelt's (1983, 1989) perceptual loop theory. It divides the task of language production into three main components: The conceptualizer, which produces a pre-verbal message; the formulator, which retrieves lexical items, builds sentence structure, and determines phonological form; and the articulator, which controls speech motor processes. Following Levelt (1989) and Sternberg, Knoll, Monsell, and Wright (1988), the articulator consists of a stage of selection (retrieving motor programs) and a stage of command (executing these motor programs). Actual speech begins when the stage of command commences.

The right-hand side of Figure 15.1 shows the processes involved in language comprehension. First, there is an auditory processing component, which constructs a phonetic representation. This representation is used by the "speech comprehension" component for word recognition, integrating the lexical representations into a sentence, and inferring the thematic roles ("who did what to whom"). Finally, the output of the language comprehension system ("parsed speech" in Levelt's terminology) is fed back into the conceptualizer.

Self-monitoring proceeds through two, largely overlapping, channels. The *external* monitoring channel consists of the perception of one's own overt

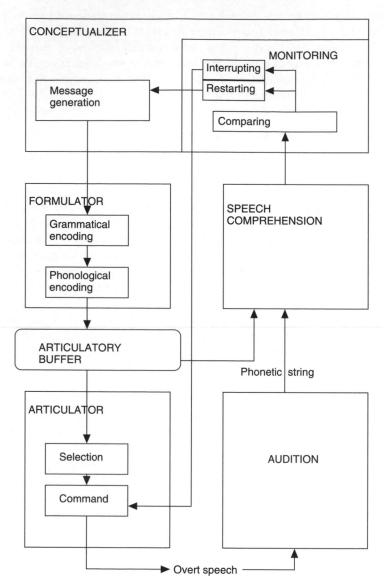

Figure 15.1 An overview of the organization of speech production and perception
stages in Hartsuiker and Kolk's (2001) computational model.

speech using the auditory processing component. The *internal* monitoring
channel consists of the phonetic plan (the output of the formulator), which
directly feeds into the language comprehension system. This is the place
where the two channels converge. The output of each of these channels feeds
in a monitoring component located in the conceptualizer. There are three

processes for which this component is responsible. First, there is a *comparison* of the intended representation with the actual representation. If there is a discrepancy between these representations, interrupting and restarting come into play. The existence of self-repairs that follow the interruption without delay (Blackmer & Mitton, 1991; Oomen & Postma, 2001b) have led us to the assumption that interruption and repair are executed in parallel. We estimate the time from error detection to the actual moment of interruption to be 200 ms (see Logan & Cowan, 1984). The speaker uses this time to initiate the repair.

The model calculates error-to-interruption and interruption-to-repair times by adding estimates (taken from the literature) for the duration of each process involved in speech production and perception. This computation takes into account that some processes cannot begin for a given word if this process is still concerned with the previous word (e.g., one cannot articulate two words at the same time, but one can plan, and buffer, the next word while the previous word is being articulated). The model produces estimates of (1) the onset of articulation of the error; (2) the moment of interruption if the error were detected through the inner monitoring channel; (3) the moment of interruption if the error were detected through the external monitoring channel; (4) the onset of the self-correction. More detailed descriptions of the model can be found in Hartsuiker and Kolk (2001).

Mapping rules

Similar to Postma and Kolk (1993), we relate the moment of interruption to disfluency types. The present "mapping rules" are:

1. If the interruption takes place after the syllable has been uttered, the disfluency will be an overt repair or a syllable repetition.
2. If the interruption takes place during the uttering of the syllable, it will lead to a prolongation, sub-syllabic repetition, drawl, or broken word.
3. If the interruption takes place just before the (hypothetical) onset of the syllable (i.e., during articulatory planning) it will lead to a block.
4. If the interruption takes place longer before the (hypothetical) onset of the utterance (i.e., after the phonological code has been compiled, but before articulatory planning), it will not lead to an observable disfluency.

Our proposal differs from Postma and Kolk's (1993) proposal in three respects. First, Postma and Kolk only considered effects of interruption at certain points within a produced syllable. The present proposal considers effects of interruption at certain stages within the *production process*, including planning stages before articulation.

Second, we map times into symptoms using a larger grain size. The main reason for using this larger grain size is that we wish to restrict the degrees of freedom in the model. Postma and Kolk's proposal would force us to incorporate many additional parameters into the model, such as the duration of individual phonemes, the average numbers of phonemes in words, the position of the wrong phoneme in phonological errors, etc. This is not necessary for our current objective of showing position effects for stuttering on words of different lexical class.

Third, we assume the existence of covert repairs without observable consequences (mapping rule 4). Notice that the model has an articulatory buffer. If a speech plan containing an error is buffered for a long time, the plan can be revised before articulatory planning of that word. In that case, the system can continue to deliver speech smoothly. It is important to reiterate at this point that there is empirical evidence in favor of this view: For example, Motley et al. (1982) observed fluent productions of two-word utterances which were, however, designed so that a slip of the tongue would lead to taboo words. Even though the taboo-word slips were unobservable, measurements of galvanic skin response (a psychophysiological measure of emotion) suggested the slip did occur.

Target utterances

The model generated three-word utterances, each consisting of one content word (C) and two function words (F_n) with the following structures: (1) Two function words, followed by one content word ($F_1 F_2 C$); (2) a content word, flanked by two function words ($F_1 C F_2$); and (3) a content word, followed by the two function words ($C F_1 F_2$). Realistic examples of such utterances are *in the garden* (F F C), *I envied him* (F C F), and *follow it up* (C F F); the model, however, abstracts away from phonological content except for the number of syllables and the function/content-word distinction.

Parameters

The parameters of the model were identical to those used in previous simulations (Hartsuiker & Kolk, 2001; see appendix), with the exception of the duration of function and content words. In order to introduce the function/content-word distinction, we concentrated on two differences between these types of words. The first aspect is the length of the word (in syllables): Content words tend to be longer than function words. We captured the length difference by (arbitrarily) assigning the function words one syllable, and the content words two syllables in the first simulation. The second aspect is the degree of automatization of function word production (as a consequence of factors such as their high frequency). We assumed that function words are processed faster than content words, and that this holds across the board (in other words, every stage is a certain proportion faster; see Hartsuiker & Kolk, 2001, for a similar approach to model variations in speech rate). In order to capture the distinction between function words and content words we introduced a single parameter that specified how much shorter a function word, and how much longer a content word was as compared to the original value in the Hartsuiker and Kolk model. (Further details about the simulation are reported in the appendix.)

Output

Model output consisted of a predicted moment-of-interruption and a predicted onset-of-speech (based on monitoring by the internal channel), for each position in the phonological word and for each type of phonological word. The difference scores (moment of interruption – speech onset) resulted in a hypothetical "error-to-cut-off" value, with a negative value indicating how much earlier the interruption occurred relative to speech onset if no error would have been made (or detected). Furthermore, the model considered at which production stage the interruption took place (roughly, before, during, or after articulation).

Results

The average hypothetical error-to-interruption times are shown in Figure 15.2, for a value of the scaling parameter of 0.3. Each line represents one of the three phonological words that we tested, and each of the three positions indicates the error-to-cut-off time, if an error were to occur at that particular position.

The figure shows a general trend towards a position effect. That is, errors at positions later in the phonological word lead to an interruption earlier relative to their onset of articulation. Function words at position 3, in particular, tend to have very large negative error-to-cut-off times. Importantly, the general position effect interacts with part-of-speech status: The error-to-cut-off time

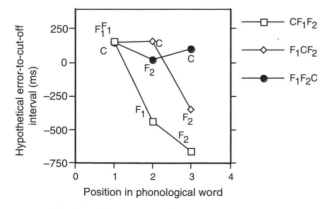

Figure 15.2 Predicted "error cut-off times", for errors in each position in each of the three phonological word structures.

for content word errors does not vary with position, but the error-to-cut-off time for function words does.

We translated the error-to-interruption times predicted by the model to predicted patterns of disfluencies, using the mapping rules described earlier. The results are presented in Table 15.2.

Table 15.2 lists the predicted symptoms if there were a covert error repair in either the first, second, or third word within each of the three phonological words (C F F), (F C F), or (F F C). For example, an error in the second unit in the phonological word C F F would be fluently repaired, but an error in the second unit of F F C would lead to a disfluency (a prolongation, repetition, drawl, or broken word). The model predicts that covert repair of *content* words will always lead to disfluencies, independent of position in the phonological word (Table 15.2). But this is not the case for function words. If two function words follow a content word (C F F), the model predicts that an error in either function word will be fluently repaired. If one function word precedes a content word, and another one follows it (F C F), the model predicts disfluencies on the first function word only. If both function words precede the content word (F F C), the model predicts disfluencies on both function words (but more whole-word repetitions and overt repairs on the first one, and more sub-syllabic incidents for the second one). Thus, if the scaling factor is set to 0.3 the model captures the basic pattern of data that Au-Yeung et al. observed. Before we discuss this in more detail, we address the generality of this finding. Variation of the scaling parameter showed that the data pattern reported in Table 15.2 holds across the entire range of that parameter (from 0 to 1). That is, even though the exact error-to-interruption times will vary with the value of the scaling parameter, this has no consequences for whether the model predicts disfluencies or not for a particular word type at a particular position.

Interestingly, the scaling factor does have a (limited) effect on the *type* of disfluency the model predicts, but only for phonological words consisting of two function words followed by a content word (F F C). In particular, for

Table 15.2 Predicted fluent or disfluent production, given a covert repair of the first, second, or third word in each of three utterance types

	Position of error		
Utterance	Position 1	Position 2	Position 3
C F F	C: Disfluent (2)	F: Fluent	F: Fluent
F C F	F: Disfluent (1)	C: Disfluent (2)	F: Fluent
F F C	F: Disfluent (1)	F: Disfluent (2)	C: Disfluent (2)

Note: C F F means that a content word occurs at the first position of the phonological word, and that there are function words in the second and third positions. Content words (C) were disyllabic, function words (F) were monosyllabic. The 'scaling factor' (S) was 0.3. Disfluent (1): Overt repair or syllable repetition. Disfluent (2): Prolongation, subsyllabic repetition, drawl, or broken word.

parameter values below 0.19, the model predicts that the interruption takes place during the stage of selection, rather than command. According to mapping rule 3, the model predicts that the predominant type of disfluency in this case is a block.

We also tested the case were all words were monosyllabic. If the scaling parameter is set to 0, the model predicts the same data pattern for each type of phonological word, since there is no distinction anymore between function words and content words. In Table 15.3 we have plotted, for each type of phonological word, how the predicted disfluency types vary with the scaling parameter.

In the baseline condition (S = 0), the model predicts disfluencies for position 1 and position 2, but not for position 3 in the phonological word, for all types of phonological word. However, it takes only a relatively small increase (S = .2) to obtain the empirical data pattern: Disfluencies on content words and function words preceding content words, no disfluencies on function words following content words.

Why does the model capture the general data pattern? The reason for the general position effect is that the predicted error-to-cut-off times depend on

Table 15.3 Relation between scaling factor and predicted interrupted stage for three types of phonological word (monosyllabic content words)

A A content word, followed by two function words (e.g. *send him off*)

Scaling factor	C	F	F
0	Disfluent (1)	Block	Fluent
0.1	Disfluent (2)	Block	Fluent
> 0.2	Disfluent (2)	Fluent	Fluent

B A content word, flanked by two function words (e.g. *I sent him*)

Scaling factor	F	C	F
0	Disfluent (1)	Block	Fluent
> 0.1	Disfluent (1)	Disfluent (2)	Fluent

C A content word, preceded by two function words (e.g. *off he goes*)

Scaling factor	F	F	C
0	Disfluent (1)	Block	Fluent
0.1	Disfluent (1)	Block	Block
0.2	Disfluent (1)	Disfluent (2)	Block
0.3	Disfluent (1)	Disfluent (2)	Block
> 0.4	Disfluent (1)	Disfluent (2)	Disfluent (2)

Note: Disfluent (1): Overt repair or syllable repetition. Disfluent (2): Prolongation, subsyllabic repetition, drawl, or broken word.

the time the phonetic plan is buffered. The longer there is buffering, the earlier the self-monitor can inspect it through the inner channel. Buffering is a device that deals with asynchronies between the articulation of the previous word and the planning of the current word. This implies first of all that there is no buffering for the first word (since there is no previous word). But the second word will have to be buffered for a while, if its planning is faster than the execution of the previous word. The third word will in general be buffered longest, because of a vicious circle effect: If the second word is buffered for a while, its articulation will be delayed. That means the third word will have to be buffered even longer: For the duration of the delay caused by the late start of word 2 and for the duration of word 2's articulation. Therefore, the monitor has the largest temporal advantage over the articulator for words at the end.

The lack of position effect for content words also follows from the model. The reason is that their planning takes relatively long, whereas articulation of function words takes a relatively short time. Thus, according to the model there is no buffering for a content word if it is preceded by one function word, and there is only a short amount of buffering if the content word appears in the third position.

Discussion

To summarize, Au-Yeung et al. (1998) observed that stuttering on a function word is more likely if this word occurs early rather than late in the phonological word, but that stuttering on content words is independent of position in the phonological word. In this chapter we showed that Postma and Kolk's (1993) covert repair hypothesis of stuttering can account for these findings, if it is supplemented with formal modeling of the time-course of the process of self-monitoring.

In our simulations, we took two properties of function words into account. First, function words tend to contain fewer syllables than content words: Therefore our first test case consisted of monosyllabic function words and disyllabic content words. Second, function words tend to be highly frequent and unstressed. Therefore, we assumed that function words can be processed faster, and that there is a gain in processing speed for each and every level of processing. We captured this gain, the extent to which content words are processed slower and function words are processed faster, using a single scaling parameter. We only allowed ourselves to vary this parameter.

The time-course predictions from our computational model were mapped onto disfluency types using a set of rules that is similar to a previous proposal by Postma and Kolk (1993). We incorporated one additional rule, namely the existence of "invisible" repairs: If the monitor detects an error long before articulation, it can filter out the error without any perceptible consequences to speech. Given this assumption, the model simulates the empirical results with respect to the effect of word class and position in phonological word on disfluency rates. For phonological words containing disyllabic content words, the model predicts this data pattern across the entire range of the scaling parameter. For monosyllabic content words, the model predicts the data pattern for values of the scaling parameter of 0.2 and higher.

Thus, both properties of function words we considered (they are shorter than content words and take less time to process than content words) have consequences for the model predictions. An interesting further prediction that can be derived from the model is that the pattern of disfluencies should be different for phonological words containing a monosyllabic content word and a multisyllabic function word (e.g., *go away*). In this case, one would expect relatively many disfluencies on the function word.

Comparison to other monitoring approaches

As outlined in the introduction to this chapter, there are several types of monitoring explanations for disfluencies. One explanation considers stuttering a *direct* effect of monitoring processes (e.g., Russell, Corley, & Lickley, this volume, Chapter 14; Vasiç & Wijnen, this volume, Chapter 13). People who stutter would be overvigilant in monitoring (certain aspects of) their own speech. Their monitor focusses too much on upcoming disfluencies or on planning problems or sets an unrealistically high criterion. As a result of this overvigilance, the monitor often interrupts speech and starts again, which paradoxically induces disfluencies rather than prevents them. This explanation is a variant of the CRH, but one where the dysfunction is in the monitor, not in the planning system. At this point, however, support for this explanation is still very limited, and not entirely conclusive. For example, Vasiç and Wijnen (this volume, Chapter 13) showed that word repetitions occurred more frequently when stuttering participants engaged in a linguistic double task (word monitoring), whereas other disfluencies became less frequent (blocks). In order to account for that difference, the authors postulated different mechanisms for different types of disfluency.

Another set of theories (Blackmer & Mitton, 1991; Clark & Wasow, 1998; Oomen & Postma, 2001a) view a specific type of disfluency, (function) word repetitions, as the result of self-monitoring. Function word repetitions result from the detection of problems in the planning of subsequent words. Repetitions are then a consequence of a strategy to gain time, whilst holding the floor in the conversation, in other words as a stalling device (e.g., Clark & Wasow, 1998). Notice that these theories invoke different monitoring channels from the ones depicted in Figure 15.1. They require monitoring systems that assess whether planning is delayed, and which then autonomously trigger a repetition (Blackmer & Mitton, 1991), or inform a central component (presumably the conceptualizer) about the delay (Clark & Wasow, 1998). This class of theories can be considered less parsimonious than the covert repair hypothesis: In order for them to work they would have to assume additional special-purpose monitoring systems.

Finally, Howell and colleagues (e.g., Au-Yeung et al., 1998; Howell & Sackin, 2000; Howell et al., 1999) made a more elaborate proposal. Like Blackmer and Mitton (1991), they hypothesize that disfluencies occur when execution of speech is too fast for the planning of subsequent speech. They propose that this is detected by a low-level mechanism, possibly located in the cerebellum, which inspects temporal synchrony between actions. If this mechanism detects asynchrony between speech planning and execution it will give an alarm signal. Subsequent to this alarm signal, either previous material is repeated (i.e., the same stalling tactic proposed by Clark & Wasow), or an attempt is made to execute an incomplete plan. Since the planning of (phonologically complex) content words is more demanding than the planning of relatively simple function words, temporal asynchrony will occur more frequently when a function words precedes, rather than follows, a content word.

The version of the covert repair hypothesis we propose shares important properties with the account of Howell and colleagues. In both accounts, the occurrence of stuttering depends on the synchrony between speech planning and execution. In the Howell et al. account, stuttering occurs because the plan for a content word is not ready in time for execution. In the present proposal, stuttering occurs when an erroneous speech plan is not buffered long enough to allow for silent revision. An advantage of the current proposal is that it explains different incidents by postulating only a single reaction to speech problems: Covert self-repair. Howell et al. postulate *two* possible reactions, which we might call *stalling* (repeating previous material) or *daring* (attempting to execute an incomplete speech plan). Thus, the current proposal can be considered more parsimonious. Further, there is no transparent relationship between executing an incomplete plan and the type of disfluencies one observes in stuttering. In order for the Howell et al. proposal to work in this respect, many additional assumptions will have to be made. Most importantly, it is unclear what executing an "incomplete plan" means. If it means the plan is underspecified for certain articulatory movements, one might expect it to lead to articulation errors and not to disfluencies. If it means only an earlier part of the word is ready, but not a later part, the type of disfluency, and indeed whether there is a disfluency or not will depend on a number of factors. For example, how much of the plan is ready when one begins executing the incomplete plan? Can planning of the second part catch up during execution of the first part? In contrast, as argued in this chapter, the CRH postulates a straightforward account of the types of disfluency: An account where the type of disfluency is a direct function of the moment in time one interrupts oneself.

Acknowledgements

Part of this chapter was previously published in B. Maassen, W. Hulstijn, R. Kent, H. Peters, & P. Van Lieshout (2001) (Eds.), *Speech motor control in normal and disordered speech. Proceedings of the 4th international speech motor conference*. Nijmegen, The Netherlands: Vantilt. We thank Pete Howell for useful comments on an earlier version of this chapter.

Note

1 We use the term 'monitor' here to denote any mechanism that signals discrepancies between intended and executed speech, irrespective of whether it produces a full analysis of the error. See Postma (2000) for an overview of postulated monitors in this broad sense.

Appendix: details of simulation

"Model time" starts at the beginning of phonological encoding. The current model predictions are based on a deterministic version of the model (Hartsuiker Kolk added random noise to each parameter). The reason is that we are now interested in *mean* times in different conditions, rather than in distributions of times. This allows us to reduce the model to the following equations:

$$Begin_{com,i} = End_{phon,i} + Max(0, End_{com,i-1} - End_{phon,i}) + \tau_{sel,i} \tag{1}$$

$$M_{int,i,IN} = End_{phon,i,} + C_{parse,i,i-1} + \tau_{parse,i} + C_{comp,i,j-1} + \tau_{comp,i} + \tau_{int,i} \tag{2}$$

Equation 1 determines the onset of overt speech for word with position i in the utterance. The onset is the beginning of the command stage for i ($Begin_{com,i}$). It depends on the end of the phonological encoding stage ($End_{phon, i}$), the time the speech plan is buffered (the temporal advantage of planning word i over the articulation of the previous word $i-1$, if there is any such advantage; otherwise 0 ms) and the time the selection stage for word i takes. Equation 2 determines the moment of interruption. It depends on the end of the phonological encoding stage, as well as on the monitoring parameters (language comprehension or "parsing", comparing, and interrupting). The symbols C are correction factors (so that a given stage cannot begin working on unit i, until it has dealt with the previous unit).

The basic parameter set was identical to the one used by Hartsuiker and Kolk (2001). That is, phonological encoding (110 ms/syllable); selection (148 ms/word); command (148 ms/syllable); comprehension (100 ms/word); comparison (50 ms/word) and interrupting (150 ms). The articulatory parameters (selection and command) were based on relatively fast speech (222 ms/syllable, including pauses).

The only parameter varied in the present simulations was a scaling factor, S ($0 < S < 1$), which determined the proportional increase of each parameter for content words, and the proportional decrease of each parameter for function words. Given a duration of τ in the basic parameter set, a function word would take $(1 - S).\tau$, and a content word would take $(1 + S).\tau$. Following Hartsuiker and Kolk (2001), we assume that the duration of interruption does not vary with linguistic factors; this parameter was kept constant at 150 ms for each lexical type.

References

Arends, N., Povel, D. J., & Kolk, H. H. J. (1988). Stuttering as an attentional phenomenon. *Journal of Fluency Disorders, 13*, 141–51.

Au-Yeung, J., Howell, P., & Pilgrim, L. (1998). Phonological words and stuttering on function words. *Journal of Speech, Language, and Hearing Research, 41*, 1019–1030.

Blackmer, E. R., & Mitton, E. R. (1991). Theories of monitoring and the timing of repairs in spontaneous speech. *Cognition, 39*, 173–94.

Bloodstein, O., & Grossman, M. (1981). Early stutterings: Some aspects of their form and distribution. *Journal of Speech and Hearing Research, 24*, 298–302.

Bosshardt, H. G. (2001). Speech-related planning as a determinant of stuttering. In B. Maassen, W. Hulstijn, R. Kent, H. Peters, & P. Van Lieshout (Eds.), Speech motor control in normal and disordered speech. *Proceedings of the 4th International Speech Motor Conference*. Nijmegen, The Netherlands: Vantilt.

Bradley, D., Garrett, M. F., & Zurif, E. (1980). Syntactic deficits in Broca's aphasia. In D. Caplan (Ed.), *Biological studies of mental processes* (pp. 269–86). Cambridge, MA: MIT Press.

Brown, S. F. (1945). The loci of stutterings in the speech sequence. *Journal of Speech Disorders, 10*, 181–92.

Burger, R., & Wijnen, F. N. K. (1999). Phonological encoding and word stress in stuttering and nonstuttering subjects. *Journal of Fluency Disorders, 24*, 91–106.

Clark, H. H., & Wasow, T. (1998). Repeating words in spontaneous speech. *Cognitive Psychology, 37*, 201–42.

Dell, G. S. (1986). A spreading-activation theory of retrieval in sentence production. *Psychological Review, 93*, 283–21.

Fayol, M., Largy P., & Lemaire P. (1994). Cognitive overload and orthographic errors: When cognitive overload enhances subject verb agreement errors. *Quarterly Journal of Experimental Psychology, 47A*, 437–64.

Garrett, M. F. (1982). Production of speech: Observations from normal and patho- logical language use. In A. Ellis (Ed.), *Normality and pathology in cognitive function* (pp. 19–76). London: Academic Press.

Hartsuiker, R. J., & Barkhuysen, P. N. (2001). The production of subject-verb agreement and verbal working memory. *Abstracts of the Psychonomic Society, 42nd Annual Meeting, 6*, 50.

Hartsuiker, R. J., & Kolk, H. H. J. (2001). Error monitoring in speech production: A computational test of the perceptual loop theory. *Cognitive Psychology, 42*, 113–57.

Howell, P., & Au-Yeung, J. (1995). The association between stuttering, Brown's factors, and phonological categories in child stutterers ranging in age between 2 and 12 years. *Journal of Fluency Disorders, 20*, 331–44.

Howell, P., Au-Yeung, J., & Sackin, S. (1999). Exchange of stuttering from function words to content words with age. *Journal of Speech, Language, and Hearing Research, 42*, 345–54.

Howell, P., Au-Yeung, J., & Sackin, S. (2000). Internal structure of content words leading to lifespan difference in phonological difficulty in stuttering. *Journal of Fluency Disorders, 25*, 1–20.

Howell, P., & Sackin, S. (2000). Speech rate modification and its effects on fluency reversal in fluent speakers and people who stutter. *Journal of Developmental and Physical Disabilities, 12*, 291–315.

Jou, J., & Harris, R. J. (1992). The effect of divided attention on speech production. *Bulletin of the Psychonomic Society, 30*, 301–304.

Kolk, H. H. J. & Postma, A. (1997). Stuttering as a covert-repair phenomenon. In R. Corlee & G. Siegel (Eds.), *Nature and treatment of stuttering: New directions* (pp. 182–203). Boston: Allyn & Bacon.

Levelt, W. J. M. (1983). Monitoring and self-repair in speech. *Cognition, 14*, 41–104.

Levelt, W. J. M. (1989). *Speaking: From intention to articulation.* Cambridge, MA: MIT Press.

Levelt, W. J. M., Roelofs, A., & Meyer, A. S. (1999). A theory of lexical access in speech production. *Behavioral and Brain Sciences, 22*, 1–75.

Logan, G. D., & Cowan, W. B. (1984). On the ability to inhibit thought and action: A theory of an act of control. *Psychological Review, 91*, 295–327.

Meyer, A. S. (1990). The time course of phonological encoding in language production: The encoding of successive syllables of a word. *Journal of Memory and Language, 29*, 524–45.

Motley, M. T., Camden, C. T., & Baars, B. J. (1982). Covert formulation and editing of anomalies in speech production: Evidence from experimentally elicited slips of the tongue. *Journal of Verbal Learning and Verbal Behavior, 21*, 578–94.

Oomen, C. C. E., & Postma, A. (2001a). Effects of divided attention on the production of disfluencies. *Journal of Speech, Language, and Hearing Research, 44*, 997–1004.

Oomen, C. C. E., & Postma, A. (2001b). Effects of time pressure on mechanisms of speech production and self-monitoring and self-repair. *Journal of Psycholinguistic Research, 30*, 163–84.

Oomen, C. C. E., & Postma, A. (2002). Limitations in processing resources and speech monitoring. *Language and Cognitive Processes, 17*, 163–84.

Postma (2000). Detection of errors during speech production: A review of speech monitoring models. *Cognition, 77*, 97–131.

Postma, A., & Kolk, H. H. J. (1993). The covert repair hypothesis: Prearticulatory repair processes in normal and stuttered disfluencies. *Journal of Speech and Hearing Research, 36*, 472–87.

Roelofs, A., & Meyer, A. S. (1998). Metrical structure in planning the production of spoken words. *Journal of Experimental Psychology: Learning, Memory, & Cognition, 24*, 922–39.

Selkirk, E. (1984). *Phonology and syntax: The relation between sound and structure.* Cambridge, MA: MIT Press.

Sternberg, S., Knoll, R. L., Monsell, S., & Wright, C. E. (1988). Motor programs and hierarchical organization in the control of rapid speech. *Phonetica, 45*, 175–197.

Timmermans, M., Schriefers, H., & Dijkstra, T. (submitted). When the white house turns red: Effects of input changes during picture naming tasks.

Wijnen, F. N. K., & Boers, I. (1994). Phonological priming effects in stutterers. *Journal of Fluency Disorders, 19*, 1–20.

Wolk, L., Blomgren, M., & Smith, A. B. (2000). The frequency of simultaneous disfluency and phonological errors in children: A preliminary investigation. *Journal of Fluency Disorders, 25,* 269–81.

Yaruss, J. S., & Conture, E. G. (1996). Stuttering and phonological disorders in children: Examination of the covert repair hypothesis. *Journal of Speech and Hearing Research, 39,* 349–64.

Part V

Conclusions and prospects

16 Phonological encoding, monitoring, and language pathology: Conclusions and prospects

Frank Wijnen and Herman H. J. Kolk

Introduction

The question that forms the backdrop of most of the work reported in this book is the following: Can the results of experimental research into normal language production, and the models based on these results, help us understand language pathology? In this concluding chapter we put this question center stage, and try to determine to what extent the empirical contributions in this volume shed light on this issue. In doing so, we also discuss a handful of issues that appear to be in need of further attention. The question just posed has a mirror image, which can be formulated as follows: Can the study of language pathology help us gain a better insight into the (neuro)cognitive architecture underlying normal language production? We address this question as well. Particularly, we point out a number of issues in the domain of phonological encoding and monitoring that the study of language pathology appears to put in a new light.

Connecting psycholinguistic research into language production with language pathology can only be fruitfully done on the basis of explicit, testable assumptions regarding the nature of the dysfunction. A problem that arises concerns (excess) degrees of freedom. If a certain psycholinguistic model and a set of pathological data do not match, it could either be the model that is failing, or the assumed parameters of the underlying dysfunction (disregarding the possibility of irrelevant or faulty data). Inspection of the relevant literature makes clear that there is no consensus concerning the assumptions on how the difference between normal functioning and dysfunction in the domain of language (production) should be modeled. The research program that gave rise to this volume[1] adopts a specific view on this matter, as already announced in the introduction to this book. We present this perspective in some detail here. In the ensuing sections, we use the materials supplied in this book, as well as previously published results, to evaluate our approach.

The perspective on pathological language production that we choose as our frame of reference is characterized by two notions: *Continuity* and *plasticity*. "Continuity" refers to the assumption that perturbations of language production that are canonically labeled "pathological" (for instance, stuttering) and those that are considered "normal" (e.g., ordinary disfluency) are not qualitatively different, but represent different points on a continuum. Importantly, it is not just the superficial resemblance between normal perturbances and pathological distortions that is at the heart of the matter, but the presupposition that both are generated by the same mechanism. In other words, in pathology the processing architecture is structurally unaltered, but some of its parameters, for example, the rate of build-up or decay of activation, or the amount of background noise, are altered (cf. Martin, this volume Chapter 4; Rapp & Goldrick, 2000).

"Continuity," as referring to the similarity of symptoms of language pathology to everyday speech mishaps, has been associated with Sigmund Freud's 19th-century work on aphasia. Buckingham (1999, p.87) writes that:

> The crucial claim of the continuity thesis is the functional postulation of some underlying psycholinguistic system, which, when disrupted under very different contextual settings, gives rise to errors that settle into similar sorts of patterns . . ., and within reason this should hold for paraphasias, slips, hysteria, sleep talk, the glossolalia of charismatics, child language errors, historical change, dialect variation, and, if we are to believe Arnold Pick, many of the errors observed in speakers of a second language.

Indeed, in the recent child language literature, the continuity thesis has been the subject of vigorous debate. In this context it represents the assumption that the full grammatical machinery linguists assume to underlie normal adult language use is present in children from birth, at least latently. Children's deficient, i.e., non-adult, language production is to be ascribed to either a limited vocabulary, or an insufficient amount of the processing resources needed to put the grammatical knowledge to use. It stands in opposition to the maturational perspective, which holds that children's early language system is qualitatively different from what it eventually will be. Analogously, the continuity perspective in aphasiology can be contrasted with "knowledge loss" approaches (Avrutin, 2001).

We now come to our second principle. "Plasticity" refers to the brain's ability to change. First of all, the brain is capable of structural change, for instance after limb amputation (e.g., Merzenich & Jenkins, 1995). Second, the brain may also change the way in which it deals with its tasks. For such cases we use the term *functional* plasticity rather than structural plasticity. In the early 1980s, Caramazza formulated a central principle for the analysis of behavioral data obtained from brain-damaged patients. According to this *transparency assumption*, "the cognitive system of a brain-damaged patient is fundamentally the same except for a 'local' modification [. . .] This assumption rejects the possibility that brain damage results in the *de novo* creation of cognitive operations" (Caramazza, 1986, p. 52; see also Caramazza, 1992). This seems logical enough, and undoubtedly most cognitive neuropsychologists take this assumption for granted (although see Farah, 1994). However, the transparency assumption may have its limitations. Brain damage may not lead to completely new operations, but something may change nevertheless. In particular, less frequently used cognitive operations could become more frequent. It is known for instance that after limb amputation major adaptations of learned motor patterns occur (see Latash & Anson, 1996, for a review). Apparently, the brain has ways to recruit motor patterns that are within its reach, but that are normally not or only infrequently used. And if the brain can do this after amputation, there is reason to assume that this same capacity can be used after damage to the brain itself, unless of course brain parts necessary for this adaptive change are also damaged.

Whether the transparency assumption works in a particular case, depends on the availability of *alternative routes* to the same ultimate goal, something referred to elsewhere as multiple-route plasticity (Kolk, 2000). Behavior appears to vary in this respect. For instance, it seems likely that there is only one way to stretch your finger, but there are certainly a number of ways to move your finger to a target. In the motor control literature, this state of affairs is referred to as *functional equivalence* or *degrees of freedom*. Functional equivalence also exists in speaking: Speech sounds can be articulated in more than one way. That the availability of alternative articulatory routes is employed for adaptive purposes is shown by the phenomenon of "pipe speech": When speakers are given bite blocks between their teeth, they immediately produce acceptable vowels or consonants, notwithstanding the fact that the normal target positions of their articulators can no longer be reached.

With respect to language behavior, functional equivalence seems abundant. Take, for instance, word reading, a popular topic for neuropsychologists. It has long been recognized that there are two ways to read aloud a word: Via the lexical and via the non-lexical route. Recent evidence suggests that the selection of one or the other route is under control of the reader (Hendriks & Kolk, 1997; Kello & Plaut, 2003). At the sentence level, many sentences can be understood largely on the basis of individual word meaning, without the use of syntactic information: aphasic patients are known to make use of this possibility (cf. Hagoort, Wassenaar, & Brown, 2003). In all these cases, there is an alternative to not changing: the impaired system *reorganizes* to exploit alternative routes to the same goal. It is this functional reorganization we refer to when we talk about plasticity.

In language production, plasticity may result in adaptive changes in spoken output in response to a deficit. So, distorted output may not be the direct result of a malfunctioning (component of the) production system, but rather of an adaptation of the system to this malfunction. In many cases the adaptation is brought about through the internal monitoring device, i.e., the component that safeguards the quality and efficacy of the output. The continuity perspective implies that the interaction between a malfunctioning encoding device and the monitor applies to both normal and pathological conditions. From this perspective, it is not only sensible, but even necessary to consider encoding and monitoring in close connection.

Kolk (1998 and elsewhere), in this connection, distinguishes between two types of pathological symptoms: *Dysfunction symptoms*, which are direct reflections of the underlying dysfunction, and *adaptation symptoms*, which result from using another system (adaptation strategy). The criterion by which to discriminate between these is normalcy. Adaptation symptoms are, essentially, normal, in the sense that they are identical to phenomena in non-pathological speech. Speaking slowly, inserting pauses etc. are normal reactions to problems in language production. Reducing the syntactic complexity of utterances, as in agrammatism, is another one. In Kolk's view, this is adapting to a failing encoding system by overusing a simplified register, which *in itself*, is fully regular (grammatical).

In an attempt to answer the questions laid out earlier, our approach is to evaluate the extent to which results reported in this volume, and elsewhere, are in line with the continuity/plasticity hypothesis. To summarize, this hypothesis holds that pathological symptoms are the results of an interaction between *encoding* and *monitoring*. Due to a processing malfunction (as opposed to damage to knowledge representations or the functional architecture), representations generated in the course of planning utterances contain errors. It is the monitor that enables the system to respond adaptively to the malfunction, by initiating repair attempts, or by initiating alternative (simplified) courses of planning.

Traditional evidence

Before we take a closer look at how the studies collected in this volume contribute to the continuity/plasticity – transparency debate, we give a brief overview of some of the evidence that has been brought to bear on the issue in the recent past. One of the language pathologies that has figured quite prominently in the discussion is Broca's aphasia, more particularly one of its characteristic symptoms, *agrammatism*.

A prominent version of the transparency view of agrammatism is that it results from loss of grammatical knowledge, such that syntactic structures that involve complex derivations are not attainable anymore. In particular, structures involving syntactic movement of various types, such as passives, clefts and sentences with displaced objects (scrambling) are affected. Hypothetical concepts such as Grodzinsky's *trace deletion* and Friedmann's *tree pruning* attempt to account for the observed dysfunction in terms of loss of grammatical components (see Avrutin, 2001 for details). Obviously, if the assumption is that the grammatical knowledge necessary to construct particular representations is gone, the prediction must be that patients will *never* produce the corresponding sentences. There is convincing evidence, however, that contradicts this prediction.

The constructions that knowledge loss hypotheses predict to be inaccessible are occasionally produced by agrammatic patients. This finding, obviously, is unproblematic under the hypothesis that avoidance of structural complexity is an adaptation to a failing encoding system (e.g., Kolk, 1995). On this view, experimental manipulations that reduce processing load are predicted to counter complexity avoidance. Priming (or pre-activating) syntactic structures is an example in point: It is supposed to help the pathologically constrained system to overcome its processing bottleneck. Indeed, Hartsuiker and Kolk (1998) demonstrated that performance of agrammatic speakers benefits from structural priming. For example, when patients were presented with a passive, and were then asked to describe the picture of a transitive event, they can use a passive. The ability to produce such sentences has not been wiped away by tissue damage.

Agrammatic symptoms in spontaneous speech can be suppressed, but it appears to come at a cost. Hofstede and Kolk (1994) compared free narratives where it is up to the patient how much detail she is willing to provide, with a picture description task in which the patient is asked to describe the picture "as well as possible". The pictures were constructed to elicit various types of grammatical morphology. The picture description tasks yielded fewer omissions of prepositions, determiners, and finiteness markers, as compared to the interview. The decrease in the number of omissions of prepositions was correlated with an increase of substitutions. In a second task, patients were presented with a set of pictures depicting spatial relationships (e.g., a red circle on top of a blue square or a yellow square in front of a green circle), and were asked describe the pictures in such a way that the experimenter could reproduce them. In this situation, there was an even more dramatic reduction of preposition omission. At the same time, substitution rate went up considerably. These results suggest very strongly that omission (of functional elements) is due to an adaptive strategy, aimed at circumventing a lexical retrieval and/or morphosyntactic encoding problem.

Not only does the continuity hypothesis predict that pathological symptoms can be suppressed, it also predicts that these symptoms can be elicited in normally functioning, neurologically intact individuals, given the appropriate (experimental) manipulations. It is important to note once again that the output generated by agrammatic speakers, although simpler than expected (elliptical), obeys the grammatical constraints of the patient's native language, for example, with respect to word order, or verb position-finiteness interactions (De Roo 1999; Ruigendijk, 2002). One could even say on the basis of these findings that "agrammatism" is a misnomer. At the same time, it must be kept in mind that if in specific tasks overuse of normal ellipses is counterproductive, we do see a substantial amount of grammatical errors in the agrammatic output.

Obedience to general grammatical principles is also found in early child language, and, more tellingly, in certain – informal or substandard – registers naturally used by intact adult speakers, characterized by a predominance of structurally simple, elliptic utterances (e.g., foreigner talk, diary register, anecdote register; Hofstede 1992; Wijnen 1998). Each of these registers seems to be used in contexts where it appears to be useful to reduce the complexity of the output. Thus, the phenomenon suggests that (normal) speakers can – more or less strategically – *decide* to reduce output complexity. In many cases, this appears to be done in the interest of the listener (who is typically not a competent language user). It is an interesting question whether speakers can also switch to an elliptic register for their own sake, possibly because it may help them cope with a performance bottleneck. If so, it may count as a point in favor of the assumption that so-called agrammatic language use in Broca's patients is an adaptive strategy, as argued by Kolk and Heeschen (1992). Speculatively, the diary and anecdote registers may be invoked in the interest of speed (to keep up with the stream of thought), or reduction of effort.

An interesting question is also whether normal speakers will revert to such reduced output (indeed, telegraphic speech) when they are put under pressure. A recent study by Kemper, Herman, and Lian (2003) indicates that normal adult speakers change their speech style when given a second task to perform while speaking. While young adults reduced sentence length and grammatical complexity, older adults – whose speech was already less complex and less fluent in single task conditions in comparison to the young adults – only shifted to a reduced rate.[2] There is also highly suggestive evidence from language comprehension. Miyake, Carpenter, and Just (1995) presented sentences of varying complexity to normal subjects by means of rapid serial visual presentation. Not only did the normal subjects start to make comprehension errors, the profile of their errors was highly similar to the error profiles of aphasic patients. Dick, Bates, Wulfeck, Utman, Dronkers, and Gernsbacher (2001) recently replicated this result not only with rapid serial visual presentation, but with other kinds of stimulus degradation as well.

Another example of language pathology for which the opposition between continuity/plasticity and transparency is quite high on the research agenda is stuttering. Non-continuity hypotheses on stuttering generally hold that, despite superficial resemblances, stuttering and normal disfluency are qualitatively different, and imply that stuttering is caused by structural damage to the language production system. Specifically, various authors have suggested that stuttering results from a (possibly innate) malfunction in the neural systems subserving articulatory programming or execution (Caruso, 1991; Webster, 1993).

By contrast, the continuity perspective on stuttering suggests that its behavioral manifestations correspond to the disfluencies that can be witnessed in all speakers, and, by implication, that there is only one process underlying both normal and disordered fluency. The continuity view is supported by much developmental research, which generally reports the absence of a clear, qualitative distinction or breakpoint between the frequently occurring disfluency increase arising at about age 3, and clinically significant stuttering, which in some cases ensues (Yairi & Lewis, 1984). As to the process underlying both normal and disordered disfluency, a coherent and parsimonious proposal is Kolk and Postma's *Covert Repair Hypothesis* (CRH) (Kolk 1991; Kolk & Postma, 1997; Postma & Kolk, 1993). This hypothesis, as is explained in several places throughout this book, holds that disfluencies – i.e., *all* disfluencies – reflect attempts of the self-monitoring device to repair errors in the speech plan before they are articulated. The difference between people who stutter and those who do not is that phonological encoding in the former fails more often, and so the monitor finds many more occasions for interrupting and repairing. Specifically, the underlying problem in stuttering is assumed to lie in the selection of phonological segments for the speech plan.

It is important to note that the CRH (and its variants, cf. Chapters 13, 15), like the continuity perspective on aphasia presented earlier, has as its key assumption that pathology does not impinge on the structure of the language-processing mechanism, or the representations it generates. Rather, disordered speech is the result of alterations to the processing dynamics of the system. The plasticity perspective has as its key assumption that the system adapts to such a change by finding new ways to optimize communication. It does so by overusing normal mechanisms of covert repair. As a consequence, as we argued before with regard to aphasia, the CRH predicts that symptoms are optional, or, in other words, can be suppressed under conditions that compensate for suboptimal settings of processing parameters. Complementarily, it should be possible to induce stuttering in persons who are considered to be normally fluent speakers.

There is empirical support – albeit preliminary and tentative in many cases – for both predictions. First, it is common clinical knowledge that the severity of stuttering varies a lot over time within patients, even up to virtual disappearance. Furthermore, significant suppression of stuttering under specific conditions has been repeatedly reported in the literature. Such conditions relate to either the manner of speaking, the nature of auditory feedback, or the social parameters of verbal interaction. Vasic and Wijnen (this volume, Chapter 13) present a more detailed overview of these observations, as well as the outline of an explanatory account that binds them together.

In the context of the continuity thesis, it is somewhat strange to speak of "inducing stuttering" in normally fluent speakers, as there is, basically, nothing special about stuttering. It is just increased disfluency,[3] and there are various ways by which disfluency in non-stuttering persons can be promoted, ranging from forcing them to speak (much) faster than they normally do to significantly increasing the complexity of the output (as in tongue twisters), to altering social parameters. Naturally, one does not have to rely solely on applying delayed auditory feedback (Goldiamond, 1965), the effect of which, incidentally, is ill understood.

Evidence collected in the present volume

Phonological encoding

Clearly, if the linguistic representations generated by a pathologically compromised encoding system were shown to deviate qualitatively from normal output, this would be a serious blow to the continuity thesis. Linguistic analyses indicate that the output generated by patients with Broca's aphasia are, on the whole, less complex than what is expected, but are nonetheless grammatical in all relevant respects. It is important to determine whether the same holds at the level of phonology. The contributions by Code (Chapter 7) and Den Ouden and Bastiaanse (Chapter 5) speak to this matter. Both show that phonological structure is essentially unaffected by aphasia (or apraxia). Similarly, Nijland, and Maassen (Chapter 8) point out that the inconsistent phonological realizations typical of developmental apraxia of speech (DAS) are indicative of a processing problem, not of a deficit at the level of phonological representation.

Code looks at non-lexical recurring utterances (i.e., reiterated, concatenated meaningless syllables), and concludes that, while they are segmentally simpler than the norm, they do not violate phonotaxis. Similarly, sonority patterns are fully regular. Code suggests that the simplifications may be due to a degradation of the articulatory buffer – a processing capacity type of explanation. It could be remarked, however, that degradation as such should lead to errors, not to simplifications. To explain simplification, it should be assumed that the system develops a bias for simpler forms, in response to the degradation.

In the same vein, Den Ouden and Bastiaanse observe that phonological constraints are upheld in phonemic paraphasias in conduction aphasia. In two of the patients discussed, patterns of omission are predicted by segmental markedness (more sonorous segments are more often dropped). The authors suggest that the primary problem for these patients lies with the construction of the phonological plan. In two others, the pattern of omission seems to be conditioned by linear order, such that final segments are most vulnerable. This is linked to a problem in maintaining phonological plans in working memory. Thus, they suggest that there may be two functionally different etiologies underlying conduction aphasia.

The markedness effects reported by Den Ouden and Bastiaanse raise the question as to whether current models of phonological encoding can accommodate them. In the spirit of Dell and Kim (Chapter 2), we might argue that the preservation of phonological structure in speech errors is a result of the encoding architecture's sensitivity to frequency and similarity. Let us try to determine how this might work in WEAVER++ (Levelt, Roelofs, & Meyer 1999; Roelofs, this volume, Chapter 3). This model assumes that segments are inserted sequentially (left to right) in phonological word representations constructed from the metrical templates associated with one or several lexical items (lemmas). Syllabification comes about automatically, as segments are mapped onto the template. The basic algorithm of this process takes the form of a production rule. Thus, the initial /k/ of the word "cat" is assigned to an onset position by production rule ONSET(k), and so on.

In order to model positional markedness effects with regard to errors, two approaches seem possible. First, one might enrich the production rule system as proposed by Roelofs, by allowing more specific rules such as ONSET-MARGIN(X) or ONSET-CORE(X). In doing so, markedness could be an automatic spin-off of the frequency with which rules are called. Since core positions (both in onsets and codas) occur more frequently than satellites or margins (because the latter are dependent on the former), the frequency with which the appropriate rules are accessed will differ correspondingly. Assuming that a high frequency of usage protects against the processing impediment resulting from brain damage (cf. Dell & Kim, this volume, Chapter 2), production rules corresponding to less marked syllable positions will less often be affected than those dealing with syllable constituents that are marked. Contrariwise, it could be that also here plasticity plays a crucial role. Considerations such as the ones given earlier may explain why marked segments or segments in marked positions give more problems, but not why they are *omitted* rather than substituted by another element. Omission suggests strategic simplification.

Alternatively, the positioning of consonants in syllable-initial or final clusters could be regulated by their phonological properties, notably sonority (Levelt et al., 1999). It is not difficult to see that the sonority hierarchy can be converted into an algorithm that takes care of consonant sequencing. It is less evident how such an approach could account for markedness effects, either positional or segmental. A third approach starts from the idea that consonant clusters are inserted as units (Levelt et al., 1999). This would readily explain markedness effects, on the assumption that simpler clusters (respectively singletons) are more frequent, and hence have a higher base rate activation than more complex clusters. This solution is similar to Stemberger's (1984) proposal that agrammatism is the result of a problem in activating relatively complex syntactic templates or frames.

The conclusion we draw from Code's and Den Ouden and Bastiaanse's observations is that phonological paraphasias are analogous to the elliptic utterances typical of agrammatism. There is a reduction in output complexity, but the relevant constraints are in place. The cause of the reduction of complexity is assumed to lie with processing restrictions, combined with strategic simplification. In her contribution, Martin (Chapter 4) gives an explicit account of what such a processing restriction might look like. She works in the interactive activation framework initiated by Dell and his colleagues (cf. Chapter 2), and hence focusses on two main parameters of information processing: Connection strength and decay rate. Simulation studies in which either of these two parameters is manipulated (reduction of connection strength, increase of decay rate) lead to distinctive error patterns that mimick those seen in patients with a variety of lesions.

One question that can be raised with regard to this approach is whether the notion of continuity should be extended in order to encompass the parametric differences between pathological and normal processing systems. What we mean is this: If you take a stringent look on continuity, you may well want to know whether the decrease of connection strength and increase of decay rate argued to exist in pathology have a counterpart in the normal situation, thus honoring the supposition that disruptions of various kinds (i.e., not only those that arise from pathology) produce similar error patterns. Martin argues that this problem might be addressed by applying identical methodological procedures to studies of pathological and normal speech. The variation in error patterns considered to be indicative of pathology are normally documented in single case studies, whereas descriptions of normal error patterns are grounded in corpora collected from a large number of different speakers. It may well be that the variation that we see in patients, which is, by hypothesis, an effect of parametric differences in the processing system, has a parallel in interindividual variation across normally speaking subjects. A good example of such a parallel can be found in the work of Just and Carpenter (1992) on sentence comprehension. A core assumption of this work is that there are inter-individual differences in sentence-processing capacity, which can be measured with a reading span test. Just and Carpenter demonstrate that these individual differences have an important impact on sentence comprehension. In their computational model, CC reader, processing capacity variation corresponds, roughly speaking, to differences in processing rate ("efficiency") and/or differences in decay rate ("maintenance"). Interestingly, Haarmann, Just, and Carpenter (1999) have extended this model to agrammatic comprehension. In summary, this work suggests that pathologically induced fluctuations and interindividual variation within the normal range are of the same type.

Martin refers to evidence that may link the purported parameter changes in aphasia to normal phenomena. Simulations show that an overall reduction of connection strength is related to predominance of perseveratory (as opposed to anticipatory) errors. In normally speaking subjects, connection weight may be related to the amount of practice (or automatization), in pronouncing complex speech patterns (tongue twisters). At the onset of training, perseveratory errors predominate, but as practicing continues, they decrease in favor of anticipations. A similar phenomenon is observed in normal speech development. Children's speech errors are more often perseveratory than those of adults (Dell, Burger, & Svec, 1997; Wijnen, 1992). This, again, suggests that changes in processing parameters that occur under normal circumstances and those that are the result of pathological conditions, are on the same continuum.

A more general question one might have concerning the approach advocated by Martin and her colleagues is whether the simulations adequately represent the pathological phenomena of interest. The work discussed in Chapter 4 focusses on how changes in model parameters (connection strength, decay rate) produce shifts in relative frequencies of error types. Thus, another, equally important aspect of aphasia may be underexposed: The absolute increase in error frequency. However, the dynamic notions we have discussed also capture this aspect, because they enable one to explain variation in *severity* between patients. Although everyone who has worked with aphasic patients knows that variation in severity exists, only rarely attempts have been made to account for it. Haarmann and Kolk (1991) were the first to demonstrate that severity variation can be simulated by varying mean decay or activation rate. In the later model of aphasic word production by Dell, Schwartz, Martin, Saffran, & Gagnon (1997), a similar relation was made between severity and the reduction of connection strength or increase in decay rate.

The issue of suboptimal processing dynamics returns in the context of stuttering in the chapter by Melnick, Conture, and Ohde (6). These authors take up the lead supplied by the Covert Repair Hypothesis, and assume that stuttering in children may be the result of a slowdown of planning processes. This temporal disruption may well be applicable to the entire planning system, but has a noticeable detrimental effect on phonological encoding, such that phonological errors occur frequently. The slowdown in activation of phonological segments that Kolk and Postma, and, in their footsteps, Melnick et al. invoke as the functional deficit underlying stuttering, is basically the same as the reduction of connection strength in Martin's modeling approach, which is argued to underlie the increase of non-word phonological errors (paraphasias). This raises questions about (and perhaps predictions on) the relations between various language pathologies that are etiologically and clinically highly diverse. We will come back to this issue later.

Monitoring

As indicated earlier, the monitor plays a crucial role in the continuity/ plasticity perspective on language pathology. The basic assumption is that the monitor is not only in place and intact, but also that it does exactly what it normally does: Compensating for problems resulting from failures in the encoding system.

Obviously, reality may turn out to be different; pathological conditions could comprise either the architecture of the monitoring system, or its functioning (cf. Postma & Oomen, this volume, Chapter 9). A preliminary question is, then, what exactly is the architecture of the monitoring system? Here we touch on the issue of production-based vs perception-based monitoring. If we, for ease of exposition, concentrate on perception-based monitoring – which is most prominent in this volume anyway – we see that there are several pieces of evidence supporting the continuity view sprinkled throughout this book. Roelofs's (Chapter 3) reanalysis of the data reported by Nickels and

Howard (1995) supports the idea that comprehension-based self-monitoring is in place in aphasia, although its efficacy may vary across individuals. The computational simulations by Hartsuiker, Kolk, and Martensen (Chapter 11) underscore this conclusion, and moreover indicate that aphasia may be associated with an increased attention for the internal feedback channel relative to the external channel, as was previously suggested by Oomen and Postma (2001; cf. Oomen, Postma, & Kolk, this volume, Chapter 12). In line with the findings on aphasia, the studies on stuttering reported in this book (Chapters 13, 14, 15), as well as Nijland and Maassen's contribution on developmental verbal dyspraxia (Chapter 8), see no need for positing a structural alteration of the monitoring mechanism. In addition to this, the evidence suggests that even the efficiency (albeit not the efficacy) of the monitor is unaltered under pathological conditions. Symptoms mentioned in this book, such as *conduites d'approche* in conduction aphasia (Chapter 5), and articulatory groping in developmental verbal dyspraxia (Chapter 8) seem to imply a monitor fully capable of supporting self-repair, if only the encoding mechanism were functioning normally.

All of this is not to say that the monitor's function does not change at all under pathological conditions. We already mentioned the relative increase of attention for the internal feedback loop at the expense of the external channel in patients with Broca's aphasia. It is not yet clear what this signifies. One possibility argued for by Oomen, Postma, and Kolk (2001) is that aphasic speakers do this because they want to prevent errors to occur in overt speech. Quite another matter is the proposal put forth by Vasic and Wijnen in Chapter 13. They say that the monitor can be overvigilant, diagnosing discontinuities that are intrinsic to speech planning and delivery as undesired incidents, warranting interruption and repair. This idea, which finds some support in dual task performance data as well as the disfluency detection study by Russell, Corley, and Lickley (Chapter 14), points to the possibility that plasticity may under some circumstances also have negative effects. A system made to detect and correct errors is subject to false alarms and may therefore sometimes produce repair behavior in the absence of any real error.

Anything in favor of non-continuity?

At the beginning of this chapter, we observed that in trying to bring insights from psycholinguistics to bear on language pathology, one needs to specify the parameters of pathology. The evidence reported in this volume appears to be at least compatible with, and in many cases plainly supportive of a continuity/plasticity perspective. The implication is that language pathology can be understood as the product of a processing architecture that is structurally uncompromised, but in which the dynamics of processing are quantitatively altered, due to a reduction of critical resources. As a result of this, various encoding tasks can no longer be performed errorlessly within a certain time frame. Within limits, the system can adapt to this new situation, and the component that plays a crucial role in this adaptation is self-monitoring.

Obviously, this conclusion may not apply invariably to all clinical populations. For one thing, knowledge loss does occur. Alzheimer patients truly seem to lose semantic knowledge progressively (e.g., Chertkow & Bub, 1991). Second, the continuity/plasticity model may reach its limits where pathological malfunction of the monitor system is at stake. The available evidence on this matter is as yet fragmentary. According to some authors, the so-called "formal thought disorders" in schizophrenia, marked by incoherent and strongly associative verbal output, are to be interpreted in this way (see Postma & Oomen, this volume, Chapter 9). We doubt, however, whether this phenomenon counts as a language dysfunction. Wernicke's aphasia may be another case in point. In contrast to the agrammatic speech of patients with Broca's aphasia, the speech of Wernicke patients is fast and full of errors, often uncorrected. Furthermore, their comprehension is severely impaired, which could make monitoring via the comprehension system difficult. By way of contrast, Haarmann and Kolk (1992) found that in a sentence-completion task, Wernicke patients were as slow and made as many grammatical errors as the agrammatic patients, which is difficult to reconcile with their being sloppy monitors of their own output. At any rate, it is conceivable that there is a principled difference between types of language pathology in which only (one of) the encoding components are (is) comprised, and types of pathology in which the monitor itself (as the component that implements plasticity) is compromised.

Challenges

At the outset of this chapter, we noted that not only the psycholinguistic study of normal language production can contribute to the understanding of language pathology, but that studying language pathology may also contribute to our understanding of the intact production system. Analyzing language pathology may cast a new light on issues that are contentious in psycholinguistics, or even bring issues to the fore that have hitherto gone unnoticed. We mention some of these, together with some more general observations that invite further study.

Architecture of monitoring

What information does the monitor have access to? Levelt, Kolk, and Postma, and many others assume that the monitor inspects the speech plan (or phonological representation) and/or realized speech for errors and infelicities. Consequently, all self-initiated interruptions of ongoing speech (overt corrections as well as disfluencies) are linked to a planning error. Other authors have proposed that particular disfluencies are related to delays in planning (Au-Yeung, Howell, & Pilgrim 1998; Clark & Wasow, 1998; Maclay & Osgood, 1959).

Hartsuiker, Kolk, and Lickley (this volume, Chapter 15) interpret the *stalling* phenomenon (repeating bits of a speech plan while waiting for its completion) as the result of a strategy (and they take their cue from Clark & Wasow, 1998). This invokes the monitor as a device that not only detects errors, but also oversees the flow of planning, and is thus capable of detecting delays. There is an alternative hypothesis, however. It is conceivable that repeating, i.e., re-issuing speech material from an underspecified and therefore not fully executable plan, is an automatic response of the encoding system when the input to a particular processor is incomplete (or: when the processor reads out its input buffer too early). Thus, in contrast to what Oomen and Postma (2001, also this volume, Chapter 9) suggest, the monitor need not have a role in this process. Under this assumption, there is no need to attribute to the monitor an eye on the progress of encoding.

How does monitoring for errors occur? Levelt's (1983, 1989) perceptual loop theory holds that in the monitoring process, two comparisons are made. First, an intended message is compared to an expressed message. Triggered by a preverbal message, the formulator generates a phonetic plan and subsequently overt speech is produced. Both the phonetic plan and overt speech are processed by the comprehension system leading to a conceptual interpretation of the utterance.

Ideally, the two conceptual structures – preverbal message and conceptual interpretation – should be identical. By comparing these two interpretations, the monitor checks whether you get out what you put in. If not, a repair follows. The other comparison entails checking whether what is said meets the standards of production: Is it syntactically and phonologically well formed, is it loud enough, fast enough and does it contain the proper prosody?

One may argue that such an elaborate process of comparison and repair would be too time consuming, given the high rapidity of running speech. It is therefore good to realize that even in the context of the perceptual loop hypothesis, the process could be simpler than this. First of all, with error repairs, an actual change of the current speech plan would not be necessary. Since speech errors are rare events, it would be sufficient to restart the production process and produce the same plan again. In the majority of the cases, this would now lead to correct output.

A second simplification is related to the fact that in many cases, error detection is possible without explicit comparison. Since monitoring parasitizes on the language comprehension system, the detection of various classes of errors may "come for free," as a spin-off of failing to interpret particular bits of input. We provide a very brief overview of some major error types and the mechanism by which they could be detected (see also Roelofs, this volume, Chapter 3):

- phonological errors resulting in nonwords → no lexical access; real-word phonological errors are treated like lexical selection errors
- lexical selection errors → grammatical and/or semantic inappropriateness in sentence context
- grammatical errors (morphology, syntax) → parsing failure
- semantic errors (e.g., scope, negation, anaphora) → infelicitousness in discourse; ambiguity.

Is it conceivable that any errors can pass through the "tests" provided by the different components of the comprehension system? The answer is affirmative: These are words that are phonologically, grammatically, semantically as well as pragmatically acceptable, yet do not conform to what the speaker intended to say. According to Roelofs (this volume, Chapter 3) such errors can be detected by verifying whether the lemma accessed in comprehension is linked to the lexical concept prepared for production.

Levelt et al. (1999) and Roelofs (this volume, Chapter 3) argue that this same procedure underlies detection of phonological errors that yield existing words, the underlying assumption being that the monitor does *not* have access to the intended phonological output. Nooteboom (this volume, Chapter 10) argues against this view, by showing that phonological speech errors resulting in existing words and those that do not, have identical distributional characteristics, which must mean that the monitor does not blindly handle the former as lexical selection errors. Furthermore, Nooteboom shows that the lexical bias effect – meaning that real-word-yielding phonological errors have a higher probability than nonword-yielding errors – occurs in overt (realized) errors, but not in self-corrections.

The lexical bias effect has been a critical issue almost since the beginning of the systematic psycholinguistic study of language production. It has become a primary battleground for advocates and opponents of bottom-up information flow in the production system. Dell and his co-workers have argued in several places (see this volume, Chapter 2) that lexical bias is due to upward spreading of activation from phonological segment nodes to word nodes. This is ruled out in Levelt's strictly feedforward model. Instead, this model suggests that lexical bias comes about as a result of editing (see also Baars, Motley, & MacKay, 1975). Starting from the assumption that the external and internal feedback loops employed by the monitor are functionally equivalent, Nooteboom argues that lexical bias should be found in overt errors as well as self-corrections, and thus his results cast doubt on the monitoring explanation of lexical bias. The difference found between overt errors and self-corrections, Nooteboom points out, can be explained by assuming some feedback leakage from the phonological to the lexical level, which would at the same time explain why real-word-yielding phonological errors are recognized as phonological errors, rather than lexical errors.

We have two problems with this account, however. First of all, it is as yet unclear how it would square with observations of contextual and strategically induced modulation of lexical bias (but see Dell & Kim, this volume, Chapter 2). More importantly, Nooteboom implicitly assumes that the lexical bias is a property of the monitoring system, both of the inner and of the outer loop. There is an alternative view however. Perhaps there is no bias within the monitoring system itself but in the input to the monitoring system. It seems a priori plausible that permutations of phonemes within a word or word string lead to nonwords more often than to words. This means that in case of a phonological planning error, nonwords will be overrepresented. Even with an unbiased monitor, the chance of nonwords being edited out would be higher than the chance of a word's being edited out. This would bring about a lexical bias in overt speech without a bias in overt repair.

Observations suggesting that internal and external monitoring apply different criteria (such as those pointed out by Nooteboom) set the stage for assuming that internal monitoring may be of a different nature than external monitoring. Conceivably, internal monitoring is (also) production based. The question is whether assuming this may help clarifying the issues touched on by Nooteboom and others in this volume, particularly direct access to the intended phonological representation.

Production-based monitoring refers to the idea that components of the production system check *their own* output, i.e., have their own in-built feedback loop, without recourse to language comprehension (see, e.g., Laver, 1980; Postma, 2000). Quite often, the notion is argued against by an appeal to Ockham's razor (cf. Postma & Oomen, this volume, Chapter 9). It would be an unparsimonious concept, as it seems to necessitate "reduplication" of processing mechanisms and knowledge representations. But such reduplication may in fact be an intrinsically necessary feature of language production. Recent investigations of speech motor control demonstrate that the capacity to configure the articulators in such a way that they produce an intended speech sound depends on the availability of two types of internal models. The first of these is the *forward model*. This is a representation of articulation-to-acoustics mappings. It predicts the acoustic outcome of a particular articulatory command or program. The forward model is complemented by an *inverse model*, which specifies the articulatory motor program that will produce a desired acoustic outcome (Wolpert, Miall, & Kawato, 1998). Possibly, these internal models emerge as a result of practicing the articulators early in life, starting with the babbling phase. We speculate that, at the level of speech sounds, a feedback loop comprising of a forward model and its complementary inverse model can function as a high-speed monitoring device, provided that articulatory control begins with a specification of how the output must sound (sound → inverse model → articulatory program → forward model → sound → match?) If we suppose for the time being that this is feasible (it is impossible to go into detail), a next question is whether forward models may exist at other levels of structure. Another language domain besides phonetics in which many-to-many mappings are ubiquitous, is the semantics-syntax (meaning-form) interface. It is an intriguing question whether linking a syntactic structure to a particular semantic structure may depend on an inverse (semantics-to-syntax) model, and whether such a model, coupled with a forward model (syntax-to-semantics) may play a role in monitoring.

Irrespective of the plausibility of this speculation, it seems quite likely that perception-based monitoring and production-based monitoring exist side by side, which is, in fact, what most proponents of production-based monitoring would argue (see this volume, Chapter 9). Interestingly, Roelofs (this volume, Chapter 3), being an ardent advocate of a strict feedforward approach, explicitly states that both production- and perception-based monitoring are for real, and in his WEAVER++ model are based on the same operation, viz verification. He points out however, that production-internal verification is different from the verification by means of the perceptual loop, in the sense that it is strictly automatic, and beyond attentional control. Indeed, there are numerous indications that, as Levelt already argued in his groundbreaking paper (1983), monitoring is an attentive, semi-conscious process. The contributions to the present volume add some new observations in support of this claim. Oomen, Postma, and Kolk (this volume, Chapter 12) and Hartsuiker, Kolk, and Martensen (this volume, Chapter 11) provide evidence that attention may determine the relative contributions of internal and external loops to self-correcting. Thus, the parameter of detection accuracy appears to be under strategic control, which is related to the "threshold" parameter introduced by Vasic and Wijnen (this volume, Chapter 13), who furthermore also argue that the attention-driven, strategic processes may impact on the *focus* of the monitor, even up to the point of being unadaptive, as in persons who stutter.

Variation in pathology

It is received wisdom in speech and language pathology that many syndromes that are distinguished in the clinic (and for good reasons, most likely) have various, even characteristic/defining symptoms in common. We need only think of the different aphasic syndromes, all of which show, for example, paraphasias and word finding problems in varying degrees of severity (Dell et al., 1997; Haarman & Kolk, 1991; Prins & Bastiaanse, 1997). From a theoretical point of view, the question raised by this observation is whether the underlying dysfunctions (i.e., at the level of the production mechanism) are similar, not only among pathologies within the same nosological categories, but in particular also across syndromes that are quite divergent in terms of (presumed) etiology. Indeed, a number of theoretical (notably modeling) contributions to this volume suggest that divergent pathologies may result from alterations to basically the same processing parameters (connection strength, decay rate, noise level, etc.). Given the overlap in symptomatology and the presumed similarity in (functionally defined) underlying dysfunction, we may ask how different "phenotypes", i.e., syndromes arise.

There are three possible options within the current framework. The first is to postulate dynamic changes to occur with respect to specific processing components only. For instance, in the original study by Dell et al. (1997), word production errors in fluent aphasia were modeled by assuming either fast decay or reduced connection strength. A later version of the model (Foygel & Dell, 2000) assumed a reduced connection strength for all patients, but occurring at different layers of the network: Either the phonological or the semantic. However, this approach is not sufficient. To explain variation between syndromes, which are supposed to have the same component damaged, we could also look at differences in additional damage. If a particular clinical population has damage in more than one component, this could affect their symptomatology. Finally, of course, we could search for differences in plasticity.

Kolk and Heeschen (1992) and Haarmann and Kolk (1992) have found similar error profiles in patients with Broca's and Wernicke's aphasia in specific tests for production of grammatical morphology. Kolk and Heeschen argued for a difference in adaptation, in that the patients with Broca's aphasia adapt to their grammatical deficit, and the patients with Wernicke's aphasia do not. Initially, it was assumed that the patients with Wernicke's aphasia would fail to adapt because of lack of error awareness, but as we saw earlier, the Haarmann and Kolk (1992) data do not support that assumption. Nevertheless, differences in strategic adaptation remain a possible source of differences between syndromes that have damage to the same component.

Perhaps developmental disorders pose a special challenge. Nijland and Maassen (this volume; Chapter 8) make an observation about the unspecificity of symptoms in developmental apraxia of speech. They point to the difficulty of distinguishing developmental disorders of spoken language on the basis of visible and audible behavioral symptoms (as contrasted with instrumental measurements). It may be that speech disorders that arise in young age are notoriously difficult to understand (and to overcome) because of the crucial interplay of perception and production necessary for the development of language and speech skills. Learning to produce spoken language crucially hinges on the perception of oneself and other speakers. Complementarily, learning to analyze and understand spoken language quite likely depends on production skills (think of the forward/inverse models mentioned earlier). The interactions that may ensue when one of the components in the perception-production chain fails are complex, and perhaps not even fully predictable. This, however, cannot be judged until we have better, more refined data and models on the development of the language-processing systems.

Notes

1 The NWO-funded research program "Phonological encoding and monitoring in normal and pathological speech", grant number 572–21–001.

2 Studies of sports commentators, who often speak under considerable time pressure, indicate that they make extensive use of precompiled utterances (fixed expressions).
3 We are disregarding non-verbal motor behavior often associated with stuttering (e.g., swallowing, lip smacking, grimacing, and other oro-facial movements, or gross movements of the head or the limbs), not because we think they are unimportant, but because we believe these are responses acquired in the course of trying to cope with the speech problem, rather than to the core symptom.

References

Au-Yeung, J., Howell, P., & Pilgrim, L. (1998). Phonological words and stuttering on function words. *Journal of Speech, Language, and Hearing Research, 41*, 1019–1030.

Avrutin, S. (2001). Linguistics and agrammatism. *Glot International, 5*, 1–11.

Baars, B., Motley, M. T., & MacKay, D. G. (1975). Output editing for lexical status in artificially elicited slips of the tongue. *Journal of Verbal Learning and Verbal Behavior, 14*, 382–91.

Buckingham, H. W. (1999). Freud's continuity thesis. *Brain and Language, 69*, 76–92.

Caramazza, A. (1986). On drawing inferences about the structure of normal cognitive systems from the analysis of patterns of impaired performance: The case for single case-studies. *Brain and Cognition, 5*, 41–66.

Caramazza, A. (1992) Is cognitive neuropsychology possible? *Journal of Cognitive Neuroscience, 6*, 80–95.

Caruso, A. J. (1991). Neuromotor processes underlying stuttering. In H. F. M. Peters, W. Hulstijn, & C. W. Starkweather (Eds.), *Speech motor control and stuttering* (pp. 101–16). Amsterdam: Excerpta Medica.

Chertkow, H., & Bub, D. (1990). Semantic loss in Alzheimer-type dementia. In M. F. Schwartz (Ed.), *Modular deficits in Alzheimer-type dementia* (pp. 207–44). Cambridge, MA: MIT Press.

Clark, H., & Wasow, T. (1998). Repeating words in spontaneous speech. *Cognitive Psychology, 37*, 201–42.

De Roo, E. (1999). *Agrammatic grammar: Functional categories in agrammatic speech.* PhD dissertation, University of Leiden.

Dell, G. S., Burger, L. K., & Svec, W. R. (1997). Language production and serial order: A functional analysis and a model. *Psychological Review, 104*, 123–47.

Dell, G. S., Schwartz, M. F., Martin, N., Saffran, E. M., &. Gagnon, D. A. (1997). Lexical access in aphasic and nonaphasic speakers. *Psychological Review, 104*, 801–38.

Dick, F., Bates, E., Wulfeck, B., Utman, J. A., Dronkers, N., & Gernsbacher, M. A. (2001). Language deficits, localization, and grammar: Evidence for a distributive model of language breakdown in aphasic patients and neurologically intact individuals. *Psychological Review, 108*, 759–88.

Farah, M. J. (1994). Neuropsychological inference with an interactive brain: A critique of the "locality" assumption. *Behavioral and Brain Sciences, 17*, 77–8.

Foygel, D., & Dell, G. S. (2000). Models of impaired lexical access in speech production. *Journal of Memory and Language, 43*, 182–216.

Goldiamond, I. (1965). Stuttering and fluency as manipulable operant response classes. In L. Krasner & L. Ullman (Eds.), *Research in behavior modification.* New York: Holt, Rinehart & Winston.

Haarmann, H. J., Just, M. A., & Carpenter, P. A. (1997). Aphasic sentence comprehension as a resource deficit: A computational approach. *Brain and Language*, *59*, 76–120.

Haarmann, H. J., & Kolk, H. H. J. (1991). A computer model of the temporal course of agrammatic sentence understanding: the effects of variation in severity and sentence complexity. *Cognitive Science*, *15*, 49–87.

Haarmann, H. J., & Kolk, H. H. J. (1992). The production of grammatical morphology in Broca's and Wernicke's aphasics: Speed and accuracy factors. *Cortex*, *28*, 97–112.

Hagoort, P., Wassenaar, M., & Brown, C. (2003). Real-time semantic compensation in patients with agrammatic comprehension: electrophysiological evidence for multiple-route plasticity. *Proceedings of the National Academy of Sciences*, *100*, 4340–45.

Hartsuiker, R. J., & Kolk, H. H. J. (1998). Syntactic facilitation in agrammatic sentence production. *Brain and Language*, *62*, 221–54.

Hendriks, A. W., & Kolk, H. H. J. (1997) Strategic control in developmental dyslexia. *Cognitive Neuropsychology*, *14*, 321–66.

Hofstede, B. T. M. (1992). *Agrammatic speech in Broca's aphasia: Strategic choice for the elliptical register*. PhD dissertation, University of Nijmegen [available as NICI technical report 92–07].

Hofstede, B. T. M., & Kolk, H. H. J. (1994). The effects of task variation on the production of grammatical morphology in Broca's aphasia: A multiple case study. *Brain and Language*, *46*, 278–328.

Just, M. A., & Carpenter, P. (1992). A capacity theory of comprehension: Individual differences in working memory. *Psychological Review*, *99*, 122–49.

Kello, C. T., & Plaut, D. C. (2003). Strategic control over rate of processing in word reading: A computational investigation. *Journal of Memory and Language*, *48*, 207–32.

Kemper, S., Herman, R., & Lian, C. (2003). Age differences in sentence production. *Journals of Gerontology. Series B – Psychological Sciences and Social Sciences*, *58*, 260–68.

Kolk, H. H. J. (1991). Is stuttering a symptom of adaptation or of impairment? In H. F. M. Peters, W. Hulstijn, & C. W. Starkwheather (Eds.), *Speech motor control and stuttering*. Amsterdam: Elsevier Science/Excerpta Medica.

Kolk, H. H. J. (1995). A time-based approach to agrammatic production. *Brain and Language*, *50*, 282–303.

Kolk, H. H. J. (1998). *Compenseren voor een taalstoornis* [Compensating for a language disorder]. Inaugural address, University of Nijmegen.

Kolk, H. H. J. (2000). Multiple route plasticity. *Brain and Language*, *71*, 129–31.

Kolk, H. H. J., & Heeschen, C. (1992). Agrammatism, paragrammatism and the management of language. *Language and Cognitive Processes*, *7*, 82–129.

Kolk, H. H. J., & Postma, A. (1997) Stuttering as a covert-repair phenomenon. In R. Curlee, & G. Siegel (Eds.), *Nature and treatment of stuttering: New directions*. Boston: Allyn & Bacon.

Latash, M. L., & Anson, J. G. (1996). What are "normal movements" in atypical populations? *Behavioral and Brain Sciences*, *19*, 55–106.

Laver, J. (1980). Monitoring systems in the neurolinguistic control of speech production. In V. A. Fromkin (Ed.), *Errors in linguistic performance: Slips of the tongue, ear, pen and hand*. New York: Academic Press.

Levelt, W. J. M. (1983). Monitoring and self-repair in speech paper. *Cognition, 14*, 41–104.

Levelt, W. J. M. (1989). *Speaking. From intention to articulation*. Cambridge, MA: MIT Press/Bradford Books.

Levelt, W. J. M., Roelofs, A., & Meyer, A. S. (1999). A theory of lexical access in speech production. *Behavioral and Brain Sciences, 21*, 1–38.

Maclay, H., & Osgood, C. E. (1959). Hesitation phenomena in spontaneous English speech. *Word, 15*, 19–44.

Merzenich, M., & Jenkins, W. M. (1995). Cortical plasticity, learning and learning dysfunction. In B. Julesz, & I. Kovacs (Eds.), *Maturational windows and adult cortical plasticity* (pp. 1–24). Reading, MA: Addison-Wesley.

Miyake, A., Carpenter, P. A., & Just, M. A. (1995). Reduced resources and specific impairments in normal and aphasic sentence comprehension. *Cognitive Neuropsychology, 12*, 651–79.

Nickels, L., & Howard, D. (1995). Phonological errors in aphasic naming: Comprehension, monitoring and lexicality. *Cortex, 31*, 209–37.

Oomen, C. C. E., & Postma, A. (2001). Effects of divided attention on the production of filled pauses and repetitions. *Journal of Speech, Language, and Hearing Research, 44*, 997–1004.

Oomen, C. C. E., Postma, A., & Kolk, H. H. J. (2001). Prearticulatory and postarticulatory selfmonitoring in Broca's aphasia. *Cortex, 37*, 627–41.

Postma, A. (2000). Detection of errors during speech production: A review of speech monitoring models. *Cognition, 77*, 97–131.

Postma, A., & Kolk, H. H. J. (1993). The covert repair hypothesis: Prearticulatory repair processes in normal and stuttered disfluencies. *Journal of Speech and Hearing Research, 36*, 472–87.

Prins, R. S., & Bastiaanse, R. (1997). Afasic: Symptomatologie en wetenschappelijke inzichten [Aphasia: Symptomatology and scientific insights]. In H. M. F. Peters, R. Bastiaanse, J. van Borsel, Ph. Dejonckere, K. Jansonius, & Sj. van der Meulen (Eds.), *Handboek Stem-, Spraak- Taalpathologie*. Houten: Bohn, Stafleu, Van Loghum.

Rapp, B., & Goldrick, M. (2000). Discreteness and interactivity in spoken word production. *Psychological Review, 107*, 460–99.

Ruigendijk, E. (2002). *Case assignment in agrammatism: A cross-linguistic study*. PhD dissertation University of Groningen.

Stemberger, J. P. (1984). Structural errors in normal and agrammatic speech. *Cognitive Neuropsychology, 1*, 281–313.

Webster, W. G. (1993). Hurried hands and tangled tongues. Implications of current research for the management of stuttering. In E. Boberg (Ed.), *Neuropsychology of stuttering* (pp. 73–127). Edmonton: University of Alberta Press.

Wijnen, F. (1992). Incidental word and sound errors in young speakers. *Journal of Memory and Language, 31*, 734–55.

Wijnen, F. (1998). The temporal interpretation of Dutch children's root infinitivals: The effect of eventivity. *First Language, 18*, 379–402.

Wolpert, D. M., Miall, R. C., & Kawato, M. (1998). Internal models in the cerebellum. *Trends in Cognitive Sciences, 2*, 338–47.

Yairi, E., & Lewis, B. (1984). Disfluencies at the onset of stuttering. *Journal of Speech and Hearing Research, 27*, 154–9.

Author index

Subject index